Blockchain in Digital Healthcare

Blockchain in Digital Healthcare

Edited by
Malaya Dutta Borah, Roberto Moro-Visconti and
Ganesh Chandra Deka

CRC Press
Taylor & Francis Group
Boca Raton London New York

CRC Press is an imprint of the
Taylor & Francis Group, an **informa** business
A CHAPMAN & HALL BOOK

First edition published 2022
by CRC Press
6000 Broken Sound Parkway NW, Suite 300, Boca Raton, FL 33487-2742

and by CRC Press
2 Park Square, Milton Park, Abingdon, Oxon, OX14 4RN

Library of Congress Cataloging-in-Publication Data

Names: Borah, Malaya Dutta, editor. | Moro Visconti, Roberto, editor. | Deka, Ganesh Chandra, 1969- editor.
Title: Blockchain in digital healthcare / edited by Malaya Dutta Borah, Department of Computer Science and Engineering, National Institute of Technology Silchar, India, Roberto Moro Visconti, Università Cattolica del Sacro Cuore Milano, Italy, and Ganesh Chandra Deka, Directorate General of Training, Ministry of Skill Development and Entrepreneurship, India.
Description: First edition. | Boca Raton : Chapman & Hall/CRC Press, 2022. | Includes bibliographical references and index. | Summary: "Health information about a patient is very critical, and currently, health records are saved in the databases controlled by individual users or organizations. As there are many malicious users, this information is not shared with other organizations due to security issues or data tampering. Blockchain can be used to securely exchange sensitive healthcare data that can be accessed by organizations sharing the same network in turn allowing doctors/practitioners to provide better care for patients. Focuses on patient-centric applications of blockchain technology Covers e-health, telemedicine and m-health advances and perspectives D iscusses impact of Blockchains on smart healthcare and blockchained platforms on B2B, B2C interactions P rovides solutions to (some) healthcare bottlenecks Analyses networking digital platforms (considering blockchains as a peculiar form of network) Includes case studies of healthcare applications for a realistic strand on the subject This book is aimed primarily at postgraduates and researchers studying blockchain technology with focus on healthcare Informatics. Software developers will also find this book helpful"-- Provided by publisher.
Identifiers: LCCN 2021032691 (print) | LCCN 2021032692 (ebook) | ISBN 9780367678616 (hardback) | ISBN 9780367678692 (paperback) | ISBN 9781003133179 (ebook)
Subjects: LCSH: Medicine--Data processing. | Blockchains (Databases)
Classification: LCC R858 .B5697 2022 (print) | LCC R858 (ebook) | DDC 610.285--dc23
LC record available at https://lccn.loc.gov/2021032691
LC ebook record available at https://lccn.loc.gov/2021032692

ISBN: 9780367678616 (hbk)
ISBN: 9780367678692 (pbk)
ISBN: 9781003133179 (ebk)

DOI: 10.1201/9781003133179

Typeset in Palatino
by Deanta Global Publishing Services, Chennai, India

Contents

Preface

Blockchain is a series of transactions *recorded in blocks, secured cryptographically*. Blockchain has unique characteristics such as being *immutable, decentralized* and *transparent*. Users within blockchain can *record transactions in blocks* in an *immutable* distributed ledger, i.e., unchangeable once recorded/published. Another advantage of blockchain is that it is *decentralized*, which eliminates the dependency on a *trusted third party* to facilitate the transactions. This enables the clients/users of the blockchain to take ownership of the data they push onto the network. Besides making the transactions, blockchain also makes them more secure as each of those clients have their own copies of the transactions.

Blockchain has proved to be beneficial for all the domains of modernization, the healthcare industry among them, as it maintains the *privacy, integrity* and *security* of healthcare data. This edited book, *Blockchain in Digital Healthcare*, provides a panoramic review of prospects of blockchain technology in the healthcare domain.

Chapter 1 discusses the potential of the blockchain technology, while Chapter 2 explores the potential of blockchain with the Internet of Things (IoT) in healthcare. Chapter 3 discusses how blockchain technology may accelerate effective data governance during the pandemic crisis of Covid-19.

Chapter 4 is about the implementation of the IoT in intelligent distributed healthcare systems. Chapter 5 illustrates the concept of smart contracts to create a decentralized application.

Chapter 6 contemplates the scope for prevention of chronological distortion of input information to detect and correct medical errors with the blockchain. A Blockchain-enabled IoT-based Healthcare Monitoring System (BIoT-HMS) can reduce unnecessary hospital visits by patients to meet with their healthcare experts. The security requirements and applications of BIoT-HMS and a summary of various existing security protocols of BIoT-HMS are covered in Chapter 7.

Chapter 8 discusses the networked P2P interactions through blockchains and how using blockchain-based networks considerably reduces the vulnerabilities of healthcare data. Chapter 9 is a case study on securing the Covid-19 pandemic data. Chapter 10 explains how blockchain-based Electronic Medical Records (EMR) makes it convenient for the patients and doctors to interact. *Ethereum* and *IPFS* are used for data encryption in this illustration. Similarly, Chapter 11 demonstrates how *Ethereum Hyperledger* may be used to build a blockchain-based insurance application.

Chapter 12 explores how the blockchain solves the challenges of the pharmaceutical sector. Finally, Chapter 13 is about applications of blockchain to various aspects of drug manufacturing and the pharma supply chain.

The editors are confident that this book will be a valuable addition to the growing knowledge base of *Blockchains in Digital Healthcare*. As *blockchain* becomes more intrusive and pervasive there will be increasing interest in this domain. It is our hope that this book will not only showcase the current state of the art and practice but also set the agenda for future directions in prospects of *Blockchains in Digital Healthcare*.

Malaya Dutta Borah
Roberto Moro-Visconti
Ganesh Chandra Deka

Editor Bios

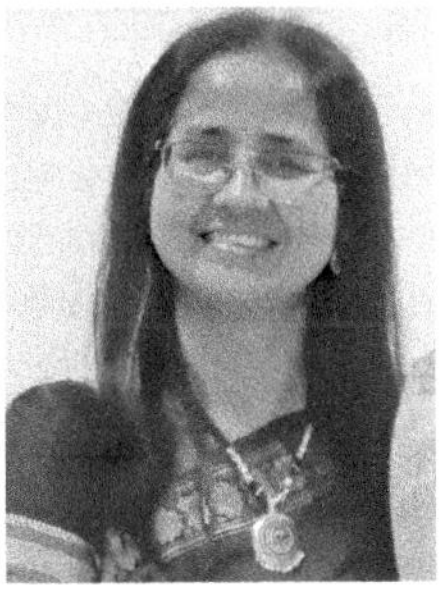

Malaya Dutta Borah is an Assistant Professor in the Department of Computer Science and Engineering at National Institute of Technology (NIT) Silchar, Assam, India.

She received her Engineering Degree (B Tech) in Computer Science and Engineering, Master of Engineering (with distinction) in Computer Technology and Applications and PhD in Computer Science and Engineering.

She has authored/co-authored around 40 research papers in national/international journals/conferences and is actively involved in research works in the fields of Data Mining, Blockchain Technology, Cloud Computing, ICT and e-governance.

As of now, she has organized three international conferences (Springer & IEEE) in India as organizing chair, finance chair and member. She is an editorial board member of the International Journal of Information Systems and Social Change, IGI-Global and reviewer for various journals and international conferences.

She is an associate member of CSI (India) and IEEE.

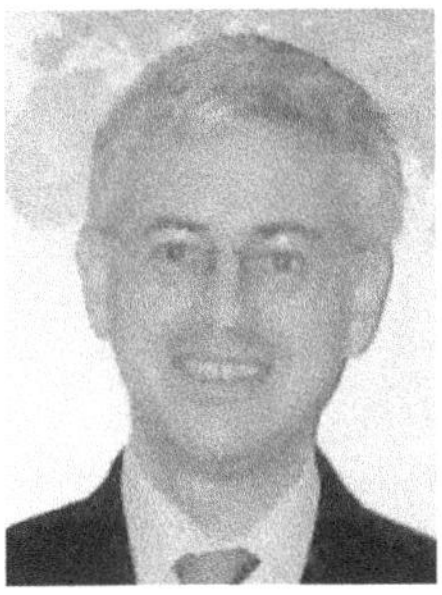

Roberto Moro-Visconti teaches Corporate Finance at the Catholic University of the Sacred Heart, Milan, Italy. He received his Bachelors degree in Economics from Catholic University of the Sacred Heart, his MA in Finance and Investment from University of Exeter, UK, and his PhD in Economics from University of Exeter. His research interests include the valuation of digital intangibles, healthcare project financing and microfinance.

He has authored more than 20 books (most recently *The Valuation of Digital Intangibles. Technology, Marketing and Internet,* Palgrave Macmillan, 2020) and around 200 research papers (available online at: https://www.researchgate.net/profile/Roberto_Moro_Visconti2. His profile can also be viewed at http://www.morovisconti.com/wp/en/home-2/ or https://docenti.unicatt.it/ppd2/en/#/en/docenti/03514/roberto-moro-visconti/profilo).

Moro-Visconti is a chartered accountant and intellectual property consultant, managing a boutique consulting firm in Milan, Italy.

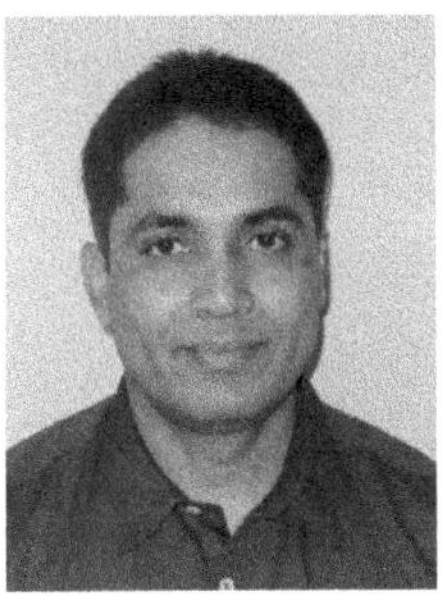

Ganesh Chandra Deka is currently Deputy Director at the Directorate General of Training, under the Ministry of Skill Development and Entrepreneurship, Government of India. His previous assignments include Principal, NSIT (W) Tura, Meghalaya (National Skill Training Institute for Women), Consultant (Computer Science), North-Eastern Regional Centre of the National Institute of Rural Development and Panchayati Raj (NIRD & PR-NERC), Ministry of Rural Development, Government of India and Programmer (World Bank Project), Directorate of Technical Education, Assam, India.

His research interests include Bigdata Analytics, Blockchain Technology, Internet of Things (IoT), Cloud Computing and NoSQL Databases.

He is the co-author of four textbooks on the fundamentals of computer science and has edited 24 books (8 with IGI Global, USA, 8 with Chapman and Hall/CRC Press, USA, 4 with Springer and 4 with Elsevier) on Bigdata Analytics, NoSQL Database, Internet of Things (IoT) and Blockchain Technology. He has also authored 14 book chapters.

He has published eight research papers in various reputed journals (IEEE 2, Elsevier 1) and more than 47 research papers in various international conferences of IEEE and Springer. To date, he has organized eight IEEE international conferences as technical chair and publication chair. He has published five special issues in international journals published by IGI Global, USA, in the *International Journal of Applied Evolutionary Computation (IJAEC)*, Volume 8, Issue 1 (*Special Issue on*: Emerging Research Trend in Computing and Communication Technologies), *International Journal of Organizational and End User Computing (JOEUC)*, Volume 29, Issue 4, (*Special Issue on* Bigdata Analytics in Business, Healthcare, and Governance), Volume 30, Issue 4, (*Special Issue on* Internet of Things: Issues, Challenges and Opportunities), *International Journal of Open Source Software and Processes (IJOSSP)*, Volume 9, Issue 3 (*Special Issue on* Prospects of Free and Open Source Software in Digital Revolution and *International Journal of Information Systems and Social Change (IJISSC)*, Volume 10, Issue 2 (*Special Issue on* Blockchain Technology: Platforms, Tools, & Use Cases).

List of Contributors

Rachit Agarwal
Department of Computer Science and Engineering
Indian Institute of Technology
Kanpur, India

Karm Veer Arya
ABV-Indian Institute of Information Technology & Management
Gwalior, India

A. Averin
Department of Electrical Engineering and Computer Science
South Ural State University
Chelyabinsk, Russia

Manorama Devi B
Department of Computer Science and Engineering
Kandula Sreenivasa Reddy Memorial College Of Engineering
Andhra Pradesh, India

Arnab Banerjee
Senior Manager, Global Supply Chain
Micron Technology
Hyderabad, India

Basudeb Bera
Center for Security Theory and Algorithmic Research
International Institute of Information Technology
Hyderabad, India

Rajib Biswas
Department of Physics
Tezpur University
Tezpur, India

Malaya Dutta Borah
Department of Computer Science and Engineering
National Institute of Technology
Silchar, India

Ashok Kumar Das
Center for Security Theory and Algorithmic Research
International Institute of Information Technology
Hyderabad, India

Manoj Kumar Dhadwal
Babasaheb Bhimrao Ambedkar University
Lucknow, India

Ujjawal Jain
Department of Computer Science and Engineering
National Institute of Technology
Silchar, India

Rajni Jindal
Department of Computer Science and Engineering
Delhi Technological University
Delhi, India

Champa Joshi
Department Information Technology
Babasaheb Bhimrao Ambedkar University
Lucknow, India

Saritha Kuppala
Independent Researcher
Hyderabad, India

Muralidhar Kurni
Department of Computer Science and Engineering
Jawaharlal Nehru Technological University, Anantapur University
Hyderabad, India

Roberto Moro-Visconti
Catholic University of the Sacred Heart
Milan, Italy

Mrunalini M
Department of Computer Application
M S Ramaiah Institute of Technology
Bangalore, India

K. Nikolskaia
South Ural State University
Chelyabinsk, Russia

Mayank Pandey
Department of Electrical Engineering
Indian Institute of Technology
Kanpur, India

Ravi Prakash Pandey
Institute of Engineering and Technology
Rammanohar Lohia Avadh University
Ayodhya, India

Agya Pathak
Department of Computer Science and Engineering
National Institute of Technology
Silchar, India

Joythish Reddy
Department of Computer Science and Engineering
National Institute of Technology
Silchar, India

K. Somasena Reddy
Jawaharlal Nehru Technological University, Anantapur University
College of Engineering, Ananthapuramu
Hyderabad, India

Yash Sarwaswa
Department of Computer Science and Engineering
National Institute of Technology
Silchar, India

Pratima Sharma
Department of Computer Science and Engineering
Delhi Technological University
Delhi India

Satyendra Kumar Shet
Department of Electrical and Electronics Engineering
NMAM Institute of Technology (VTU Belagavi)
Nitte, India

Vinayaka B Shet
Department of Biotechnology Engineering
NMAM Institute of Technology (VTU Belagavi)
Nitte, India

Raj Shree
PI (CST-UP) Department Information Technology
Babasaheb Bhimrao Ambedkar University
Lucknow, India

Sameer Shrivastava
Department of Computer Science and Engineering
National Institute of Technology
Silchar, India

Ashwani Kant Shukla
Department of Information Technology
Babasaheb Bhimrao Ambedkar University
Lucknow, India

Sandeep K Shukla
Department of Computer Science and Engineering
Indian Institute of Technology
Kanpur, India

Vivek Shukla
Department of Information Technology
Babasaheb Bhimrao Ambedkar University
Lucknow, India

Ranjana Sikarwar
Department of Computer Science and Engineering
Amity University
Noida, India

Devesh Pratap Singh
Department of Computer Science and Engineering
Graphic Era University
Dehradun, India

Nishchal K Verma
Department of Electrical Engineering
Indian Institute of Technology
Kanpur, India

Mohammad Wazid
Department of Computer Science and Engineering
Graphic Era University
Dehradun, India

1

An Overview of Emerging Updates in Blockchain Technology: Analysis and Recommendations

Champa Joshi, Karm Veer Arya, Ashwani Kant Shukla, Raj Shree, Ravi Prakash Pandey, Vivek Shukla and Manoj Kumar Dhadwal

CONTENTS

DOI: 10.1201/9781003133179-1

1.1 Introduction

In recent decades, blockchain technology has revolutionized the world in various sectors such as banking, finance, healthcare, etc. (Zhang, 2016). The blockchain concept gained momentum in 2008 with the introduction of the cryptocurrency bitcoin by Satoshi Nakamoto. Blockchain-powered bitcoin became the first electronic payment system, which works as a decentralized network (Anjum et al., 2017). Earlier, in online commerce, various financial entities have been working as the third party and the structure of commerce was totally trust-based. Even though that structure works well for some kinds of electronic payments, they still have some drawbacks as there are no proper ways to convince the customer about the verification and validation of all transactions by a trusted unbiased third-party financial entity. In addition, there are cost and payment uncertainties, which fluctuate with mediation costs as well. Therefore, the idea of Bitcoin came to mitigate the mistrust and lack of transparency of the third party. To reduce the drawbacks in conventional transaction methods, the system needed an electronic payment method with cryptographic proof. Generally, the use of digital signatures, which are a string of bits and tether with particular rules and parameters, make transactions successful. Digital signatures help in the verification of a signatory's identity and the data but are not reliable in cases of double-spending (Botta et al., 2016). Therefore, Satoshi Nakamoto proposed a solution to the issue of double-spending using a peer-to-peer type of electronic cash system and proposed direct online payments from one person or party to another without any third-party intervention (Zhang, 2016). Blockchain technology is, specifically, a cryptographically secured chain of blocks, in which each block includes a hash of previous blocks, a timestamp and transaction data in a distributed ledger or database. This secures transactions and brings transparency to the digital transactions by hashing them into an ongoing chain of hash-based proof-of-work, forming a record that is tamper-proof (Zhang, 2016). Bitcoin protocol uses the principle of blockchain technology, which is a digital database for storing information in groups of blocks and is also known as digital sheets or digital ledgers. These ledgers are approved by a digital signature which validates three-purpose authentication, non-repudiation and integrity of any transaction which cannot be removed or deleted and thus are immutable in behavior. The information of transactions is a series of blocks which can hold the complete information of a total transaction or information exchanged and therefore it works like a public ledger blockchain that has only one initial parent block called a genesis block. The size of the block depends on the information it contains, such that the bigger the block the more information it contains. The authentication of the information transfer or any kind of transaction is validated by the asymmetric cryptography mechanism and is traceable. The typical digital signature algorithm used in blockchains is the elliptic curve digital signature algorithm (Fan et al., 2018). This review explores the specific characteristics of blockchain technology (BT), its operation, architecture, main platforms and its various applications in different sectors.

1.2 Background to Blockchain

There are certain things that help to provide immutability, anonymity, security and robustness to blockchain transactions, for instance hashing, which links the blocks to one

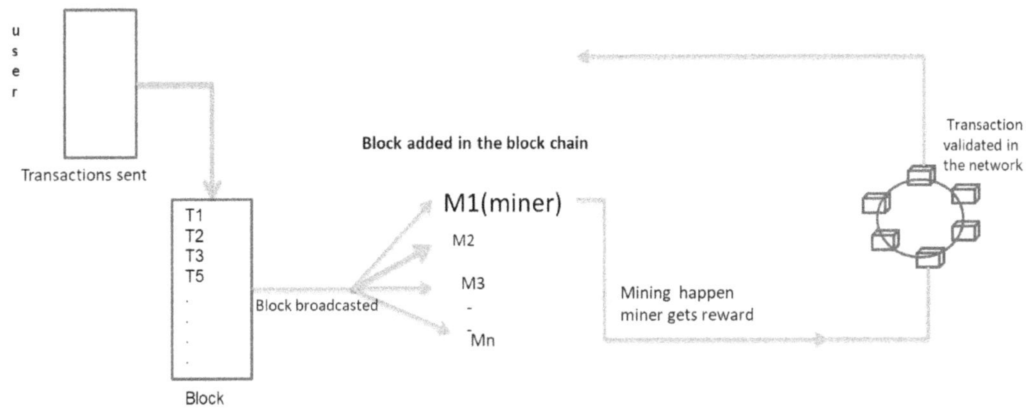

FIGURE 1.1
Depiction of blockchain transaction: 1–Request for a transaction is made by a user; 2–Block is created (record of transitions); 3–Block is broadcasted in the network; 4–Transactions (blocks) are validated by nodes in the network; 5–New block is added in already present block chain; 6–Transaction is complete

another with metadata property and each new block contains hashed data of the previous block. Any changes in one block could result in changes in the whole blockchain so tampering with data is not possible. The validation of a new block depends on the information of all previous blocks; if it is valid then only the new block gets space in the chain.

The architecture of blockchain is depicted in Figure 1.1. In the request for a transaction, a block is created which represents a transaction and then that block is broadcasted in the network and it is validated by nodes in the network. Finally, the new transaction, such as blocks, is added into the pre-existing block chain which completes the transaction.

1.2.1 Nonce

This is a random number which is used in blocks to make cryptographic communication secure and to provide authentication to the transactions. It prevents replay attacks (Crosby et al., 2016) and works as a one-time password in the network in Figure 1.2.

1.2.2 Timestamping

Timestamping plays a role in the authorization of any document and it proves possession of any document for a particular time period. It is a legal certificate, which assures the existence

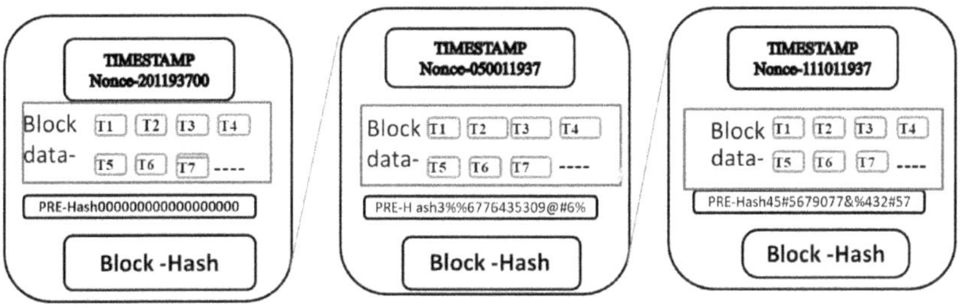

FIGURE 1.2
Cryptographic functions in the blockchains: Cryptographic hash.

of a particular transaction period. The important attributes, such as time and date, provide time signatures to any document to prove ownership. Timestamping by a third party presents a chance of manipulation by its authority, but distributed timestamping in blockchain helps get rid of manipulation and network delay conflict. Here, each node gets its own stamp to prove the transaction. Timestamping increases the reliability of blockchain, gives an anonymous solution to generate trust and is tamper-proof (Casino et al., 2019) in Figure 1.2.

1.2.3 Hashing

A cryptographic hash is an important component of blockchain technology, as shown in Figure 1.2. Hashing is a process in which an input transaction value can be any size or length but the output comes as a fixed-length hash value (digest), for instance it has one character input value and one line input sentence or a whole library of books produce the same hash value length. Practical loading, a document or a book in blockchain will take a lot of space and time but if we convert it into a fixed-size hash value it takes far less space and time. Also, anyone can individually input any value and get and secure that value for checking any tampering of that data in the near future. In a hashing system two inputs, which produce the same output are not feasible such as the value a, b, hash(a)=hash(b) is not possible (Fanning et al., 2016). It is helpful to protect data integrity. There are no chances of data modification here. Bitcoin cryptocurrency runs with hashing security (Tan et al., 2018).

1.3 Essences of the Blockchain Technology

1.3.1 Merkle Tree

Every block in the blockchain has many transactions, and each transaction has its hash value, but we need one hash value for the entire block to get rid of space problems. Getting one out of many hashes is possible through the Merkle tree. It is a binary tree which helps combine all the hashes of the transaction or we can say one hash value for the entire block in Figure 1.3. Each block in the blockchain usually contains more than a thousand transactions, and each transaction has its hash ID which takes a minimum of 256 bits. According to that, we will need a lot more space in the block for all transaction IDs. Merkle came up with the idea which can reduce the memory space of transactions t1, t2, t3, t4, etc., representing the transaction and h1 to h12 where h1 is the first hash and h12 is the final hash for the block (Tan et al., 2018).

Merkle trees benefit both users and miners on a blockchain. Users can verify individual parts of the blocks and can also check transactions by using hashes from other branches of the Merkle tree. Miners can calculate hashes progressively as they receive transactions from their peers.

1.3.2 Decentralization

In a centralized network, one single entity has control over the whole network, but in decentralized network, the power of decision-making depends on all the users in the network and the distributed system must ensure consistency; that is, when a transaction occurs using the information supplied by one of the nodes, it must be correctly reflected

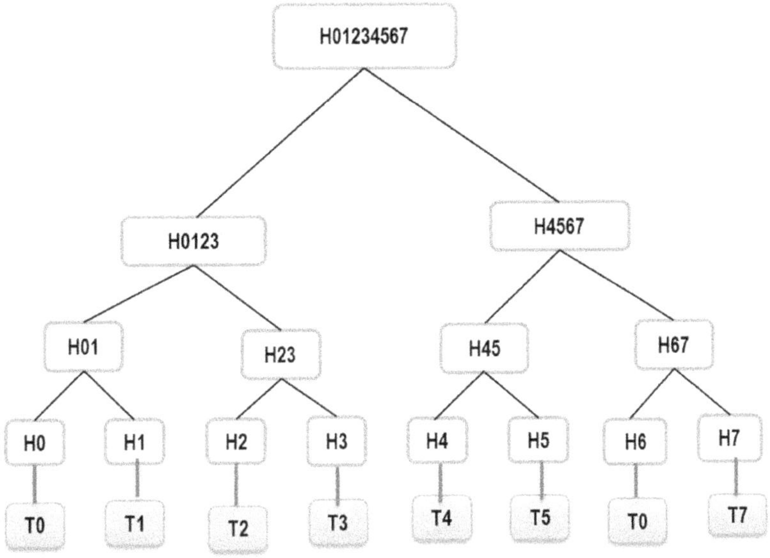

FIGURE 1.3
Depictions of a Merkle tree.

in all other nodes. Decentralization is also known as distributed ledger technology, which aims to provide privacy, security and reliability to users. In this system all transactions are monitored and confirmed by all nodes in the BT network and are tamper-proof. In contrast to the centralized system, BT does not need the involvement of a third party and consensus algorithms play an important role in maintaining data integrity.

1.3.3 Ledger

A ledger is a public record of transactions. Until now pen, paper and the electronic version of sheets have been used to track various kinds of transactions. The ledger generator or holder has maintained the authority of all the information within the ledger, but the distributed nature of the ledger provides all information, including the number of participants in the network as well as all the transactions ever done. If a block proves the authentication, non-repudiation and integrity, then it adds in the blockchain as a new block and the chain continues to grow. In the network, the same copy of the ledger is available to each participant instantly. Therefore, there are almost no chances of modification in any transaction and hence it is immutable in nature.

1.3.4 Mining

Blockchain mining is the addition of new transaction events in the distributed ledger among all users of a blockchain. Mining involves creating a hash of a block that cannot be modified by any single entity in the transaction that thus protects the integrity of the blockchain.

1.3.5 Smart Contracts

Smart contracts are programs that run on BT which are digitally written as codes and represent an agreement between two people and are similar versions of traditional agreements.

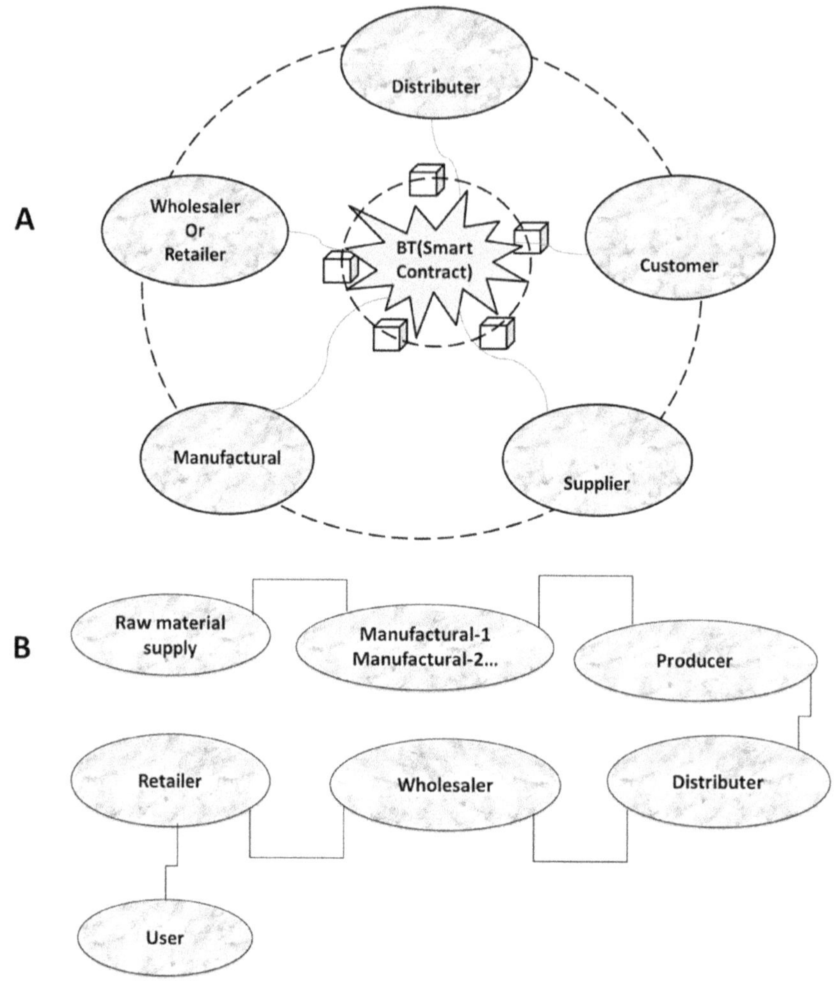

FIGURE 1.4
Smart contracts: A–BT-based smart contracts; B–Traditional smart contracts.

These smart contract programs are written on Ethereum-like platforms. Smart contracts have helped in the ease of doing business. By providing unmatched security, scalability, transparency and performance at a much lower cost as well as eliminating the middleman, they can profoundly impact industries like insurance, banking, government, financial services and health work (Figure 1.4).

1.4 Consensus Model and Achievement

Consensus achievement is a method of identifying the valid order of a transaction. Every miner can build their own blocks with different transactions and a generated block could be validated, and which block should be added to the global network first is decided by the consensus algorithm, but the consensus algorithm should be powerful enough to verify the nodes.

If verification is done, that means consensus is achieved. The consensus model defines the success and failure of the blockchain network to make the BT network secure; many consensus models have been introduced such as Proof of Work (PoW), Proof of Stake (PoS), Delegated Proof of Stake (DPoS), Round Robin, Proof of Authority, Proof of Elapsed Time (PoET).

1.4.1 Proof of Work (PoW)

PoW is one out of many consensus mechanisms in the network. PoW is a validation of work and verifies a new block in the existing blockchain. In PoW, each node of the network calculates a hash value of the constantly changing block header. The consensus requires that the calculated value must be equal to or smaller than a certain given value. In the decentralized network, all participants have to calculate the hash value for different nodes to validate the blocks continuously by using the correct nonce (Tang et al., 2018). Bitcoin uses a PoW algorithm to validate transactions.

1.4.2 Proof of Stake (PoS)

PoS is likely similar to a consensus algorithm which is used to achieve distributed consensus. By PoS in the block chain, new block adder is selected with a combination of random selection and possession of digital coins. PoS does not rely on a nonce in an unlimited space but is based on the ownership of the amount of currency by the users to avoid possible attack by the miners (Tapscott et al., 2017).

1.4.3 Delegated Proof of Stake (DPoS)

DPoS is an alternative to the PoW consensus protocol and its robustness and flexibility provide additional power to the blockchain network (Wang et al., 2018). DPoS was introduced and developed by Daniel Larimer. In this algorithm, stakeholders elect their delegates to generate and validate a block to avoid malicious attacks. DPoS uses minimal nodes to quickly validate and confirm the blocks, making the transactions easy. In addition, dishonest delegates can be removed easily by consensus voting. DPoS has been used by Lisk, Steem, EOS (Wang et al., 2018), Bitshare, etc.

1.4.4 Round Robin

This consensus model works for permission BT networks. It gives a fixed slice of time to each node for publishing blocks, removes standstill situations in the network and provides efficiency and fairness to each node. Public BT networks will not benefit from it because trust between nodes plays important role in Round Robin consensus. Its implementation is multi-chain (White, 2017).

1.4.5 Proof of Authority

This consensus model depends on a permission prerequisite. As per the consensus model only identity-proven nodes can publish a new block and preapproved nodes do not need further verification; that way, this model introduces an energy saving method in comparison to PoS and PoW, and in this model nodes have to make a reputation in order to get chances to publish a new block. It works as an improved decentralized version of the earlier semi-centralized models. A private blockchain network can use this model and most likely the financial sector can benefit from this kind of consensus. Its implementation is Ethereum Kovan Testnet (Xu et al., 2018).

1.4.6 Proof of Elapsed Time (PoET)

The goal of a PoET consensus algorithm is to provide distributed consensus. It was introduced by Intel with software guard extension (SGX) technology which especially helps the developer to protect specific code and data. SGX is helpful in preventing the tampering of data and protects code from revelation by using enclaves or protected areas of execution in the memory. PoET is a more economical and energy efficient consensus model and has found use in permission blockchain (Yang et al., 2018).

1.5 Salient Blockchain Platforms

1.5.1 Ethereum

Ethereum is a platform which provides a means to build simple and efficient decentralized applications. There are some decentralized applications which are functional and built on the Ethereum platform such as Chainlink, MakerDAO, DAI, CryptoKitties, Cent and Bitcoin.

1.5.2 Hyperledger

Hyperledger is an open-source common project in which communities of developers from different sectors like finance, aviation, banking, technology, supply chain and many more are working together toward a common goal and making blockchain frameworks and platforms. It started with a small group of developers with a piece of code, which is constantly modifying and redistributing the hyperledger and covers many blockchain technologies like graphical interfaces, distributed ledger frameworks, smart contract engines (Ying et al., 2018).

1.5.3 R3-Corda

An enterprise software company, R3, developed Corda. It is a distributed ledger platform helping in the financial sector and is an open-source blockchain platform which mainly focuses on businesses and provides them with scalability, interoperability and much more, with smart contracts. It also reduces excessive costs in business and has a blockchain application firewall, which provides security to any kind of business, like supply chain, healthcare, insurance; the digital identity language, Java, can be used to write CorDapps.

1.6 Emerging Applications of Blockchain Technology

Blockchain technology has been steadily finding use in many sectors and has transformed the business world. In the financial sector, blockchain technology has enhanced asset management systems such as cryptocurrency transactions and portfolio management. Encryption features have further simplified the process of claim verifications in the insurance sector. In addition, online money transfer has become more secure and efficient through the use of blockchain technology. Various sectors such as entertainment, government and healthcare, voting, online music, crowdfunding, forecasting, real estate, insurance, energy management, the Internet of Things (IoT) and many more use it in making smart contracts which facilitate easy maintenance of records in the form of blocks and help prevent fraud in the network. Blockchain technology offers safety for digital IDs without using physical identification and is the safest method for preventing identity theft. One of the major uses of blockchain is in IoT-connected devices, which are very secure, fast and interconnected. The information flow in the IoT is recorded as blockchain and hence is immune to fraud. Furthermore, the transfer of big data is easy and can be shared for efficient analysis and which is available for immediate use. BT offers promising possibilities for use in science.

BT-based solutions are emerging as a global financial regulating market with an estimate of about US$11.7 billion by 2022 and is believed to increase to US$20 billion by 2024. Currently, there are more than 42 million blockchain wallet users in the market. Most of the banks (about 90%) in Europe and North America have already started exploring the possibilities of using BT that can cut about 30% of the cost of bank infrastructure. Financial companies can also save about US$12 billion per year by adopting BT, therefore, by 2018 the financial sector had invested US$552 million in BT. It is estimated that by 2025, more than 55% of healthcare applications will be using BT. Common devices that will run on the IoT are also projected to reach US$50 billion in coming years.

1.6.1 Financial Sector

The first cryptocurrency, bitcoin, has utilized blockchain technology and now its application range is increasing, the contribution of this technology in the finance sector has revolutionized the world. The financial sector uses it in asset settlement and risk management as well as reducing expenses in trade and many more places; cross-border transactions will be much safer and less expensive with transparent, systematic technology. Deployment of BT can short out existing financial sector problems easily like a real-time payment problem. For instance, international transaction processes have to pass through many stages and are time-consuming, therefore the transfer from one gateway to another causes delays in reaching the final destination. On the other hand, blockchain offers the direct path of node-to-node delivery, therefore it consumes less time in reaching the final destination. In addition, high transaction fees are another problem associated with a long-range path destination and can be significantly reduced by using the direct path of node-to-node delivery in BT. The banking system works in a centralized way and sometimes authority is given to a third party; what if there is a problem in the third-party management system? Here, there are many chances of fraud in a transaction and only one corrupted node can help a hacker to manipulate records, but BT offers a distributed ledger with timestamps so it enhances the security of the data. Overall, in the current existing financial system, we have many more irregularities that can be handled by deployment of BT.

1.6.2 Internet of Things (IoT)

The IoT is a network of smart devices like refrigerators, air-conditioners, TVs, phones and many more, the interconnection between them makes human life easier, but there are many challenges in the interoperability of these devices, the benefit of the IoT can be realized only if we are able to mitigate the challenges. Every company is making its own devices with different features, therefore compatibility and security issues are arising. Similarly, fields like hospitals, agriculture, banks and many more are facing similar security issues with interconnectivity. Therefore, we need a profound solution to solve these challenges and hence BT is seen as a solution as it follows the secure distributed ledger system.

1.6.3 Healthcare Sector

These days every industry wants to improve its services using the latest technology. In the healthcare industry there are many problems such as the accessibility of patient data, providing clinical data to the researcher, securing sensitive data records, retrieving information from the electronic health record (EHR), data sharing between healthcare providers and care institutions, securing drug-related information, data breaches and many more aspects in this system. These critical issues need to be taken care of in a systematic way and the immediate challenges need urgent attention like access control, data integrity and data provenance. In addition, many times a patient is operated on by more than one doctor and therefore the health record data are scattered and it takes a lot of time to access all the health data from different doctors and at the same time the patient is not able to get proper care because of this. In a worst-case scenario, in the case of an accident requiring urgent attention and care in a clinic where the patient receives treatment but had not visited before, the current doctor has no prior knowledge of the patient's health. Therefore, the doctor prescribes a range of tests for proper diagnosis before proceeding to the operating theater. Here, BT can prove very helpful as a distributed ledger keeps all previous records of the patient. An EHR can be enhanced by the Graphics Environment Manager (GEM) operating system. GEM is an infrastructure and proprietary technology which can be deployed in blockchain to automatically reconcile the medical data of providers, healthcare payment systems and more (Yli-Huumo et al., 2016).

1.6.4 Supply Chain

Supply chains depend on transparency, witnesses, beliefs and agreement, and blockchain strengthens this simple idea with a direct connection between buyer and seller and gives encrypted security. Currently many companies use the ABRA application to reduce human labor; it is based on blockchain and it links orders, offers, appointments, invoices and acceleration of sales, etc. and every document gets stored in batches with serial numbers and it provides automation at every stage.

BT can help in improving the supply chain process for better performance and will work on all sizes of goods transportation from one place to another with a transparent path from the place of origin to the destination point. In the current scenario, Walmart, an American company, uses this BT for its inventory management system as well as shipment tracking. If we wanted to record the process of how a particular grocery item gets to the store we needed to record all the processes in the traditional management system or in an excel sheet in a physical manner. It costs money as well as being time-consuming, but with the distributed ledger system it is quite easy to know the current position of the product and help to save money and time. IBM is also fully involved in it. The World Trade Organization is claiming 5% GDP growth worldwide by using this technology. With BT, a transaction can take place in a decentralized fashion. As a result, blockchain can save costs and improve efficiency.

1.6.5 Electronic Voting Machines (EVMs)

Nowadays, in the government sector different parties are questioning the validity of counting votes through electronic voting machines (EVMs). Even though there is no reported proof of data breaches by EVMs, and they are a better solution than the earlier paper voting system, computer experts believe that a voting system can be rigged, and results can be manipulated by cybercriminals. On top of that, we have other problems like how to maintain EVMs and how to save time in voting. Here, BT shows capability in enhancing security to voters at voting time, reducing the time it takes to declare results and the possibility of increasing remote voting too.

1.6.6 Energy Sector

The power sector is an important system where power generators, power transmission networks and power distributors operate at various levels, are not integrated and therefore a lot of cost is associated with this multi-tiered system. BT can certainly provide a decentralized system to make it more efficient and cost effective. Using BT, all these multiple levels can be directly linked to each other and therefore producers can directly interact with consumers as per their requirements. Consumers can avail the billing system in the energy sector by using BT. Here legally binding smart contracts can be made in this system.

1.6.7 Real Estate

Traditionally, the recording of property rights takes place in the government system and employees play an important role in storing ownership-related data. The system works as a third party and data go into a central database and public directory. Later on, a public directory is the only source for data recovery in cases of property disputes and claims. Also, the data recovery process can be time-consuming and error-prone, a minor human error while making a data record can put ownership in jeopardy, but on a blockchain network data storing goes with proper verification. It provides an easy way of scanning or tracking historical data with a distributed ledger system, so BT is very helpful in securing property rights.

1.6.8 Intellectual Property Rights

Intellectual property is a product of the human intellect that only the creator can hold or have possession of, and property rights make clear that property belongs to a particular person for a certain period of time. Blockchain has been used to protect property rights. According to Manual Araoz, a developer from Argentina developed a site name "proof of existence" which is based on blockchain and allows the user to submit their original data and get it processed and encrypted without revealing the identity of the real author. The copy of the work gets verified by many nodes in the network (Yoo et al., 2018).

1.7 Conclusion

With the property of decentralization, audibility and immutability, BT has proven its potential to revolutionize the world in all types of secure communications. This chapter shows deployment of BT in many fields (banking, IPR, finance, IoT, electronic voting, etc.) redefines these fields from better to best. The categorization of BT is showing its best use in different scenarios. Nowadays many blockchain platforms are available which support different languages for different applications; some are defined in this chapter. This review has explored the overall operation, characteristics, architecture, potential market value and its various applications. Furthermore, we have discussed some potential drawbacks in BT which might breach security (Zhang et al., 2017). However, the field of BT continues to gain popularity and is still unexplored and is expected to find application in many untouched fields; it has the potential to revolutionize the world.

Although BT has many characteristics which make it secure, recent breaches in its security have raised eyebrows about its security. In 2018, a Japanese exchange, Coincheck, lost US$500 million of cryptocurrency which was transferred to another Coincheck account. Yet another problem is the disk space which needs to be clear after each transaction. The major problem that BT faces is the governance challenge, as many private and closed ledgers are run by consortium companies. Another problem that BT faces is the high energy consumption because of validating the transactions by the miners and in the process of signature validations (Zhang et al., 2017). There are other challenges called the forks, which set new rules for the users and may not support the earlier transactions in the block if it violates the new rule (Zeilinger, 2018).

References

Anjum, A, Sporny, M and Sill, A. (2017). Blockchain standards for compliance and trust. *IEEE Cloud Computing* 4:84–90.

Botta, A, De Donato, W, Persico, V and Pescape, A. (2016). Integration of cloud computing and internet of things: A survey. *Future Generation Computer System* 56:684–700.

Crosby, M, Pattanayak, P, Verma, S and Kalyanaraman, V. (2016). Blockchain technology: Beyond bitcoin. *Appllication Innovation* 2:6–10.

Casino, F, Dasaklis, KT and Patsakis, C. (2019). A systematic literature review of blockchain-based applications: Current status, classification and open issues. *Telematics and Informatics* 36:55–81.

Fan, K, Ren, Y, Wang, Y, Li, H and Yang, Y. (2018). Blockchain-based efficient privacy preserving and data sharing scheme of content-centric network in 5G. *IET Communication* 12:527–532.

Fanning, K and Centers, DP. (2016). Blockchain and its coming impact on financial services. *Journal of Corporate Accounting & Finance* 27:53–57.

Tan, AWK, Zhao, Y and Halliday, T. (2018). A blockchain model for less container load operations in China. *International Journal of Information Systems and Supply Chain Management* 11:39–53.

Tang, CM, Zhang, YL and Yu, X. (2018). Design of vehicle networking data exchange system based on BlockChain. *Journal of Tianjin Polytechnic University* 37:84–88.

Tapscott, D and Tapscott, A. (2017). How blockchain will change organizations. *MIT Sloan Management Review* 58:10–13.

Wang, J, Li, M, He, Y, Li, H, Xiao, K and Wang, C. (2018). A blockchain based privacy-preserving incentive mechanism in crowd sensing applications. *IEEE Access* 6:17545–17556.

White, GRT. (2017). Future applications of blockchain in business and management: A Delphi study. *Strategic Change* 26:439–451.

Xu, Q, Aung, KMM, Zhu, Y and Yong, KL. (2018). A blockchain-based storage system for data analytics in the internet of things. *Studies in Computational Intelligence* 715:119–138.

Yang, C, Chen, X and Xiang, Y. (2018). Blockchain-based publicly verifiable data deletion scheme for cloud storage. *Journal of Network and Computer Applications* 103:185–193.

Ying, W, Jia, S and Du, W. (2018). Digital enablement of blockchain: Evidence from HNA group. *International Journal of Information Management* 39:1–4.

Yli-Huumo, J, Ko, D, Choi, S, Park, S and Smolander, K. (2016). Where is current research on blockchain technology?–A systematic review. *PloS one* 11:1–27.
Yoo, M and Won, Y. 2018. Study on smart automated sales system with blockchain-based data storage and management. *Lecture Notes Electrical Engineering* 474:734–740.
Zeilinger, M. (2018). Digital art as 'monetised graphics': Enforcing intellectual property on the blockchain. *Philosophy & Technology* 31:15–41.
Zhang, N, Zhong, S and Tian, L. (2017). Using blockchain to protect personal privacy in the scenario of Online taxi-hailing. *International Journal of Computers Communications & Control* 12:886–902.
Zhang, J. (2016). Walks trajectory tracking of shared information based on consortium blockchain. *Revista de la Facultad de Ingenieria* 31:8–17.

2

Blockchain for IoT-Enabled Healthcare Systems

Ranjana Sikarwar

CONTENTS

2.1 Introduction

The application of Blockchain and the Internet of Things (IoT), has emerged as the most captivating concept of the technological era, transforming the future of the digital world. IoT- enabled objects are smart and capable of sharing data online. IoT devices connecting and communicating through the internet send data to a centralized storage system, like a cloud server for exchanging information, which may pose threats to the security of the system due to cyberattacks and may violate the privacy of the large responsive data produced. So blockchain technology provides a confidential mechanism for exchanging information in order to accomplish privacy, and authentication (Thakore et al., 2019). Blockchain

DOI: 10.1201/9781003133179-2

is an open distributed ledger where data is resistant to modification, typically managed by a peer-to-peer network using an inter-node communication protocol and validating new blocks in the chain. IoT applications can now be seen in digital healthcare and also for the personalized healthcare of patients. Patients can wear smart bands, smart-watches or non-wearable devices like blood pressure monitors, glucose level monitors, lung function monitors, etc. to record their body activity. Such smart devices can collect patients' body information and could also sense environmental conditions like temperature, humidity, pressure, etc. These devices are connected to the internet to provide continuous monitoring of all patient-related health parameters. This approach is very useful in the healthcare industry as doctors can now monitor and track the patient's health in real-time when they are away from the patient. This application of the IoT in healthcare also helps to prevent unnecessary tests, thus reducing costs and saving time. In the blockchain-based IoT systems, nodes deployed in the blockchain technology are likely to be the devices connected in the IoT systems network. Blockchain-enabled IoT systems facilitate the ease of business processes, enhancing transparency for improved customer experience.

2.1.1 IoT Companies Using Blockchain

- **Helium** - Helium is a San Francisco, California-based company, and recently demonstrated its first successful blockchain transaction. The company uses radio technology to empower its wireless internet infrastructure (blockchain-based) (Daley, 2019, March 16).
- **Chronicled** - It uses the combination of blockchain-based IoT devices for a point-to-point supply chain solution. The company uses IoT-based consignments with embedded sensors to produce real-time shipping information for the pharmaceutical and food supply industries. Groups of people which are part of the medical industry, or a food supply shipping task are updated on the custody chain by using blockchain in their IoT devices.
- **ArcTouch** - The company has developed and built blockchain-based software for wearables, smart TVs, voice assistants, etc. ArcTouch has developed decentralized apps (DApps) for many companies using IoT devices (Daley, 2019, March 16).
- **HYPR** - HYPR is located in New York and uses decentralized networks to provide security for ATM machines, cars, locks and homes. The systems of centralized databases, with millions of passwords, are more susceptible to cyberattacks.

Let us first understand the basic concepts of the IoT and blockchain before going into the details of the transformation caused by the merging of the two most popular technologies in the healthcare industry.

2.2 IoT and Blockchain in Healthcare

2.2.1 What is the IoT?

To understand the basics of the IoT consider the example of a smartphone which can now be used for many purposes like listening to music online, playing games, watching movies, mobile banking, checking emails, sharing data with peers, online reservation, etc. But a few years back cell phones were used only for the purpose of making calls and sending text messages. They were not smart because they were not connected to the internet. But cell phones have become smart phones because they can send or receive data through the internet. This is the indispensable theory of how objects or devices can become smarter using the internet.

Classification of the IoT can be done as follows:

- **Devices that collect data and act on it.**
  Things like smart cars, connected medical devices, watches, etc. that receive data from sensors and act in response to that data.
- **Things that aggregate and send data.**
  For example, sensors for monitoring the temperature, moisture and gas that detect and respond to changes in an environment.
- **Things that perform both functionalities.**
  Dielectric soil moisture sensors used in IoT farming collect data on moisture levels to know the amount of water required by the crops.

2.2.1.1 IoT Architecture

IoT systems need to follow a definite process framework, enabling the devices involved in the IoT network to sense the physical environment and respond to the stimuli from the real-world without the intervention of humans. Thus, the IoT framework is built for IoT systems comprising four stages or layers.

Stage 1 (Sensors/Actuators) - Devices involved in the IoT network must be embedded with sensors and actuators (Balraj, 2018).

Stage 2 (Data Acquisition Systems) - Acquisition systems collect data from the sensors and transform them into digital streams for further processing and analysis.

Stage 3 (Edge IT/Analytics) - After the IoT data are aggregated and digitized by the data acquisition systems further processing and analysis are needed before being transferred to the data center or cloud. The hardware and the software gateways in the edge IT network pre-process and analyze the data before entering the data center.

Stage 4 (Data Center) - For deep processing of the data they are transferred to the data center for further analytics, management and security control of devices.

2.2.2 Challenges in Current IoT Solutions

As current IoT architecture is centralized there is a need for proper authentication, trust and standardization to ensure security in the IoT ecosystem in which a vast volume of data is generated by the IoT devices. The IoT ecosystem has a centralized architecture where all data is stored and analyzed in cloud servers, thus making data more prone to major failure. Thus, performance of the system is affected due to the increasing number of devices in the network, leading to operational delays and redundant data transfers. Blockchain can be used to keep a record of data produced by the sensors and avoid duplication with any other malicious data. In a blockchain network, no third party is employed for establishing trust (Thakore et al., 2019). To overcome such challenges for the IoT a decentralized architecture will lower all such costs, reduce redundancy, improve services and be; resistant to major faults. In an IoT-based architecture the cloud is the center for storing all the data and a single point of failure which can bring down the whole network. Blockchain uses a distributed ledger and removes the single source of failure in the network.

2.2.2.1 Why Does IoT Need Blockchain?

The IoT network comprises many devices connected to the internet exposed to cyberattacks and hacks. According to a Gartner Research report, there will be around 20.4 billion IoT devices by the end of 2020, this means these devices will be more vulnerable to cyberattacks without blockchain. Blockchain is the best solution to protect the IoT against hacks and cyberattacks as it records the transaction and overcomes the challenge of reliability, single point of failure, trust and security. The IoT needs to implement blockchain for many reasons like security, automation and cost reduction as billions of IoT devices send data to the centralized cloud architecture currently and in the coming years. As traditional IoT systems send data to the centralized architecture, which has limited reliability, it hampers network safety. Blockchain makes all the transactions directly and records them all cryptographically so that they are not changed or altered once recorded. In digital healthcare an electronic health record (EHR) has shown many benefits for storing patient's sensitive health data and making it personalized for patients and concerned doctors only. But due to the lack of security in this approach many hospitals hesitate to embrace this application. Currently hospitals follow a centralized approach for storing health records which are difficult to exchange between various health centers. Thus, blockchain is the solution to provide security for storing sensitive data in an EHR. Using blockchain technology it would be difficult for hackers to hack sensitive health data as a patient is in control of their own EHR.

2.2.2.2 Automation to Reduce Costs

As the technology is growing quickly nowadays there is no need to perform certain tasks manually; blockchain enables the automation to complete those processes. A smart contract is one of the aspects of blockchain which can be used for automation in the industrial sector. Once created in the blockchain network, smart contracts make it possible for all the devices to execute their tasks independently by creating agreements governed, upheld and carried out by the blockchain instead of an individual person. Also, they define the rules and forfeits of an agreement. It allows peer-to-peer communication, can automatically deduct monies owed and handles transactions without human intervention. Like a traditional contract, it defines rules and regulations and enforces obligations.

2.2.3 Applications of the IoT

The top trending applications of the IoT are as follows:

Digital healthcare - IoT devices constantly collect the health data of patients and at times of emergency cases valuable time can be saved. An electronic health record (EHR) is used to store the patient's collected health data for future insights and diagnosis. An EHR is patient-specific and personalized for the patient and the concerned doctor and depersonalized for others like pharmacy institutions, other doctors, etc. Patients cannot delete or modify sensitive data from their EHR, the data are controlled fully by the EHR.

Smart homes - Smart home products consist of different appliances like air conditioners, washing machines, refrigerators, etc. which promise to save time, energy and money. This enhances the security of the house and makes life easier, for example, it detects windows and doors opening to prevent intruders (Pavithran et al., 2020).

Wearables - Wearable IoT devices are small in size, embedded with sensors and software, which track and collect data and later pre-processes to extract important insights about the user. These devices broadly cover health monitoring, fitness and entertainment. Wearable applications need to be highly energy-efficient and; small in size as a prerequisite for IoT technology.

Smart cities - A smart city is another powerful application of the IoT equipped with devices capable of sending and receiving signals through the internet. Smart surveillance, automated transportation, smart energy management systems, environmental monitoring, etc. are IoT- enabled applications for smart cities (Suter, 2019).

Smart metering - Smart grids, tank level monitoring, water flow measurement, monitoring and optimization of performance in solar energy, etc. are all applications of real-time IoT applications (Lambrechts and Sinha, 2016).

2.2.4 What is Blockchain?

The term blockchain was first coined in 1991 by a group of practitioners who wanted to invent a tool for time-stamping digital documents so that they were not altered or backdated. Nowadays blockchain technology is gaining popularity after the invention of Bitcoin, the first digital currency. Blockchain was introduced in 2008 by a person or a group named Satoshi Nakamoto after the invention of cryptocurrency, Bitcoin ("Bitcoin: A P2P Electronic Cash System") (Nakamoto, 2008). Typically, it is a type of a payment trail, a chain of blocks or growing record lists linked together using cryptography. Blockchain is composed of two parts: Blocks, consisting of a set of transactions and Chains, consisting of blocks in a specific sequence linked to hash values of previous blocks, a timestamp and transaction data represented in the form of a Merkle tree. Blockchain keeps track of the transactions in chunks of blocks which are linked using cryptography. Cryptography is a technique in which data communication is made secure by encrypting it, thus preventing third parties from accessing the private messages. Some of the challenges that the IoT faces are decentralization, poor interoperability, privacy and security vulnerabilities, which can be overcome by blockchain technology. Blockchain, technically, is a distributed ledger, cryptographically secured to a decentralized database which enables protected data transfer and records every transaction made on a network. The ledger is distributed over a network of nodes which can either be a public network or a private network.

Blockchains allow peer-to-peer transactions, dispensinging with the need for intermediaries.

The two fields that are going to be influenced by it are:

- A decentralized system with peer-to-peer interaction that eliminates the necessity for central servers.
- Full transparency and open access to all databases that prevents overwriting of data by individuals using it for their own work.

This technology basically has four elements.

Consensus: It is an agreed-upon protocol by all participating members of the network. Provides the proof of work (PoW) and verifies the ledger updating in the networks.

Ledger: Provides a detailed system of transaction records within networks.

Cryptography: Ensures encryption of data in ledger and networks and maintains data integrity, also only an authorized user can decrypt the information.

Smart contract: Also known as chain code, it is used to verify and validate the participants' terms of business agreement on the network (Kohad, 2020).

2.2.4.1 Designing Optimized Blockchain for the IoT

The architecture of the blockchain in the IoT must be designed to regulate the traffic generated by the nodes in the network. A blockchain system must provide security to protect the data from threats and cyberattacks. It must be designed to provide scalability, transparency, concurrency, etc. (Ali et al., 2019).

Wireless Sensor Networks - A large collection of sensors in a communication network called nodes, with each individual node capable of communication, sensing, actuation and; computing with constrained power requirements.

Agent Node - A special node in blockchain responsible for deploying the smart contract in the network.

Blockchain Network - A tiered coordinated blockchain system.

2.2.4.2 Cryptographic Algorithms Used

To maintain privacy in the network, a transaction is decrypted by the nodes containing the sender's public key. To keep up the integrity of data, changes or any kind of manipulation may refuse exact decoding. The use of private keys will provide security. Some of the most secure and powerful PKC schemes used are RSA and Elliptic Curve Diffie-Hellman Exchange recommended by NIST. RSA is considered to be energy draining for nodes, steady and; computation-intensive, thus inappropriate to use. Also, Ephemeral Key Exchange has heavy overhead and computation, thus not suitable for deployment. So, considering the above limitations a simplified RSA, Elliptic Key cryptography is used which shows comparatively enhanced performance on resource-constrained devices. A weak mathematical model used can easily tear down the system. The hash functions used in blockchain are very important in their work. A powerful hash function needs heavy computation, time, resources and energy which the IoT network lacks. As an example, the popularly used hash functions for consensus algorithms are SHA-256d by Bitcoin, Gridcoin, Peercoin, etc.

2.2.4.3 Types of Blockchain

There are two types of blockchain, primarily private and public. Other variations are also available like hybrid and consortium blockchains, as shown in Figure 2.1.

- **Public Blockchains** - A public blockchain is an open-source, non-restrictive system where everyone can read or write data. Anyone can become an authorized node of the network by signing into a blockchain platform through the internet.

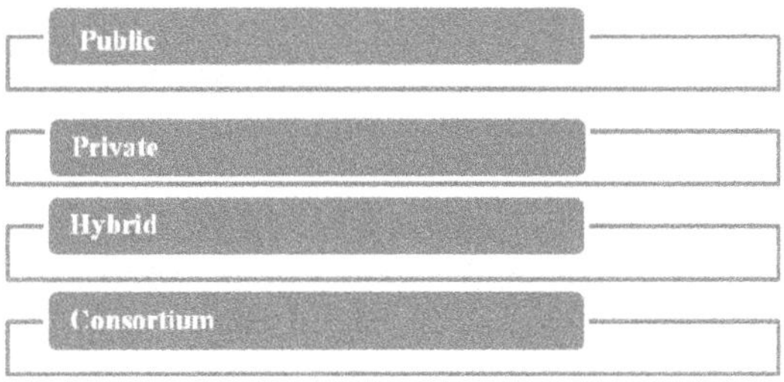

FIGURE 2.1
Types of blockchain.

All transactions are fully transparent which means that any participating node in the blockchain network is authorized. Public blockchains are used basically for mining and exchanging cryptocurrencies. Examples are Bitcoin, Ethereum, and Litecoin (Wazid et al., 2020).

- **Private Blockchains -** A private blockchain is restrictive or permissioned where all the participants are known and trusted. This is useful when blockchain is used within an organization or enterprise where all participants belong to the same network. Examples - Hyperledger and R3 Corda mainly used in supply chain management, voting, asset ownership, etc. (Fabric, Sawtooth, Corda, etc.).
- **Hybrid Blockchains -** They use the features of both public and private blockchains. Only selected data or records from the blockchain can be made public while others are kept confidential in the private network (Wazid et al., 2020). Examples include Dragon Chair, a hybrid blockchain.
- **Consortium Blockchain -** A consortium blockchain is a semi-decentralized type governed by a group rather than a single entity. Participants in a blockchain consortium may include banks, government organizations, etc. Examples of consortium blockchains are Energy Web Foundation, R3, etc.

2.2.4.4 Advantages of Using Blockchain Technology

1. Allows for scalability, data is resistant to malicious attacks because data is on a distributed network of nodes, greater automation.
2. Security of the network is maintained due to the decentralized, cryptographically-secured network.
3. There is no single point of failure, thus it does not bring the whole network down, in contrast to a centralized network when a single point of failure disables the entire network.

2.2.4.5 Advantages of Using Blockchain in the IoT

Blockchain technology when integrated with the IoT offers many advantages like improved interoperability, enhanced security, privacy, and complements the IoT with reliability and scalability. The combination of blockchain and the IoT provides the following merits:

- **Interoperability** across IoT systems, smart devices, machines, and industrial sectors where interoperability means exchanging information between IoT systems and interacting continuously with them.

- **Build trust** - Blockchain is an open distributed ledger, reduces the risk of tampering and builds trust between parties involved. There is no central controlling entity or organization over the enormous amount of data generated by the IoT devices.
- **Improved security** - Blockchain integrated with the IoT provides security against cyberattacks. Real-time threat detection can be detected using machine-learning approaches.
- **Data exchange for digital currency** - Data is exchanged for the digital currency in a more reliable way using blockchain with the IoT.
- **Reduced costs** - Blockchain allows IoT companies to reduce costs by removing the processing overheads of IoT gateways.
- **Increased speed of transactions** - Blockchain ensures fast processing of transactions and increased interaction among billions of connected devices.

2.3 Blockchain-based IoT Platforms

1) **IoT chain**

This platform, also known as ITC, is specifically designed for IoT devices and uses distributed ledger technology to solve IoT security to operate as a decentralized network. In the coming years most electronics will have some level of smart technology embedded in them to connect and share data. To communicate within the network these devices will require an IoT operating system. This technology can be implemented at the chip level with an IoT chain to become a good-to-use platform for such devices in the IoT ecosystem. The IoT chain is a digital token of the project and wanted to be the basic network for the IoT. This project was established by the Chinese team of developers who started in 2017, emphasizing the processing of micro-operations. The project was initiated with the notion of creating platforms for the communication of "smart devices."This type of network is used in the area of artificial intelligence.

2) **IOTA**

IOTA is the first blockchain-based IoT platform (crypto project) using directed acyclic graphs (DAG) specifically made for the IoT which provides a data transfer layer for connected devices with transaction settlement. This project completely eliminates the idea of paying a miner's fee. IOTA is distributed ledger technology (DLT) and in an IOTA network a new transaction will be added to the chain only ahead of the last two transactions.

An IOTA tangle platform is a decentralized, blockless network integrated with Hyperledger Fabric systems which are cryptographic where users validate the transactions of other users instead of verification by the third party. It is advantageous as it provides scalability and avoids the payment of transaction fees. Such features are beneficial where billions of micro-transactions are processed between the devices, regularly extending to feel-less payments, encrypted transaction payload and public/private message chains. When a smart contract is executed, a call is made to this platform to save the output of its execution and for the transactions between the IOTA wallet holders.

3) **Walton chain**

The word Walton in Walton chain is derived from the name of Charlie Walton who was the inventor of RFID technology. The term Walton can be elaborated as WALTON = Wisdom, Alters Label, Trade, Organization. One block in a Walton chain can accommodate up to 255 transaction records. The communication mode used in IoT devices is RFID and the electronic transaction is carried out on the blockchain architecture. This combined technology tracks the products using RFID identification at every step of distribution and production. The data linked with each item are stored on an immutable blockchain which in turn promises its accuracy. The Walton chain gave the idea of value to the IoT to introduce the merged concept of their proprietary RFID chips with blockchain technology. The software used is the Walton chain protocol and another one is Walton coin.

2.4 Use cases of blockchain in the healthcare industry

The overall vision of blockchain in healthcare is to create a network of healthcare information databases for clinical data exchange. In this blockchain-based network doctors, nurses, hospitals, etc. can access data considering the privacy issues and type of medical software used. Blockchain-based smart contracts facilitate access to patients' records between different healthcare providers.

2.4.1 Master Patient Index

A database is used to store the demographics of patients. Using Master Patient Index different organizations with this software can easily access important patient-related data files. A blockchain-based smart contract allows storage of the patient's critical information (personal files) ensuring security and restricted access.

2.4.2 Electronic Health Record (EHR)

An Electronic Health Record is the most flexible application which uses blockchain technology and smart contracts to store all medical records (doctor's reports, laboratory tests, prescriptions, etc.) in a distributed ledger making interoperability easier. When thinking about interoperability and using a blockchain platform, the EHR is the first application that will come to mind.

2.4.3 Provider Directory

Blockchain and smart contracts are also used to store the healthcare providers' directories ensuring interoperability among different providers. Verification of important credentials of the doctors' like their licenses, doctoral degrees and qualifications with a smart contract.

2.4.4 Medical Insurance Claims

Automation of medical insurance claims between different providers and patrons is possible with the help of smart contracts. Smart contracts and blockchain enforce fast and flexible interoperability amongst healthcare establishments and financiers.

2.5 Applications of blockchain in the IoT

- **Pharmaceutical industry**

  The challenge faced by the pharmaceutical sector is the counterfeiting of medicines. The use of blockchain technology with the IoT protects the drug manufacturing process by allowing the stakeholders to keep the blockchain network updated with real-time on-going activities in the manufacturing process. As blockchain works as a distributed, transparent ledger it is easy to observe and watch the drug manufacturing process and supply. One of the real-life applications of blockchain and IoT is Medi Ledger that can keep track of all the legalities involved in the medicines. It is an open decentralized network for the pharmaceutical industry. The Mediledger network helps the pharma industry to keep record of transactions and data to exhibit adherence to the regulations and enhances security. It provides permission-based private messaging for the exchange of data between the business partners. It protects business intelligence so that industry is shielded. It imposes cross industry business rules without disclosing confidential private data.

- Smart homes industry

  The use of blockchain technology in the IoT used in smart homes enhances the security of the data generated by the IoT devices which are operated remotely from smartphones.

  Blockchain used in the IoT can enhance the security of smart homes overcoming the drawbacks of centralized infrastructure. As an example, an Australian telecommunication and media company has implemented biometric security to protect the data generated by the smart devices at home from being manipulated. By injecting blockchain technology into IoT devices, data is accessed only by authorized persons.

- **Supply chain and logistics**

  The supply chain and logistics industry face a lot of issues in the delay in the delivery of items as there are a number of partners involved in the supply chain network. IoT-enabled devices are used to keep track of the transport of products at every stage. Transparency of the whole transaction is maintained with blockchain. IoT sensors (for example, motion sensors, GPS, temperature sensor, etc.) collect and keep record of the shipment status. The data collected from the IoT sensors are stored in the blockchain network as useful information for transparency to provide updates to all the participating members in the smart contracts, so that they can get real-time updated information. The combination of blockchain and the IoT adds reliability to the supply chain network. Also, they improve the traceability of the goods.

- **Automotive industry**

  The automotive industry also uses digitization like other sectors. Therefore, industries promote fully automated vehicles with IoT-enabled sensors in them. These vehicles are IoT and blockchain-enabled which help different involved users to share sensitive information easily and fast. For example, NetObjex is a blockchain automated traffic control. It works in collaboration with PN which is a parking sensor company that performs real-time vehicle detection and searches for vacant available parking slots in the parking area. Also, the payments of these are done using crypto wallets.

- **Cooperatively owned self-driving cars**

  A blockchain-based service can be used in self-driving vehicle-sharing among a group of individuals who can enter into an agreement regarding vehicle-sharing and its maintenance among themselves. Cooperative groups can form contracts with other groups and share usage of vehicles with other peer groups.

2.6 Conclusion

This chapter discusses the concepts of the IoT and blockchain along with their applications in digital healthcare. Blockchain is considered secure by design and unravels cryptocurrency-related double-spending problems. It can reshape and elevate the global infrastructure of the technologies connected with each other through the internet. In healthcare applications, when used in combination the IoT and blockchain can store the patient's sensitive health data securely and do real-time monitoring of the patients. Many companies will exploit the integration of blockchain-based IoT systems in the near future as blockchain is more commendable.

References

Toqeer Ali, Ali Alzahrani, Salman Jan, Muhammad Shoaib Siddiqui, Member, IEEE, Adnan Nadeem and Turki Alghamdi. (2019). A Comparative Analysis of Blockchain Architecture and Its Applications: Problems and Recommendations. *IEEE Access*, 7: 1–11.

Balraj. (2018). Crypto Currency: Everything You Need to Know About It. Retrieved May 2020, from https://pepnewz.com/2018/02/24/cryptocurrency-everything-need-know.

Blockchain and the Internet of Things: The IoT Blockchain Opportunity and Challenge. Retrieved 13 May 2020 from https://www.i-scoop.eu/internet-of-things-guide/blockchain-iot.

Sam Daley. (2019). Blockchain and IoT: 8 Examples Making Our Future Smarter. Retrieved 13 May 2020 from https://builtin.com/blockchain/blockchain-iot-examples.

Hemlata Kohad. (2020). Scalability Issues of Blockchain Technology *International Journal of Engineering and Advanced Technology*, 2020.

Johannes Lambrechts and Saurabh Sinha. (2016). Micro Sensing Networks for Sustainable Cities: Pollution as a Key Driving Factor. Retrieved from https://link.springer.com/chapter/10.1007/978-3-319-28358-6_1.

S. Nakamoto. (2008). Bitcoin: A Peer-to-Peer Electronic Cash System. Retrieved from http://bitcoin.org/bitcoin.pdf

Chrisjan Pauw. (2018). How Significant Is Blockchain in the Internet of Things? Retrieved from https://cointelegraph.com/news/how-significant-is-blockchain-in-internet-of-things.

Deepa Pavithran, Khaled Shaalan, Jamal N. Al-Karaki and Amjad Gawanmeh. (2020). Towards Building a Blockchain Framework for IoT. *Cluster Computing*, 23(9). DOI:10.1007/s10586-020-03059-5

Amandeep Suter (2019). How is the Internet of Things Making Life Safer? Retrieved 13 May 2020 from https://techstory.in/internet-of-things-making-life-safe.

Riya Thakore, Rajkumar Vaghashiya, Chintan Patel; and Nishant Doshi. (2019). "Blockchain - based IoT: A Survey" Proceedings of the 2nd International Workshop on Recent advances on Internet of Things: Technology and Application Approaches (IoT-T&A 2019) 2019, Halifax, Canada.

Mohammad Wazid, Ashok Kumar Das, Sachin Shetty and Minho Jo (2020). A Tutorial and Future Research for Building a Blockchain-Based Secure Communication Scheme for Internet of Intelligent Things, *IEEE Access*, 8: 88700–88716. https://doi.org/10.1109/access.2020.2992467

3

Role of Blockchain Technology: Pandemic and Insight into Data Analysis for Covid-19

Satyendra Kumar Shet and Vinayaka B Shet

CONTENTS

3.1 Introduction

The unexpected pandemic situation posed various challenges globally. Even with suitable technological advancement, many countries struggled in handling the pandemic situation effectively. Eventually, most countries opted for lockdown as the only primary option to control Covid-19. However, lockdown is not the solution. Even though the challenges of the pandemic situation were not anticipated earlier, society is now forced to learn the lessons. The root cause of the Covid-19 outbreak is still a mystery, in addition to the lack of effective data management with the highest biosafety level. Post pandemic situations are also challenging to identify the viral genome, tracing infected people, symptoms, treatment, clinical trial management, development and distribution of vaccines and making policy for the future. Hence, it is evident that data integrity, prevention of data tampering and instant information sharing are also very much essential to successfully manage the pandemic situation. Integration of blockchain technology will certainly accelerate effective governance during a pandemic crisis.

DOI: 10.1201/9781003133179-3

The rapid spread of infectious diseases to the community in a very short time is termed an epidemic. It is restricted to a city or region or country. The occurrence of an epidemic worldwide within a minimal period of time is known as a pandemic. Bacteria or viruses are responsible for spreading infectious diseases. Depending on the pandemic situation, the mode of transmission to humans will differ. Based on understanding the mechanism of transmission, precautionary measures will be adopted to prevent the spread of such a disease. During the outbreak of a pandemic such as Covid-19, the collection of accurate data by the government plays an important crisis management role. The logistics required, such as testing centers, quarantine facilities, creation of isolation wards, personal protection equipment, additional medical equipment for handling the situation, enhancing hospital capabilities, creating quarantine facilities, estimating the peak of the pandemic and projecting the span of the pandemic wave can be estimated on the basis of primary data. However, the existing conventional methods are not efficient for the collection of accurate real-time data and during the Covid-19 pandemic governments were forced to adopt the lockdown option to handle the crisis. The decisions taken changed dynamically due to the prevailing uncertainty; hence, conventional methods were not result oriented because of a lack of accurate real-time data and analysis. The uncertainty in such a situation created a challenge in decision-making to prevent the further spread of the pandemic.

3.2 Existing Methodology

The primary source of information on pandemic patients is gathered from hospitals, clinical laboratories and government-approved testing centers. The approved testing mechanisms to identify the pandemic may provide false positive results. The data obtained may not be reliable due to the lack of monitoring, negligence in the labeling of the sample, lapses in the preservation of samples until testing, delays from the time of sample collection to the testing, may include false positive cases and unintentional flaws during the process. As the screening drive for the pandemic in the mass population was initiated, the chances of lapses also increased, thus making real-time data unreliable. In the existing approach, the data will normally be stored in ledgers or computer systems and the information will be passed on to the competent authority. This data declared by competent authorities may not be dynamic because of the delay incurred in the testing of collected samples from the individual. As a result, the declared data may not be realistic. Also, during data entry, flaws such as a negative test report might be entered as positive which will add to the total cases reported. Because of the time lapses in the generation of actual reports, patients who were already infected might have traveled to different places and tracing such patients with primary contacts and secondary contacts within a number of days/weeks became a challenging task. Drawbacks of the existing method are depicted in Figure 3.1.

3.3 Data Generation and Analysis

3.3.1 Viral Genome

The virus responsible for the disease is to be isolated and its genomic information can be gathered using genome sequencing methods. The anatomy of genomic data will help to

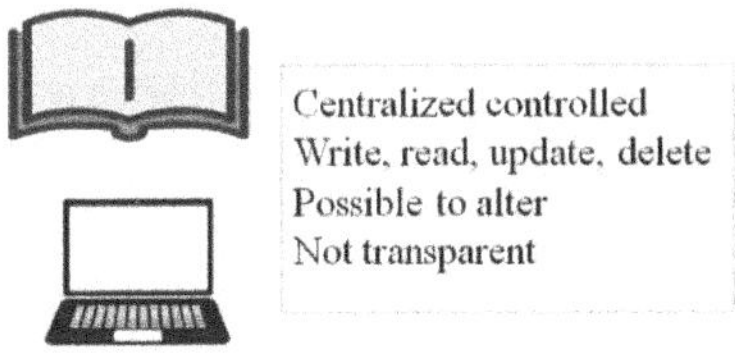

FIGURE 3.1
Drawback of existing methods.

decode the information. The virus isolated from the different geographical regions will reveal similarities based on the sequence analysis technique and insights into mutations occurring in the virus can be detected. Covid-19 is reported to have the largest genome (26.4–31.7 kb) among all the RNA viruses. Genomes are responsible for the expression of the coat protein of the virus. Genomic data are made available to the public domain by the National Center for Biotechnology Information (NCBI) database. Genome sequence analysis will reveal the relationship between different genome sequences reported from the geographical region, similarity, rate of mutation, virulence. This information will be the basis for the competent authority to develop standard operating protocol guidelines and to take preventive measures to combat the disease.

3.3.2 Infected People

The data of infected people are collected from hospitals and government-approved testing labs. Infected patients will be housed in quarantine facilities for the stipulated period of time (maximum 30 days) and treatment will be initiated. The data recorded during the monitoring period of the patients will assist the doctors to understand the symptoms, time required for recovery and type of food to be provided to overcome the situation.

3.3.3 Contact Tracing

As appositive case of the pandemic is reported, in order to prevent further spreading primary and secondary contacts will be identified and subjected to quarantine for a stipulated period. Tracing primary and secondary contacts become quite a challenge due to the time delay of availing the test report. The contact tracing concept is shown in Figure 3.2. The testing of more samples will consume time depending on the type of testing method adopted. The polymerase chain reaction (PCR) based detection will take more time compared to the antigen/antibody (rapid detection) based methods. To a greater extent, based on the cell number, tracing and mobility of the patient monitoring were successful. However, there are a few loopholes in the existing methodology to tamper with the data (Marbouh et al., 2020).

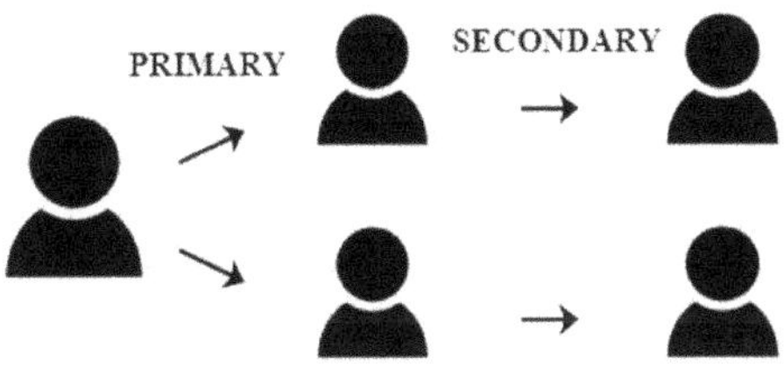

FIGURE 3.2
Contact tracing.

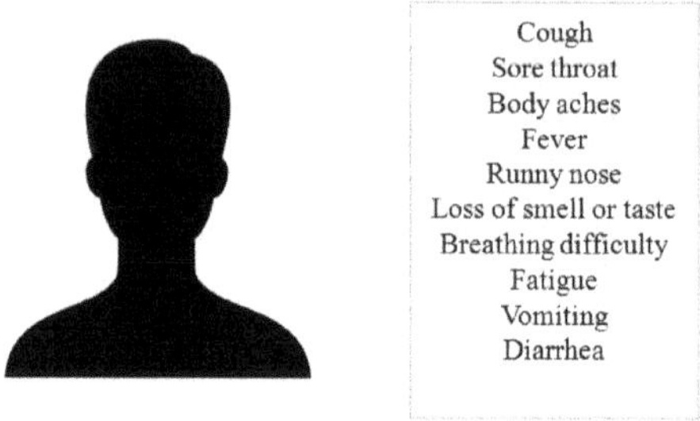

FIGURE 3.3
Symptoms prevailed during Covid-19 infection.

3.3.4 Symptoms

The symptoms of the pandemic will vary from person to person. The Covid-19 symptoms reported are cough, runny nose, fever, sore throat, body aches, loss of smell or taste, headache, breathing difficulty, fatigue, vomiting, diarrhea and an effect on the body's metabolism. Patients may have only a few of the symptoms listed, as depicted in Figure 3.3. Children, adults and senior citizens with serious medical conditions such as diabetes, heart, lung, liver or kidney disease are very much prone to be at higher risk of developing complications due to Covid-19. Complications further include blood clots, heart problems, organ failure, pneumonia and infections leading to loss of life (Marbouh et al., 2020).

3.3.5 Treatment

Based on the symptoms and their stages, different types of treatment are to be provided. For fever, medication will be recommended to reduce the temperature; oxygen will be supplied to patients with severe breathing problems. Adequate rest, intake of warm water or fluid and nutritional food is prescribed to the infected patient. In practice, a citrus fruit, protein diet is suggested. In certain cases, patients with bacterial infections are given anti-bacterial medication. The data of patients who have recovered from the symptoms are to be recorded and a percentage recovery rate has to be calculated. The treatment and diet suggested are depicted in Figure 3.4.

FIGURE 3.4
Treatment and diet.

3.4 Blockchain Technology

3.4.1 Basic Concept

Blockchain is a distributed ledger technology consisting of different blocks with data that are connected to each other.

Each block will contain data, hashes, and a hash of the previous block. Depending on the category of blockchain, the data will be stored in the respective block. The hash is unique for the individual block. The content and the blocks are identified by the hash. As and when the new block is included in the network, the corresponding hash is automatically calculated. Any changes incorporated in the contents of the block will create the changes in the respective hash. The hashes of the earlier blocks will efficiently develop chain of blocks which makes the blocks highly secures shown in Figure 3.5. The first block created is termed a genesis block. Bringing changes to the block will make the subsequent blocks invalid due to the change in hash. In order to make the blockchain valid, hashes of all the blocks have to be recalculated. The proof of work is the mechanism that slows down the creation of new blocks into the chain. This type of mechanism is quite difficult to tamper with. In order to tamper with a block, proof of work has to be recalculated for all the subsequent blocks. The security aspects of blockchain technology depend upon the creation of hashes and acceptance of the changes created in the block. Blockchains are distributed instead of managed centrally, use peer-to-peer networks and permit relevant individuals to join the blockchain network. The individual will get a copy of the blockchain whenever they join. When a new block is created, it will be sent to everyone in the network. The collection of data/records is distributed, decentralized and linked with the others involved in the network (Sharma et al., 2020)

3.4.2 Role of Blockchain Technology

Blockchain technology will play a major role during the pandemic in controlling disease, contact tracing, treatment, monitoring quarantine facilities, the recovery phase, decision-making, supply chain management, efficient governance and clinical data management (Marbouh et al., 2020; Iyengar et al., 2020). These data, collected and stored, are not possible to tamper with at any stage. As a result, real-time dynamic data will be made available to the competent authority for suitable decision-making (Govindan et al., 2020). Comparison between the existing method and blockchain technology is highlighted in Table 3.1.

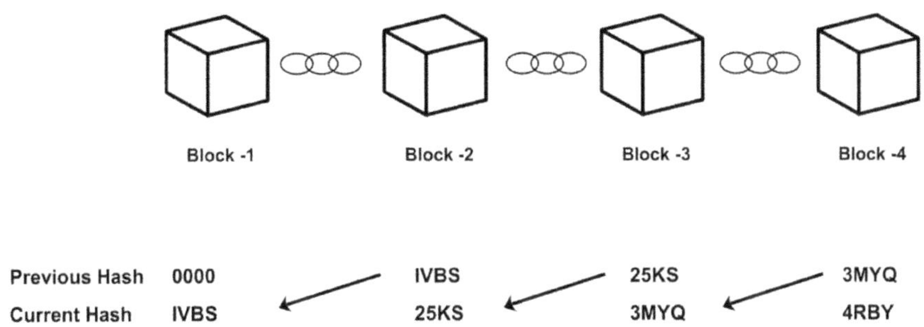

FIGURE 3.5
Basic concept of blockchain technology.

TABLE 3.1
Comparison between Existing Method and Blockchain Technology

Component	Existing Method	Blockchain Technology
Competent authority	Centralized controlled	Decentralized
Handling of data	Write, read, update, delete	Write, read
Integrity of data	Possible to alter	Immutable
Privacy	Prone to cyber attack	Secure due to cryptography technique
Transparency	Not transparent	Transparency achieved through distributed network
Quality of data	Administrator authenticates the data	Data can be traced from the origin
Fault tolerance	No	Yes
Cost	Implementation and maintenance are certain	Uncertainty in maintenance
Performance	More transactions per second can be handled and provide scalability	Limited transactions per second and scalability are challenging due to nascent stage of technology

3.5 Proposed Method

3.5.1 Application to Pandemic Data

Viral genome sequence data: Sequencing information should be shared with researchers throughout the world to analyze the sequence. Genome sequence analysis will provide information on the relative strain and coat protein-coding region. Sequence information collected from different countries and different geographical locations within the country will provide the information on the mutation that has occurred, and the virulence. Further genomic data will help in generating protein sequences and their structure essential for the drug development process.

Hospitals and recognized clinics need to update the data on the number of people screened, positive cases and negative cases. The details of infected people have to be shared, with the competent authority taking appropriate decisions. Comprehensive information on symptoms and the treatment given has to be included. Adopting blockchain technology at different stages will enhance the reliability and accuracy of the collected data.

Details of primary and secondary contacts should be made available to health officials and staff to screen them for the virus. The location of infected people should be made available on the platform accessible to the public without disclosing their personal details. The information will provide real-time data on the infected zone and enable competent authorities to make suitable precautionary decisions (Sharma et al., 2020; Govindan et al., 2020).

3.5.2 Clinical Data Management

The drug or vaccine developed will undergo clinical trials. Clinical trials are conducted in four phases. The clinical phase of the trial involves volunteers or patients in a large number and makes the process challenging. The clinical trials need to be operated efficiently, hence there is a need for a data management system to maintain integrity and transparency. Adopting blockchain technology will ensure the privacy and safety of volunteers. It will also keep track of every individual who has accessed the set of data. The information generated cannot be tampered with and transparency is maintained throughout the process. Regulatory compliance can be attained for the different phases of clinical trials. The data on the number of volunteers taking part in the clinical trial, and the dose, side effects, etc. should be available on a single platform.

3.5.3 Vaccination Drive

The data required for the supply chain for a vaccination drive is crucial. The information on hospitals involved in a vaccination drive, the number of people to be vaccinated and dosage requirements should be shared with the competent authorities. Blockchain technology offers management and sharing of the decentralized databases from multiple parties. An overview of the pandemic management process using blockchain technology is depicted in Figure 3.6.

3.5.4 Policy-Making

The blockchain technology will assist tremendously in framing the policy based on real-time data to combat pandemic situations. The real-time data on infected people, recovery and number of deaths will help the concerned authorities to make policy decisions, such as seal down, lock down, declaring the area as a containment zone, etc. The data will facilitate an understanding of the stage (imported cases, local transmission, community transmission, epidemic) of the pandemic and frame the policy for effective administration to contain the disease. Blockchain technology will provide the basis to formulate policy for the vaccination drive.

Acknowledgments

The authors would like to thank the president and Management (Nitte Education Trust, Mangaluru), Principal, N.M.A.M.I.T, Nitte, Mrs Asha S Shet, Mr Prashanth Raikar and Mr Mayur Shet for providing the necessary support to prepare the chapter.

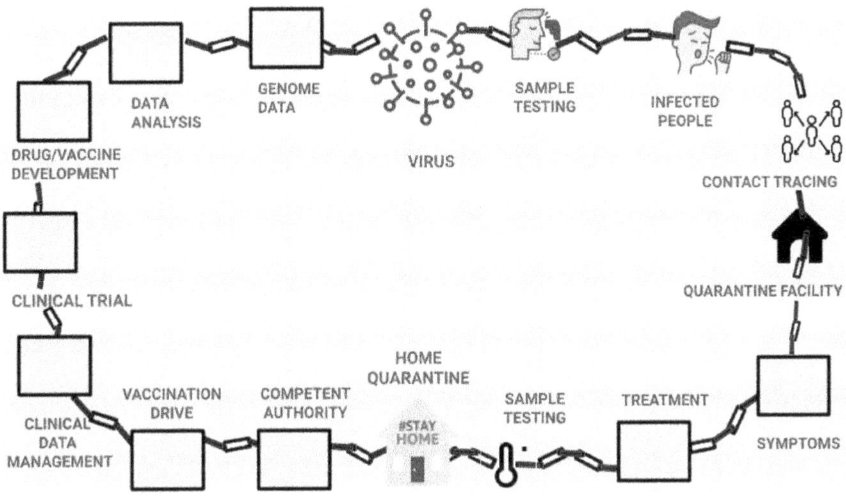

FIGURE 3.6
Overview of pandemic management process using blockchain technology.

References

Govindan, Kannan, Hassan Mina and Behrouz Alavi. (2020). A decision support system for demand management in healthcare supply chains considering the epidemic outbreaks: A case study of coronavirus disease 2019 (COVID-19). *Transportation Research Part E: Logistics and Transportation Review*, 138: 101967.

Iyengar, Karthikeyan P, Raju Vaishya, Shashi Bahland Abhishek Vaish. (2020). Impact of the coronavirus pandemic on the supply chain in healthcare. *British Journal of Healthcare Management*, 26, no. 6: 1–4.

Marbouh, Dounia, Tayaba Abbasi, Fatema Maasmi, Ilhaam A Omar, Mazin S Debe, Khaled Salah, Raja Jayaraman and Samer Ellahham. (2020). Blockchain for COVID-19: Review, opportunities, and a trusted tracking system. *Arabian Journal for Science and Engineering*, 45: 1–17.

Sharma, Abhishek, Shashi Bahl, Ashok Kumar Bagha, Mohd Javaid, Dinesh Kumar Shukla and Abid Haleem. (2020). Blockchain technology and its applications to combat COVID-19 pandemic. *Research on Biomedical Engineering*, NA: 1–8.

4

A Blockchain-Based Secure Healthcare Application

Pratima Sharma, Rajni Jindal and Malaya Dutta Borah

CONTENTS

4.1 Introduction

The Internet of Things (IoT) is a new and innovative technique that links substantial smart appliances to the web, where sensors gather and share information to benefit persons, track and respond to changes to enhance effectiveness [1, 2]. Presently, it has already been implemented in several areas, such as automotive systems [3], the intelligent grid corporation [4] and the smart home sector [5], where smart healthcare has gained growing recognition by utilizing IoT techniques. An IoT-based medical system has been introduced to significantly enhance precision, overcome geographical constraints for remote tracking [6], perform disease risk assessments [7] and develop disease prediction methods [8]. IoT tools, such as wearable sensors, continue to gather physiological information from users in the intelligent medical system, like electrocardiogram (ECG), temperature and blood pressure. This clinical information is sent to the customer's local gateway for further information processing and then issued for treatment to a medical professional so that users may well understand their state of health. Nevertheless, miniaturization and low energy utilization of these intelligent medical appliances result in minimal processing and storage space [1]. Smart medical devices thus need additional procedures for helping with processing and storage. The outsourcing of private medical information and Electronic Health

DOI: 10.1201/9781003133179-4

Records (EHRs) to cloud storage is a simplified approach [7]. The cloud-based medical system increases accuracy and lowers costs compared to conventional healthcare systems. However, it should be remembered that the cloud-based system still has several disadvantages. Smart, widescale medical solutions offer high cloud computing and storage capacities on servers. Because cloud repository services and networks may also be perceived as central to some degree, all users may be affected once the cloud servers are collapsed or targeted. Healthcare data must be protected from unauthorized access. The cloud server may share the user data with trusted third parties for commercial benefit [9].

Blockchain technology provides a robust distributed ledger that Nakamoto [10] initially proposed. It is used in cryptocurrency transactions for validation or verification purposes, such as Bitcoin [10] and Ether [11]. The blockchain network offers shared resources without a single point of failure, therefore removing the central point bottlenecks. A transaction stores the information a user intends to connect to a ledger and transmits new transactions to other nodes. Some participants gather new transactions into a block. The consensus mechanism determines the method by which a block is added to a blockchain. The blockchain cannot be forked, and all developers are continuing to work on its extension.

This chapter proposes a blockchain-based application that protects healthcare data. In the proposed application, users can submit and distribute the medical information obtained by IoT devices as a regular transaction. Doctors or medical analysts can evaluate IoT information any time and distribute the analysis as a transaction. Also, there will be wide-scale medical information with the rapid growth of IoT devices, and this medical information will keep increasing. It is not sufficient to document full customer information on the ledger, as the resource specifications will be incredibly high for each device on the blockchain. The blockchain would otherwise be too complicated to preserve, browse and confirm. Due to the node's limited capacity, we used an InterPlanetary File System (IPFS) that is an information-addressable, shared document system for high integrity and durability data storage [12]. The IPFS framework assigns a unique hash to the uploaded document. In the proposed architecture, the generated hash sequence of the uploaded document is saved in the blockchain. Healthcare architecture thus promotes the collection of large-scale healthcare data and has excellent usability. Apart from the massive data storage burden, one of the major hurdles is information protection and user safety. Consumers use health data from accredited medical professionals, such as doctors or health analysts. Therefore, medical information must be encoded for users, and access control over encoded information must be carried out. Only licensed healthcare professionals may collect medical data for specific users. The principal contributions of the work are defined as follows:

1) This work proposes a distributed application for the protection of large-scale health data based on blockchain. The proposed application allows publication or storage of IoT and healthcare data of patients and doctors. Additionally, it is impossible to manipulate or alter the IoT information and treatments to prevent diagnostic conflicts.
2) The proposed application encodes and processes healthcare data in IPFS that reduces the processing overhead while maintaining healthcare data protection.
3) The integrity and privacy of healthcare records should be secured not only against outside threats but also against illegal networks. Threats (e.g., data theft or alteration) may be deliberate and unintended, and such attacks can penalize or convict organizations. Therefore, the proposed application ensures the privacy of the healthcare data with the help of blockchain technology.

The remainder of the chapter is structured as follows. Section 4.2 presents the related work. The proposed architecture, the model of the application, and the interaction model included in Section 4.3. Section 4.4 gives the specifics of the implementation process of the proposed application. Section 4.5 presents the results, performance evaluation and comparison study. Finally, this chapter concludes in Section 4.6.

4.2 Related Work

Blockchain was initially suggested to create a shared public ledger for bitcoin transactions [10]. After that, several areas of research concentrate on the main issues of the blockchain itself, like improving performance [13, 14], overcoming the double-spending threat [15, 16] and building effective decentralized consensus methods [17]. In the meantime, several other studies concentrate on building potential applications focused on blockchain. It can also be incorporated into several IoT settings, as well as serving as the technologies for cryptocurrency frameworks [11]. For example, Bhalaji et al. [18] proposed a blockchain-based solution to protect health-related IoT data, which can be achieved through cryptographic algorithms. The authors proposed an encryption algorithm without involving key management with the help of random numbers, AND operator and modulus operator. Blockchain utilized to store IoT data maintained data integrity and authentication of the users. Srivastava et al. [19] proposed a novel blockchain model to provide security and privacy features to the existing IoT-based remote patient monitoring system. It provided a reliable model that used a double encryption scheme on the blockchain-based network and improved healthcare data security. Shahnaz et al. [20] introduced a framework that deployed blockchain technology in the EHR system. It implemented a role-based access control and provided a solution for the scalability issues using off-chain record storage. Yanez et al. [21] suggested a new context-aware data allocation method determining each IoT data request's ranking value based on various context parameters to determine its allocation on-chain. The mechanism used a data controller based on fuzzy logic to extract data request context parameters, e.g., data, network and quality. It determines the allocation rating value used as a threshold measurement to determine which data request should be stored in the blockchain or allocated off-chain, i.e., cloud database. Ni et al. [22] used consortium blockchain technologies to launch HealChain, where user-uploaded healthcare data are explicitly stored in a shared way, with security assurances. It introduced a hierarchical architecture for facilitating HealChain's network functionalities. The framework is handled by three layers, which are for data collection, verification and storage. The proposed protective interactions between HealChain involved agencies and develop an operational process to handle healthcare data to satisfy protection and privacy criteria.

Numerous studies have shown that a blockchain is indeed a viable tool for achieving the security of personal medical details and safety in recent years. Many research efforts [23–25] are dedicated to discussing the benefits of blockchain-based intelligent medical systems and proposing frameworks but lack specific details on deployment. Other literature, such as [26] and [27], concentrates on fine-grained access control of user-collected IoT information. Nevertheless, they may not recognize the doctors' privacy protection that created Electronic Medical Records (EMRs). Furthermore, specific systems [31–35] committed to using blockchain to allow patients to monitor their EMRs, which are centrally managed. In [28], healthcare data privacy-based blockchain solution ensured the security, fine-grained access control and effective revocation of users. In [29, 30] implemented an integrated blockchain and framework to provide privacy in healthcare data. Al Omar et al. [31] proposed MediBchain, a client-based information protection system called healthcare protection. Consumers encode confidential medical information in MediBchain and save it on the approved blockchain. Only consumers with the right password can access MediBchain information. Besides, MediBchain is prone to off-line dictionary assaults and replay threats. After this, Zhang and Poslad [32] used the secret exchange of Shamir to validate clients and physicians for fine-grained access permission. Also, EMRs held in a database in the system of Zhang et al., and the blockchain is kept in a trustworthy cloud, leading to centralization. The same issue arises in the framework of Yue et al. [33]. References [34, 35] may accomplish user-controlled medical data, but as the number of users and medical data increases, due to the small block size such systems contribute to unacceptable delays in identification and processing. In [34], health records stored in remote repositories and read rights established in a smart contract to minimize overhead storage for the user and improve the efficiency of the blockchain. In [35], the authors' blockchain's efficiency blocks to save the hash sequences of health documents while transmitting the authentic query connection details over HTTPS during a private transaction. This approach is, however, prone to DoS attacks. In addition to the issues mentioned above, access control, security, scalability and storage of medical/IoT data also pose difficulties. Therefore, we propose an application, which not only supports access control, security, and encryption of healthcare data but also uses decentralized storage to provide secure storage of medical and IoT data. In smart healthcare, not just the IoT details of patients, but also the treatment of physicians, should be covered for the protection of information. From the users' viewpoint, even though the patient may be anybody, the doctors who treat patients need to be tested for eligibility to assure the health of the users. Table 4.1 summarizes the strengths and weaknesses of the related work compared to the proposed application.

4.3 Proposed Distributed Application Architecture and Design

4.3.1 Proposed Application System Model

Figure 4.1 depicts the model for the proposed application. It shows all the functionalities of the proposed application layer-wise and explains the data flow between them. The top layer, the application layer, contains IoT devices, users and the application interface for user interaction [36]. The next layer is the blockchain layer. The proposed application is built on the Ethereum platform, and the blockchain user utilizes the platform's functionalities. A smart contract is designed to govern all necessary functionality of the application. The third layer is the connectivity layer, which ensures data transmission and communication between different modules. It also manages the security and authenticity of the users. It controls the data security and ensures that the patients' data is not publicly available by encrypting the data before uploading, and only authorized users can view the data hash [37]. The public-private keys of each user are used to manage access control. Users can also send the request to the network to check the integrity of a document. The proposed application checks the integrity by recalculating the hash of the document and

TABLE 4.1

Strengths and Weaknesses of Related Work

Work	Off-chain storage	Throughput	Privacy	Distribution of IoT data	Distribution of personal data	Distribution of medical data	Remarks
[18]	✘	Not mentioned	✓	✓	✓	✘	The system achieves privacy by using the cryptographic algorithm and blockchain.
[19]	Not mentioned	Not mentioned	✓	✓	✓	✘	The system supports by using the proposed double encryption scheme.
[20]	✓	✓	✓	✘	✓	✓	The system supports scalability with the help of off-chain storage. Privacy is achieved by using access control rules.
[21]	✓	Not mentioned	✓	✓	✓	✘	The system supports storage with the help of the cloud layer. The encryption algorithm supports privacy.
[22]	✓	Not mentioned	✓	✓	✓	✘	The system uses off-chain storage. The system supports the privacy feature by using cryptographic methods and digital signatures.
[28]	✓	Not mentioned	✓	✓	✓	✘	The system supports the privacy feature with the help of key management and encryption techniques.
[29]	✘	✓	✓	✓	✘	✘	The system supports the privacy feature by using a ledger.
[30]	✘	Not mentioned	✓	✓	✓	✓	The system supports privacy with the help of a double encryption algorithm.
[31]	✘	Not mentioned	✓	✘	✓	✓	The system supports patient data management. It provides privacy by using cryptographic functions.
[32]	✘	Not mentioned	✓	✘	✓	✓	The system focuses on the access control mechanism for EHRs.
[33]	✘	Not mentioned	✓	✘	✓	✘	The system focuses on patient health data and supports privacy features with the help of encryption and access control mechanisms.

(*Continued*)

TABLE 4.1 (CONTINUED)

Strengths and Weaknesses of Related Work

Work	Off-chain storage	Throughput	Privacy	Distribution of IoT data	Distribution of personal data	Distribution of medical data	Remarks
[34]	✘	Not mentioned	✓	✘	✓	✘	The system supports privacy with the help of authentication, accountability, and data sharing.
[35]	✘	Not mentioned	✓	✘	✓	✓	The system focuses on the ownership rights of the patients and supports access control.
Proposed work	✓	✓	✓	✓	✓	✓	The system supports off-chain storage with the help of IPFS. The privacy feature is achieved with the help of authentication, authorization, and integrity functions. It also supports the storage of IoT, personal, and medical healthcare data with the distributed application's help.

Off-chain storage: ✓ -> storage of healthcare data on decentralized storage to solve the scalability problem.
Privacy: ✓ -> privacy of data achieves through cryptographic methods, encryption, authentication, integrity checking and data access management.
IoT data: ✓ -> healthcare data collected from IoT devices (wearable devices).
Personal data: ✓ -> patient's private records like prescription, individual reports, medical records, lab reports, etc.
Medical data: ✓ -> medical records maintained by doctors, medical professionals, healthcare analysts, etc.

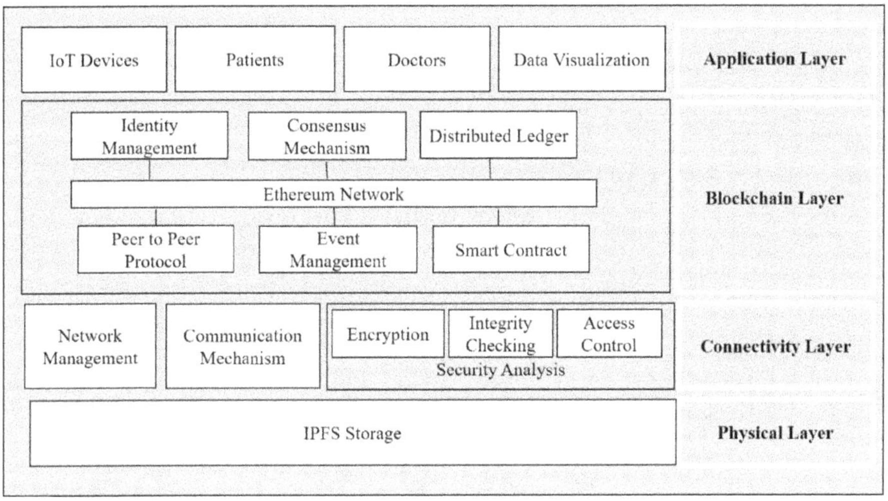

FIGURE 4.1
Proposed application system model.

compares it with the stored hash; if both are matched, integrity is maintained, otherwise it notifies the user. The last layer is the physical layer, which consists of the IPFS storage layer on which the actual patient's data is stored. It is using the Advanced Encryption Standard (AES) algorithm for encrypting the user data before storing it on IPFS. The IPFS is a decentralized storage system that shares and store user data in a peer-to-peer network. IPFS uses a global namespace for information addressing that uniquely identifies the data. It provides a robust data processing and exchanging system that allows users to store data in a distributed manner without involving a centralized authority or third parties.

4.3.2 Conceptual Scenario of the Proposed Application

Figure 4.2 represents the proposed application's overall design, which comprises IoT devices, users (patients/doctors), smart contracts and IPFS storage connected to form a peer-to-peer blockchain network. Through various IoT devices, users may collect their health data. These devices can be any device that the user has and do not need to be any specific device—the patient data from the smart devices records and stores on the proposed application in the form of files. The users may upload the data manually or can set a time after which the data will upload. The data encoded uses the AES encryption algorithm before uploading on IPFS. After the data is uploaded, it responds with a unique hash that points to the data on IPFS, and this hash is stored on the blockchain (smart contract), on which the users can check the data. The smart contract module connects the application with the blockchain and all the back-end functionalities. The smart contract provides services to create records, transfer data and funds between doctors and patients. The users may view and fetch their IoT data, prescriptions and account balance using the application, which is the center module that connects all the other modules. An architecture model of the application, as shown in Figure 4.2, is categorized into several parts, as described below.

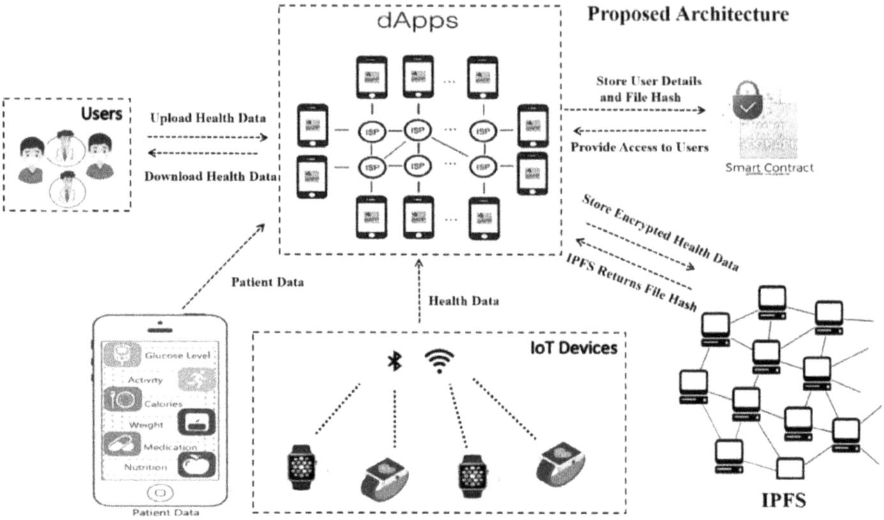

FIGURE 4.2
Proposed application architecture.

IoT gadgets: IoT devices can be handheld sensors or embedded sensors. IoT apps monitor user health factors such as weight, body temperature, calories consumed, sleep patterns, sugar levels, etc. IoT devices regularly send various collected health information to the user node. IoT devices have low power and limited processing and storage capacity. Therefore, they do not directly participate in the blockchain.

User nodes: Each user involved in the application can be only a real doctor or patient. Doctors or patients can register at the application portal by providing valid details. Then, they can use the utilities of the application. All users are allowed to upload health data using the application portal. All information is saved on the IPFS repository. Patients are allowed to access the application to collect IoT data or share their health data with the selected registered doctors of the application. Doctors may provide prescriptions to the patients through the application.

Storage nodes: They collectively store the fully encrypted data of users' and physicians' prescriptions authenticated in a distributed way [38]. Throughout this chapter, we imagine that this node is dependent on IPFS, and its framework is maintained and controlled by the blockchain network. IPFS utilizes a method of addressing the content in which location is extracted from the document's contents. The hash of each file derives from the sequence of the hash and is unique to locate the document.

Main chain: It is a blockchain that is used by authorized users to release data. Only registered users can enter the main chain to view transactions, submit requests and mine anytime. The main chain is a set of user blocks and increases over time. Each user block includes the user hash and user-generated transactions preceding it.

4.3.3 Interaction Model of the Proposed Architecture

Figure 4.3 depicts the overall flow of the proposed application and shows the user interactions and the functionalities of the application. As shown in the figure, the user first

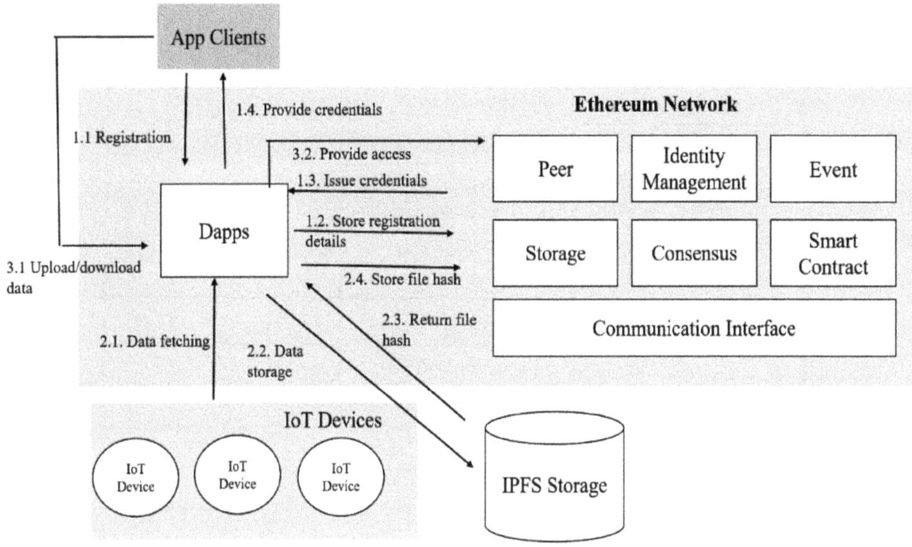

FIGURE 4.3
Overall flow of the proposed application.

signs up on the dapp and obtains credentials from the network. After the registration, the user details are saved on the Ethereum platform using smart contract functionality. The user may manually collect the data from the IoT device and send it on the dapp portal by uploading them in files. Users can store the data on IPFS anytime, anywhere and obtain the unique hash associated with it. The user can share the unique data hash with the doctor. Once the doctor receives the file hash they send the prescription to the user accordingly. During the communication between the patient and doctor, the smart contract stores the tokens from the patient's account as per the doctor's fees. It transfers it to the doctor's account when the user receives the prescription. The prescription is uploaded in the same manner, and the user gets the file hash of the prescription. Once the user gets the prescription hash, the doctor receives the fee.

As shown in Figure 4.4, the patient registers on the dapp, and their data is stored on a smart contract. The Ethereum unique address is used for the authentication purpose on the network. After registration, the user uploads data using the dapp interface. Firstly, the data is encoded to provide security. After encryption, data is bifurcated into multiple parts and saved in the IPFS decentralized storage. In response, the user receives a unique hash corresponding to the uploaded file, which is further utilized by the user to share the data with the doctors or to access the data. All the user-related or file-related information is maintained by using a smart contract. A registered patient may utilize the application portal to seek diagnosis/prescription from the doctors available on the application. The user refers to the doctor list and shares the individual health data unique hash to the selected doctor.

As shown in Figure 4.5, the doctor registers on the dapp with a valid ID. When the doctor registers, the data is stored on a smart contract. A doctor's unique Ethereum address is used to identify the validity of the doctor. The patients can send their data files to the doctors. Then, doctors will be able to view those files using the file hash, upload the prescription and receive fees in the form of tokens.

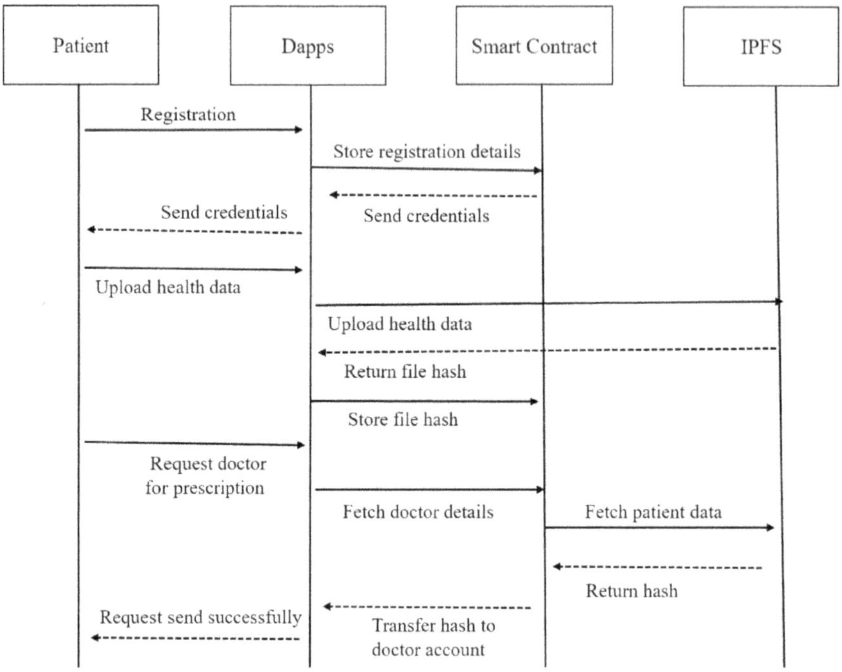

FIGURE 4.4
Sequence diagram for patient user.

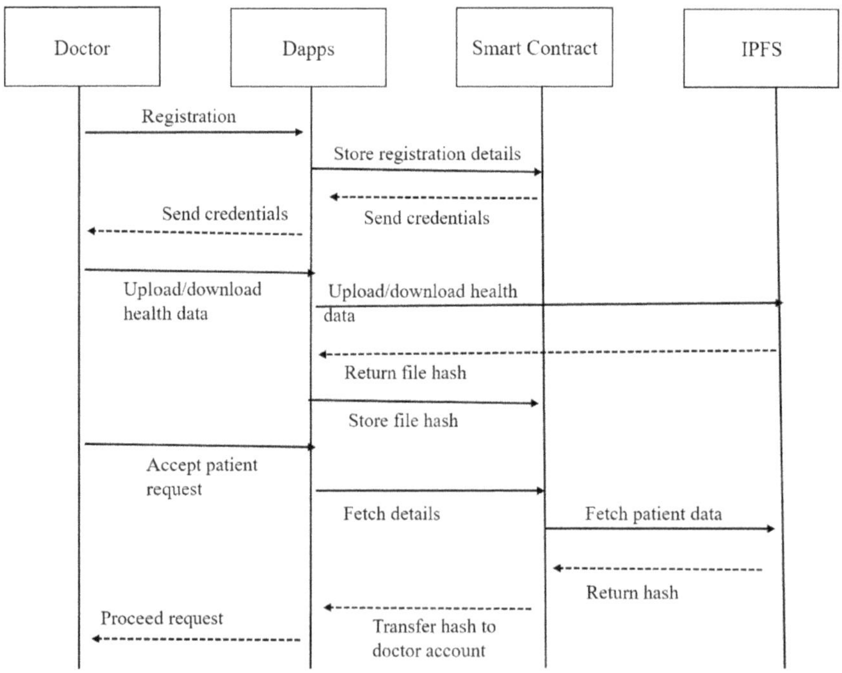

FIGURE 4.5
Sequence diagram for doctor users.

4.4 Implementation of Proposed Application

The smart contract executes on every node in the network independently and automatically, depending on the initiating operations' information. As all communications occurred via signed messages on a blockchain, all participants in the network would get an intimation of authentication trace of the smart contract's operations. The smart contract provides numerous features for reliable, efficient and safe recognition of legitimate customers. The blockchain publishes all activities, which are performed using the smart contract. The smart contract in a proposed architecture comprises the various functions: Fetching data from IoT devices, registering a new user, uploading, accessing, sending a request to registered users and checking integrity. This section presents smart contract algorithms for the patient and doctor. It explains all the functions that are being performed and various conditions associated with them.

Algorithm 1 describes the operations of the smart contract for patient users. This algorithm has five functions: To assign an address, add, access, transfer data and check integrity. The application's users execute these operations. The first function presents the registration process through which the application assigns the address to the new user. It contains two parameters, new user and new address; these would be utilized to register new users and map the details with the unique address. This function also allocates 1,000 free tokens to the user to request feedback from the doctors. The second function is to add a patient file, and the registered patients of the application execute it. This function also checks that the operation is being executed by the authenticated assigned address and not by any other malicious user. In this function, the "msg.sender" term is used in Solidity programming language in the Ethereum framework to identify the user's address. After the validation process, the authentic patient can add the healthcare data in the form of a file, and after this patient obtains the unique file hash from the IPFS storage. The third function is to access the patient file, and it needs the patient ID for authentication purposes. After the checking process, with the help of a file hash a patient may access the stored data. The fourth function is to send patient data to the registered doctors of the application. First, this function checks the patient identity and availability of the required tokens, then only allows the file transfer. By using the application portal, patients may access the registered doctors' list. After selecting the doctor, the patient uses this function to send the data to a particular doctor. The "send data" function deducts the tokens from the patient account according to the selected doctor's fees and transfers the data. The last function is used to check the integrity of the stored files. It recalculates the hash of the requested file and then matches it with the stored hash. If both are same, then integrity is maintained; otherwise it is not.

```
Algorithm 1: Patient Smart Contract
Add Patient: function Add Patient (New User, New Address)
    add new user and map account
    allocate tokens
end
Add File: function Add Patient File (parameters)
    if( msg.sender==patient ) then
        upload file/IoT data to IPFS storage
    return file hash
    else terminate session
    end if
end
```

```
Access Data: function Access File (patient id, file hash)
    if ( patient id==true)then
    retrieve data from specified account
    return (patient File) to the requested account
    else terminate session
    end if
end
Send Data: function Send Patient Data (parameters)
    if ( msg.sender==patient ) then
    if (amount==doc_fee) then
       transfer file to the selected doctor and deduct the required
       tokens
    return successful transfer
       elsereturn failure
    end if
     end if
end
Integrity check: function Integrity check (parameters)
    if ( msg.sender==patient || msg.sender==doctor ) then
           recalculate hash of file (rehash)
           if (rehash==file hash) then
              integrity maintained
    else return failure
    end if
    else return failure
    end if
end
```

Algorithm 2 describes the operations of the smart contract for doctor users. This algorithm has four functions: To assign an address, add, access and transfer data. The first function presents the registration process through which the application assigns the address to the new user. It contains two parameters, new user and new address; these would be utilized to register new users and map the details with the unique address. The second function is to add files like prescriptions, medical reports, healthcare documents, IoT data, etc. This function checks that the operation is being executed by the authenticated assigned address and not by any other malicious user. After the validation process, the authentic doctor can add the healthcare data in the form of a file and obtain the unique file hash from the IPFS storage. The third function is the access file, and it starts with the authentication process. After the verification process, the doctor accesses the stored data with the help of the file hash. The last function is to send prescription data to the patient of the application. First, this function checks the doctor's identity and then only allows the file and token transfer.

```
Algorithm 2: Doctor Smart Contract
Add Doctor: function Add Doctor (New User, New Address)
       add new user and map address
end
Add File: function Add DoctorFile (parameters)
      if ( msg.sender==doctor ) then
             add file/IoT data to IPFS storage
            return file hash
```

```
else terminate session
end if
end
Access Data: function View DoctorFile (doctor id, file hash)
if ( doctor id==true)then
access file from the account
return (doctorFile) to the requested account
else terminate session
end if
end
Send Data: function Send Prescription (parameters)
if ( msg.sender==doctor) then
   transfer file to the selected patient and add the tokens to the
account
return successful transfer
else return failure
end if
end
```

4.5 Performance Evaluation and Comparison

This section is validating the proposed application efficiency and viability. The section is further split into four parts. The first subsection presents the usage scenario of the distributed application. In the second subsection, we evaluate and analyze the app's privacy and security specifics. The next subsection analyzes the application's performance on the basis of processing time, computation time and throughput. In the last subsection, we compare the proposed architectures with the existing frameworks by using various parameters.

4.5.1 Usage Scenario of Proposed Application

Figure 4.6 presents the usage scenario of the proposed application. The application mainly has two entities: Patient and doctor. The first task would be to assign an address to the users of the application. Every user of this application would have a unique address to

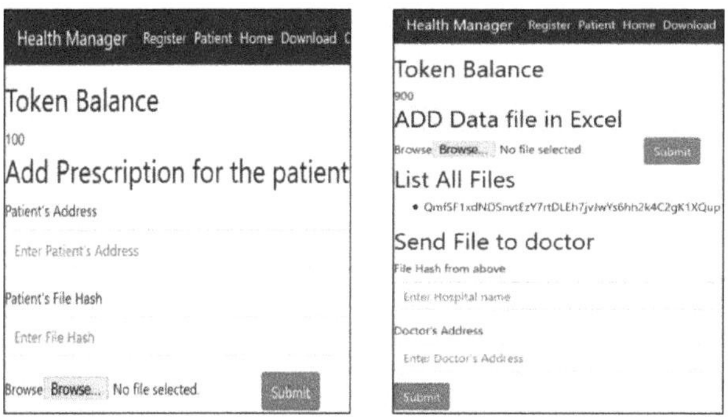

FIGURE 4.6
Proposed application portal.

access the services. All the user registration details are stored in the smart contract and utilized for validation purposes in later steps. After the registration process, when a user wants to perform some proposed application operations, s/he would at the first request to execute them. The application checks the user authentication and mapped account from the stored data. It then allows them to perform the operations after verification return success. After the operations are executed, the application would store the Ethereum and blockchain information and would perform transactions for that information. Once the transaction is confirmed, the application receives the success message from the blockchain that users can view on the dapp portal on which the whole proposed system is visible.

Registered patients would directly upload the health data using the dapp portal or upload the data from the wearable IoT devices with Bluetooth or Wi-Fi. After uploading or sharing the health data, patients can access the registered doctors' list for health-related advice. Patients are allowed to share the uploaded health data with the selected doctor and, in return, receive the response. For each registered user, the network provides 1,000 free tokens to send a request to the doctors. All registered doctors provide valid license details and fee-related information at the time of the registration process. After registration, doctors access the portal to address the queries intimated by the users. Doctors are allowed to share the response to the shared query. After completing the request, the network deducts the tokens from the patient account per the doctor's registered fees, as depicted in Figure 4.6.

4.5.2 Performance Evaluation

To evaluate the proposed architecture's performance in real-life scenarios, we conducted the performance analysis using Apache Jeter version 5.1.1 and Apache Version 2.00. Apache JMeter is a performance testing tool used for analysis and testing applications [39]. The evaluation metrics include processing time, computation time, throughput and cost estimation of the proposed application. These are described as follows.

1) **Processing time** is defined as the time duration (in seconds) between the transaction request for uploading documents and its execution in the blockchain network.
2) **Throughput** refers to the amount of data that could be transferred from one location to another in a unit amount of time.
3) **Computation time** is the average time taken to execute the users' series of transactions.

4.5.2.1 Processing Time

The processing time would include the time required for upload process. For this test, we used different sized health files and noted the time for each file uploading process, as shown in Table 4.2. These are approximate times, and these solely depend on the number of peers and the internet connection speed.

TABLE 4.2

Processing Time

File Size (f)	Time (in seconds)
F < 2 MB	~0.03
2 MB < f < 20 MB	~0.2 -- ~3
20 MB < f < 200 MB	~3 – ~18
200 MB < f	<~18

4.5.2.2 Computation Time

The computation time increases with the number of transactions. The proposed architecture supports two types of transactions, i.e., data transactions and access transactions. These transactions are executed for the smart contract's various operations, whose algorithm is defined in Section 4.2. For the particular user, the data transactions include functions like "add patient," "add a patient file" and "access transactions" include the functions "view patient file" and "send patient data." The average computation is calculated separately for each type of transaction, as shown in Figure 4.7.

4.5.2.3 Throughput

Algorithms 1 and 2 explain different operations, which are defined in the proposed application's smart contract. By utilizing JMeter, we simulated the number of users in the range of 100–500 who access the application and execute its different operations. In JMeter, the data/time (KB/sec) units indicate the throughput. We simulated the users during the experiment and evaluated the system performance. On the proposed application, these simulations are executed, and, in the end, the throughput is assessed. The application throughput is represented in Figure 4.8. During this experiment, it is observed that as the number of users and requests increases, the throughput of the application increased linearly. This linear increment in throughput indicated the efficiency of the proposed application.

4.5.3 Comparison

This section presents the proposed platform's comparative analysis with some of the related works. A comparison survey was conducted to illustrate the proposed platform's performance and flexibility, and the findings of the assessment are summarized in Table 4.3.

The proposed application provides a better approach to manage healthcare data compared with existing solutions for the following reasons:

1) **Distributed application**: The proposed application allows the users to use the application's services anywhere, anytime, using gadgets/smartphones. The designed application is extremely user-friendly since the users can be of any age.

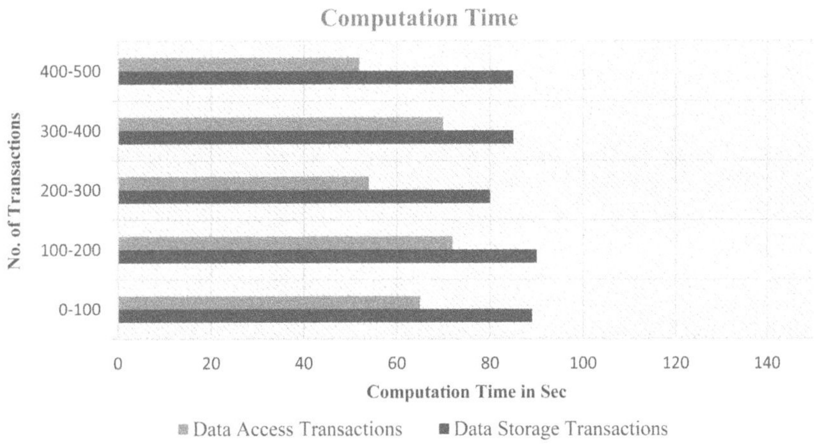

FIGURE 4.7
Computation time required for completion of transactions.

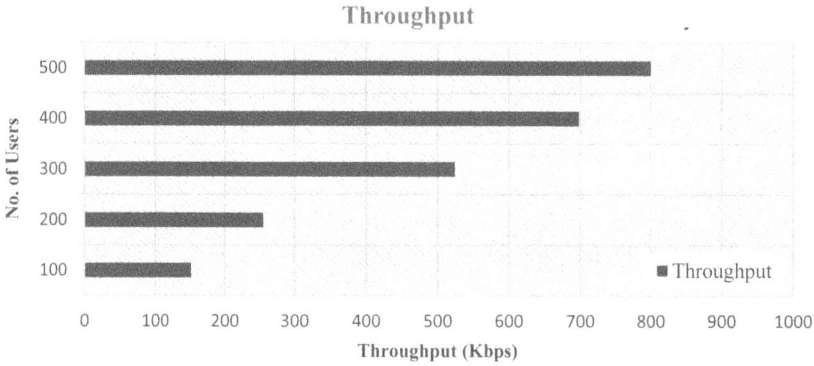

FIGURE 4.8
Throughput of the proposed application.

2) **IPFS storage:** IPFS is peer-to-peer network storage. It incorporates a cryptographic identifier that secures the data from unauthorized manipulations. Any attempt to make alterations to the data stored on IPFS could be made by updating the identifier. It is unique and is used for locating the stored data on the IPFS. This secure feature of the IPFS system makes it a favorable selection for storing private data. The generated cryptographic hash sequence is stored on the dapp to reduce the computational overhead. The existing approaches used the external or static database to store data, which causes the scalability issues. The proposed application uses off-chain storage (IPFS) for securely saving users' files and solve the scalability issues.
3) **Tokens:** The proposed application designs tokens to provide services to users. During the registration process, 1,000 free tokens are allocated to the user account. The user is allowed to use the application's services by spending the allocated tokens or buying new tokens. This feature of the proposed application provides a more secure environment because it always incurs costs to access the smart contract's function, thus preventing malicious activities.
4) **Smart contract:** A smart contract is a piece of code used to perform any task on the blockchain. It runs directly on the blockchain, thus making it secure from any kind of tampering and alterations. The proposed application uses a smart contract to store user-related/token-related information during the communication between the patient and doctor.
5) **Security:** The proposed application supports the authentication mechanism, access control and integrity-checking feature. Thus, it ensures that each individual's health data can only be accessed by him/herself and his/her approved qualified doctors.

4.6 Conclusion

This chapter proposed a distributed application for secure authentication and access control of broad-scale health data. We also incorporated the application to ensure that patients'

TABLE 4.3

Comparative Analysis

Reference	Cryptocurrency used	Mining required	Smart contract	Blockchain platform	Client support	File storage	Type of application
[28]	No	Yes	No	Permissioned/ permissionless	Yes	IPFS	—
[29]	No	No	Yes	Permissioned	Yes	Couch DB	Web app
[30]	No	Yes	Yes	Permissioned	Yes	Cloud storage	—
[31]	No	No	No	Permissioned	Yes	Blockchain as storage	—
[32]	No	No	No	Permissioned	Yes	Blockchain cloud	—
[33]	No	No	No	Permissioned	Yes	Blockchain cloud	Smart app
[34]	Yes	Yes	Yes	Permissioned	Yes	Database gatekeeper	—
[35]	No	Yes	Yes	Permissioned	Yes	EHR DB	—
Proposed Application	Yes (tokens)	Yes	Yes	Permissioned	Yes	IPFS	Distributed app

medical records are covered to avoid diagnostic collisions, taking into account the IoT's resource limitations. We developed a smart contract for the authentication process, access control, file sharing process and integrity checking process to obtain stable and scalable healthcare data protection. Also, to ensure protection and privacy at any moment, users can verify the credibility of records.

References

1. G.A Akpakwu, BJ Silva, G.P Hancke and AM Abu-Mahfouz. (2018). A survey on 5G networks for the Internet of Things: Communication technologies and challenges, *IEEE Access*, 6, 3619–3647.
2. Y Mehmood, F Ahmad, I Yaqoob, A Adnane, M Imran and S Guizani. (2017). Internet-of-Things-based smart cities: Recent advances and challenges, *IEEE Communications Magazine*, 55(9), 16–24, Sep.
3. L Zhu et al. (2018). PRIF: A privacy-preserving interest-based forwarding scheme for social Internet of vehicles, *IEEE Internet of Things Journal*, vol. 5, no. 4, pp. 2457–2466, Aug.
4. S Li, K Xue, Q Yang and P Hong. (2018). PPMA: Privacy-preserving multisubset aggregation in smart grid," *IEEE Transactions on Industrial Informatics*, 14(2), 462–471, Feb.
5. T Song, R Li, B Mei, J Yu, X Xing and X Cheng. (2017). A privacy-preserving communication protocol for IoT applications in smart homes, *IEEE Internet of Things Journal*, 4(6), 1844–1852, Dec.
6. A Redondi, M Chirico, L Borsani, M Cesana and M Tagliasacchi. (2013). An integrated system based on wireless sensor networks for patient monitoring, localization and tracking, *Ad Hoc Network*, 11(1), 39–53.
7. C Zhang, L Zhu, C Xu and R Lu. (2018). PPDP: An efficient and privacy-preserving disease prediction scheme in cloud-based e-Healthcare system, *Future Generation Computing Systems*, 79, 16–25, Feb.
8. Z Guan, Z Lv, X Du, L Wu and M Guizani. (2019). Achieving data utility-privacy tradeoff in Internet of medical things: A machine learning approach, *Future Generation Computing Systems*, 98, 60–68, Sep.
9. C Zhang, L Zhu, C Xu, K Sharif X Du, and M Guizani. (2019). LPTD: Achieving lightweight and privacy-preserving truth discovery in CIoT, *Future Generation Computing Systems*, 90, 175–184, Jan.
10. S Nakamoto. Bitcoin: A Peer-to-Peer Electronic Cash System. (2008). [Online]. Available: http://www.bitcoin.org/bitcoin.pdf
11. G Wood. (2014). Ethereum: A secure decentralised generalised transaction ledger, Zug, Switzerland, Ethereum Project, Yellow Paper, 151, 1–32,
12. N Nizamuddin, HR Hasan and K Salah. (2018). "IPFS-blockchain-based authenticity of online publications," in Proc. International Conference on Blockchain, 199–212.
13. K Nikitin et al. (2017). "CHAINIAC: Proactive software-update transparency via collectively signed skip chains and verified builds," in Proc. 26th USENIX Security Symposium, 1271–1287.
14. EK Kogias, P Jovanovic, N Gailly, I Khoffi, L Gasser and B Ford. (2016). "Enhancing bitcoin security and performance with strong consistency via collective signing," in Proc. 25th USENIX Security Symposium, 279–296.
15. GO Karame, E Androulaki and S Capkun. (2012). "Double-spending fast payments in bitcoin," in Proc. ACM Conference on Computer and Communications Security, 906–917.
16. T Ruffing, A Kate and D Schröder. (2015). "Liar, liar, coins on fire: Penalizing equivocation by loss of bitcoins," in Proc. 22nd ACM SIGSAC Conference on Computer and Communications Security, 219–230.

17. J Chen, S Yao, Q Yuan, K He, S Ji, and R Du. (2018). "CertChain: Public and efficient certificate audit based on blockchain for TLS connections," in Proc. 37th IEEE International Conference on Computer Communications (INFOCOM), 2060–2068.
18. N Bhalaji, PC Abhilashkumar and S Aboorva. (2019). "A blockchain-based approach for privacy preservation in healthcare IoT, " in Proc. ICICCT 2019 – System Reliability, Quality Control, Safety, Maintenance and Management, 465–473.
19. G Srivastava, J Crichigno and S Dhar. (2019). "A light and secure blockchain for IoT medical devices," in Proc. IEEE Canadian Conference of Electrical and Computer Engineering (CCECE).
20. A Shahnaz, U Qamar and A Khalid. (2019). Using blockchain for electronic health records, *IEEE Access*, 7, 147782–147795.
21. W Yanez, R Mahmud, R Bahsoon, Y Zhang and R Buyya. (2020). Data allocation mechanism for internet of things systems with blockchain, *IEEE Internet of Things Journal*, 7(4), 3509–3522,
22. W Ni, X Huang, J Zhang and R Yu. (2019). "Healchain: A decentralized data management system for mobile healthcare using consortium blockchain," In Proc. of the 38th Chinese Control Conference, 6333–6338.
23. Z Shae and JJP Tsai. (2017). "On the design of a blockchain platform for clinical trial and precision medicine," in Proc. 37th IEEE International Conference on Distributed Computing Systems (ICDCS), 1972–1980.
24. C Esposito, A De Santis, G Tortora, H Chang and K-KR Choo. (2018). Blockchain: A panacea for healthcare cloud-based data security and privacy? *IEEE Cloud Computing*, 5(1), 31–37, Jan/Feb.
25. T-T Kuo, H-E Kim and L Ohno-Machado. (2017). Blockchain distributed ledger technologies for biomedical and health care applications, *Journal of the American Medical Informatics Association*, 24(6), 1211–1220,
26. A Ouaddah, AA Elkalam and AA Ouahman. (2016). FairAccess: A new blockchain-based access control framework for the Internet of Things, *Security and Communication Networks*, 9(18), 5943–5964,
27. O Novo. (2018). Blockchain meets IoT: An architecture for scalable access management in IoT, *IEEE Internet of Things Journal*, 5(2), 1184–1195, Apr.
28. J Xu, K Xue, S Li, H Tian, J Hong, P Hong and N Yu. (2019). Healthchain: A blockchain-based privacy-preserving scheme for large-scale health data, *IEEE Internet of Things Journal*, 6(5), 8770–8781, October.
29. L Hang and DH Kim. (2019). Design and implementation of an integrated IoT blockchain platform for sensing data integrity, *Sensors*, 19(10), 1–26.
30. AD Dwivedi, G Srivastava, S Dhar and R Singh. (2019). A decentralized privacy-preserving healthcare blockchain for IoT, *Sensors*, 19(2), 1–17.
31. A Al Omar, MS Rahman, A Basu and S Kiyomoto. (2017). "MediBchain: A blockchain-based privacy-preserving platform for healthcare data," in Proc. International Conference on Security, Privacy and Anonymity in Computation, Communication and Storage, 534–543.
32. X Zhang and S Poslad. (2018). "Blockchain support for flexible queries with granular access control to electronic medical records (EMR)," in Proc. IEEE International Conference on Communications (ICC), 1–6.
33. X Yue, H Wang, D Jin, M Li and W Jiang. (2016). Healthcare data gateways: Found healthcare intelligence on blockchain with novel privacy risk control, *Journal of Medical Systems*, 40(10), 218.
34. A Azaria, A Ekblaw, T Vieira and A Lippman. (2016). "MedRec: Using blockchain for medical data access and permission management," in Proc. International Conference on Open and Big Data (OBD), 25–30.
35. GG Dagher, J Mohler, M Milojkovic and PB Marella. (2018). Ancile: Privacy-preserving framework for access control and interoperability of electronic health records using blockchain technology, *Sustainable Cities and Society Journal*, 39, 283–297, May.
36. J Sengupta, S Ruj and SD Bit. (2019). A comprehensive survey on attacks, security issues and blockchain solutions for IoT and IioT, *Journal of Network and Computer Applications*, 149, 1–20.

37. Q Feng, D He, S Zeadally, MK Khan and N Kumar. (2018). A survey on privacy protection in blockchain system, *Journal of Network and Computer Applications*, 126, 45–58.
38. NZ Benisi, M Aminian and B Javadi. (2020). Blockchain-based decentralized storage networks: A survey, *Journal of Network and Computer Applications*, 162, 1–10.
39. M Niranjanamurthy, K Kumar S, A Saha and DD Chahar. (2016). Comparative study on performance testing with JMeter, *International Journal of Advanced Research in Computer and Communication Engineering*, 5(2), 70–76.
40. G Wood. (2017). Ethereum: A secure decentralised generalised transaction ledger. EIP-150 revision, *TechnicalReport Rep.*, 33.

5

A Brief Appraisal of Blockchain-Assisted Secured Healthcare

Rajib Biswas

CONTENTS

5.1 Introduction

The healthcare system has recently seen a large surge in patient records. With increasing numbers of hospitals, clinics and pharmacies the amount of data generated is enormous; this goes through phases such as creation, dissemination, storage, daily access, etc. When a patient undergoes a test, the initial step emerges as generation of data. These generated data are then passed on to the data operator (such as, analyst, radiographer, clinician, etc.) and eventually to the physician. Data gets stored with accessibility to other physicians within the hospital network. With the advent of technology [1–5], the healthcare system is bolstered so that efficient allocation of resources is executed as per demand, thereby providing quality care to the patient concerned. Accordingly, there arise some key terms in e-healthcare, namely, Electronic Medical Records (EMR), Health Information Services (HIS) and Electronic Health Records (EHR), etc. EMR includes the medical and clinical data of a patient. Taking EMR as the primary group, a solution-based service provides knowns as HIS which take care of creation, sorting as well as retrieval of EMR on demand. Now, the addition of portability along with sharing leads EMR, accompanied by HIS, to formulate EHR which can be accessible at multiple points. Along with large EHR as well as sensor nodes, the security and authenticity of data are gradually given top priority. In order to avoid malicious activity or third-party invasion, it becomes imperative to have a secure transaction and dissemination as well as storage of data. As such, there is a new paradigm of rules which we refer to as blockchain (BC) to effectuate secure health data management. It can be stated as one of the innovative technologies which has completely changed the

DOI: 10.1201/9781003133179-5

concept of secured transactions. It has greatly impacted the healthcare segment endowing it with more security and tamper-proofing, accompanied by effective management of data transmission. This chapter briefly deals with BC-based smart healthcare. Apart from this, the concept of smart contracts, which can perform advance level scripting to create a BC network to provide a platform for the development of decentralized applications is also touched upon. Additionally, the challenges of BC-based healthcare are also outlined along with recent applications. Accordingly, the chapter has been divided into three sections. The first (5.2) dwells upon BC-based healthcare architecture. The second section (5.3) introduces smart contracts. The third section (5.4) overviews the challenges associated with BC technology.

5.2 Blockchain-Based Smart Healthcare

In 2008, there was a white paper by Satoshi Nakamoto, who introduced the concept of BC for the first time [3]. His objective was to assist a digital cryptocurrency called bitcoin. BC technology bridges undefined and non-reliable bases through the incorporation of smart health devices in the form of different sensors. It totally suppresses the concept of a centralized system which is the basis of cloud computing architecture. Accordingly, BC technology is based on an indisputable ledger rooted in the public domain. This public ledger holds records of data that are shared among the collaborators. In principle, it comprises of data blocks which are linked together with hashes. The blocks are, in general, distributed in a decentralized way, to multiple nodes belonging to an infrastructure. The hash of blocks can be said to be the fundamental entity for BC technology. Hashing refers to creation of a value or values taken from a string of texts through the use of a suitable mathematical function. It thus impinges security and ensures transmission solely to the intended recipient, thereby making it tamper-proof. Such features make BC invulnerable to malicious activities. Accordingly, the key features owned by BC technology include transparency in data and excellent security followed by a decentralized system.

Figure 5.1 portrays the implementation of BC technology with the Internet of Things (IoT). It is evident that the patient's data can include various data arising from various sensors. These health records remain in the repository of the hospital the patient attends for treatment. Now, these records may also appear as a component of the IoT. Within a framework, there may be multiple hospitals that may seek shared use of a patient's data. In such cases, the sharing can be executed with the incorporation of blocks which are linked together by a set of cryptographic hash keys, thereby warranting secured transmission to desired recipients in a decentralized way. As can be seen, each block is again a repository of information which can be termed as electronic health records. In order to remove the redundancy of a third-party intermediary, a smart contract is introduced which has been detailed in the next section. In principle, BC permits accruing of data from various sources via an audit log which ensures due accountability as well as transparency during the exchange of data. With the assurance of data integrity, there remains anonymity as well as impervious storage.

As a recent example of BC technology [4], it has been used to deal with the current Covid-19 pandemic. As per reports, Ernst & Young had been instrumental in improvising BC with a view to assisting employers, governments and airlines. The objective was to

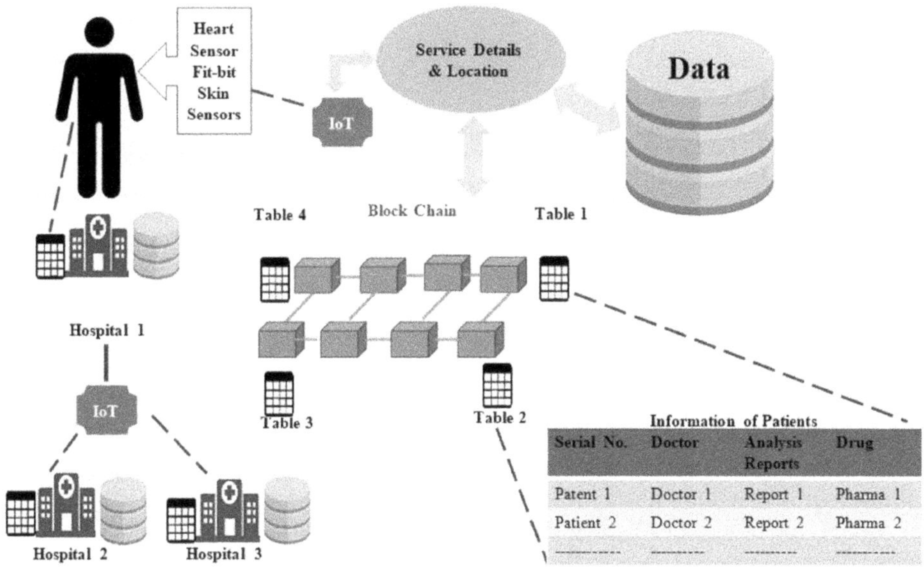

FIGURE 5.1
Schematic of blockchain architecture.

trace people having developed antibodies for immunity against SARS-COV-2. In the same note, other parties namely hospitals, made ample use of BC for equipment and others keep track of people who have had antibody tests and could be immune to the virus. Likewise, China has implemented BC technology to hasten health insurance payments to healthcare providers and patients [3–4].

5.3 Smart Contracts

The immense growth of sensor nodes puts constraints on computation time as well as a huge consumption of energy as far as e-healthcare is concerned. To tackle this, BC is integrated with the Internet of Medical Things (IoMT) which can reduce the consumption of energy as well as computation time. To further bolster it, automated codes, namely smart contracts (SCs), which are self-reliant, can be embedded in the IoMT so as to monitor the contracts. The main goal is to have effective management of assets, which, when entrenched with SCs, can be deterministically defined as required. Upon extending to the IoMT, there emerge automated functionalities resulting in the desired efficacy [5–9].

As shown in Figure 5.2, SCs engage two models, viz, transaction-based, and account-based. In the former, stress is laid on conducting transactions and variables are assigned as input to these transactions. On the contrary, SCs own an account and accordingly can take a custodial right on all assets under account on the BC.

In a BC network, one can root Supply Chain Management [SCM] being characterized by sole addresses. In conformity with the input criteria of SM, the code starts execution. In addition, invoking SCM by directly addressing the transaction is also possible. As the nodes are connected on the chain the same set of instructions can be extended to all nodes,

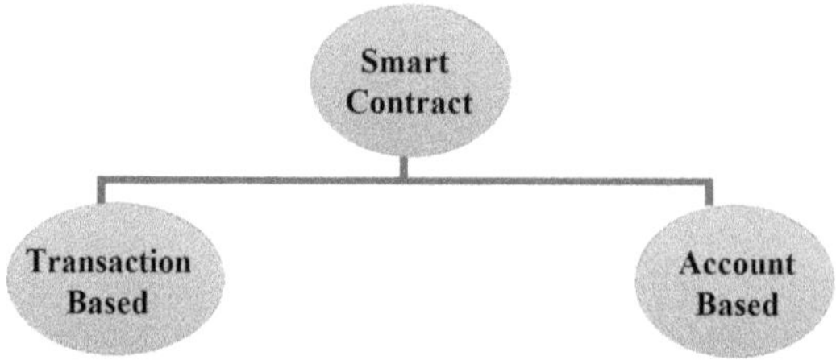

FIGURE 5.2
Types of models used in smart contracts.

resulting in independent and irrevocable transactions which are tamperproof too. SCM in other words helps in the effective management of a large volume of data.

In essence, SCs can be referred to as scripts of code which have the capability of self-authentication as well as being tamper resistant. Besides running independently, the merits accompanying SCs include augmented security, elimination of a reliable intermediary as well as cost-effectiveness [9-13]. SCs, being self-sufficient with predictable behavior allows complete transparency in the overall system which is further assisted by BC towards ruling out the need for an intermediary.

The important link known as a hash plays a very important role. A hash is in principle a unique number which has the ability to identify the block. Similarly, in a chain within blocks is the hash of the previous one. As, for instance, a patient seeks medical assistance, the medical record of the patient gets stored in each block [10–11].

In case there is malicious activity where someone seeks to tamper with data, the alteration of the next hash is inevitable. This altered hash comes under direct inspection which immediately alerts of the malicious activity. Supposing that successful tampering has taken place, it requires a change of all hashes linked to blocks, which is impractical. Thus, SCs play a pivotal role. Commensurate with this important role, a plausible algorithm is provided as shown in Figure 5.3 which depicts a simple BC-based smart contract.

Initially, an input variable in the context of delay and energy is set. It is then followed by setting the threshold values for energy for blocks. Now, suppose data are fed whose energy for blocks nearly equals the defined threshold value. Consequently, a hash is simply added to that block thereby authenticating its linkage with the next chain. Otherwise, a hash added previously gets compromised and removed thereafter. Thus, it allows a secure transmission of data with BC-based SCs. This simple algorithm may prove beneficial for transmission where security of data is prioritized the most.

5.3.1 Blockchain Risks

Although BC turns out to be a very effective solution for the management of data in e-healthcare, there are certain risks which can be totally eliminated. When an organization introduces BC technology, it must be ready to cope with the frequently encountered risks that accompany it. The most important of them include risks associated with information security, functional risk, data confidentiality, risk linked with suppliers, etc. Looking at these varying risk factors, the organization should be equipped with an effective management plan to combat these risks.

BC suffers from certain risk factors which can be categorized as standard risks, risks associated with smart contracts and risks associated with value transfer.

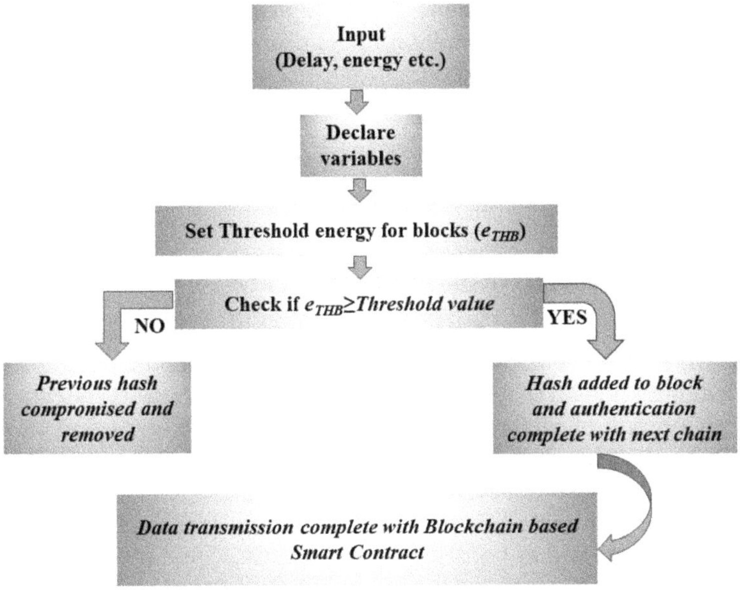

FIGURE 5.3
A plausible implementation of an SC algorithm.

5.3.2 Standard Risks

This risk involves the participants and the products being developed. Along with less time consumption as induced by BC, the assorted businesses should be capable of rapid response and recovery time in the event of failure. Furthermore, data transactions are secured with BC. However, the saddest part is that no assurance of security for an account is provided by BC technology. Additionally, the use of BC in tandem with legacy systems results in scalability as well as accountability issues.

5.3.3 Smart Contract Risks

The dependency of BC on an Oracle base leads to this risk. BC is fully sustained by the Oracle base for its operation. Again, SCs such as business processes, contacts and ancillary financial details are directly linked to BC. As such, if the Oracle base comes under threat, then it jeopardizes the entire BC.

5.3.4 Value Transfer Risks

In essence, BC is a completely decentralized system meaning that it possesses no central authority. This leads to undeterred transfer of value in the participating nodes or peers. If not managed properly, there is likelihood of a value transfer breach.

Coming with many unique features, BC technology is not without challenges. The unique features of BC include integrity in data as well as distributed storage or access of healthcare data. These unique features are assisted by certain bottlenecks such as immutability. As strong data integrity is the backbone of BC, as such, it is nearly improbable that data alteration or deletion can be executed once stored. Again, as we are talking about healthcare data, then it comes under the prerogative of privacy laws which impose limitations for perpetual storage. On the same note, it can be pointed out that the Organisation for Economic Cooperation and Development renders users the right to erase their data. Once a user is inclined to use BC to store data, it becomes obligatory for him/her to execute erasure of data if required.

5.4 Challenges of Blockchain-Based Healthcare

BC technology in general is meant for handling transaction data. These transactions data happen to be small and linear. Accordingly, the need in such cases is to trace back the original deal leaving aside all other ancillary issues. On the contrary, healthcare data comprises of a large amount of information covering imaging, analysis and treatment plans, history of patients, etc. The consequent enormity, as well as relationality, might put BC in the back seat in the absence of an organizational plan.

Despite electronic health records being aided by BC, we cannot say that BC is immune to challenges. As BC is regarded as boosting the healthcare sector, the service providers may encounter hindrances arising from access control and ownership factors [10]. It is pertinent to mention here that the traditional norm is that patients' information remains accessible only to the owner of most of the healthcare providers. Further, the segments spanning elderly people as well patients with mental health conditions cannot self-manage their health records, thus sidelining the use of BC to its fullest extent [11]. Importantly, BC also suffers from scalability issues. As we know that each node engaged in BC possesses the medical data of a patient, as such, it is quite likely that problems related to bandwidth usage and data shortage may arise [10–12].

Table 5.1 lists the limitations/challenges faced by BC technology. It is quite evident that there are certain parameters which need measures in order to make BC technology more effective. As stated in earlier sections, scalability, as well as ready availability, turns out to be one of the major limitations of BC. On the same note, operational computational cost is another bottleneck faced by BC technology.

Considering these challenges, experts suggest use of off-chain saving of data. In off-chain, the data will be stored outside BC in a traditional way. However, the hashes of the off-chain data remain inside BC. While doing so, it serves a dual purpose such that the health data stored off-chain can be secured as well as erased as per appropriation.

TABLE 5.1

Limitations of Various BC Technology

Serial No.	BC Technology	Data Type	Limitations	Reference
1	Private BC	HER and PHR	Skipping of scalability and availability	13
2	Proof-of-stake Private BC	Image data	There is no referral for data searching	14
3	Ethereum and Hyperledger Fabric platform	Transaction records	Absence of surety over tracing of off chain falsified drugs	15
4	Public BC	Sensor data	Excess computational cost	16
5	Private BC	Medical records	Inadequate treatment scenarios	17

Simultaneously, the health data stored on-chain tagged with immutable hashes can be scrutinized for the authentication and accuracy of the off-chain medical records.

In a recent paper by Nagasubramanian et al., 2020 [18], there has been a proposition of implementing a Keyless Signature Infrastructure (KSI) framework ensuring secure patient records. This can be exemplified as follows: A physician attending a patient intends to access health via his/her own ID as well as the private key of the patient. The accessed data remain saved in the local repository. This process gets accredited in an Access Control List (ACL) through verification of the ID provided by the user. After user authentication at the initial stages, adoption of KSI becomes suitable in order to make the whole framework more secure, as well as ascertaining data integrity. This is then followed by onward transmission to BC for further validation, thus effectuating the novel KSI blockchain. Accordingly, this KSIBC aids the easy addition of new records. Furthermore, the KSIBC turns out to be way more inexpensive than the existing data storage systems so far, as far as the recovery of data is concerned.

5.5 Final Remarks

With the advent of a growing IoT, the healthcare sector has undergone a radical change. Accordingly, smart healthcare has emerged, enabling speedy data transactions. However, there is the possibility of getting invaded by issues such as security threats and challenges. As a savior for these issues, there is recent growth in BC technology which ushers a new epoch in the healthcare domain so far as security and privacy are concerned. This chapter provides a brief glimpse of this evolving BC technology. Starting from the architecture of BC technology, the concept of smart contracts has been outlined along with a plausible algorithm. Apart from this, the risks associated with BC technology in the healthcare domain is overviewed. It is then followed by how the various stages of challenges encountered by BC technology are also specified along with novel measures such as KSIBC to address these issues.

References

1. Biswas, R. (2021). An Application Overview of IoT Enabled-Big Data Analytics in Health Sector with Special Reference to Covid-19. *Preprints*, 2021020203. doi:10.20944/preprints202102.0203.v1.
2. Biswas, R. (2021). BIG Data Analytics: A Boon for SMART Healthcare. *International Journal on Engineering Technologies and Informatics*, 2(1), 15–16. doi:10.51626/ijeti.2021.02.00006
3. Satoshi, N, Nakamoto, S. Bitcoin: A Peer-to-Peer Electronic Cash System. *Bitcoin* 2008, 9.
4. EUBlockathon|EUIPO(europa.eu), https://euipo.europa.eu/ohimportal/en/web/observatory/blockathon (Assessed on 20 April 2021).
5. Esposito, C, De Santis, A, Tortora, G, Chang, H, Kwang, K and Choo, R. (2018). Blockchain: A Panacea for Healthcare Cloud-Based Data Security and Privacy? *IEEE Cloud Computing*, 5, 31–37.
6. Khezr, S, Moniruzzaman, Md, Yassine, A and Benlamri, R. (2019). Blockchain Technology in Healthcare: A Comprehensive Review and Directions for Future Research. *Appl. Sci.*, 9, 1736. doi:10.3390/app9091736

7. Sharma, A, Sarishma, R, Tomar, N, Chilamkurti, and Kim, BG (2020). Blockchain Based Smart Contracts for Internet of Medical Things in e-Healthcare, *Electronics*, 9, 1609. doi:10.3390/electronics9101609
8. Tariq, N, Qamar, A, Asim, M and Khan, FA. (2020). Blockchain and Smart Healthcare Security: A Survey, *Procedia Computer Science*, 175, 615–620.
9. Bonomi, F, Milito, R, Zhu, J Addepalli, S. Fog Computing and Its Role in the Internet of Things Characterization of Fog Computing. In Proceedings of the First Edition of the MCC Workshop on Mobile Cloud Computing, Helsinki, Finland, 17 August 2012; 13–15.
11. Polyzos, GC and Fotiou, N. Blockchain-assisted Information Distribution for the Internet of Things. In Proceedings of the 2017 IEEE International Conference on Information Reuse and Integration (IRI), San Diego, CA, USA, 4–6 August 2017; 75–78.
12. Swan, M. (2016). Blockchain Temporality: Smart Contract Time Specifiability with Blocktime. In International Symposium on Rules and Rule Markup Languages for the Semantic Web; Springer: Cham, Switzerland, 184–196.
13. Yue, X, Wang, H, Jin, D, Li, M and Jiang, W. (2016). Healthcare Data Gateways: Found Healthcare Intelligence Onblockchain with Novel Privacy Risk Control. *J. Med. Syst.*, 40, 218.
14. Fan, K, Wang, S, Ren, Y, Li, H and Yang, Y. (2018). Medblock: Efficient and Secure Medical Data Sharing via Blockchain. *J. Med. Syst.*, 42, 136.
15. Sylim, P, Liu, F, Marcelo, A and Fontelo, P. (2018). Blockchain Technology for Detecting Falsified and Substandard Drugs in Distribution: Pharmaceutical Supply Chain Intervention. *JMIR Res. Protoc.*, 7, e10163.
16. Saia, R. Internet of Entities (IoE): A Blockchain-based Distributed Paradigm to Security. arXiv 2018, arXiv:1808.08809
17. Wang, S, Wang, J, Wang, X, Qiu, T, Yuan, Y, Ouyang, L, Guo, Y and Wang, FY. (2018). Blockchain-Powered Parallel Healthcare Systems Based on the ACP Approach. *IEEE Trans. Comput. Soc. Syst.*, 5, 942–950.
18. Nagasubramanian, G, Sakthivel, RK, Patan, R, Gandomi, AH, Sankayya, M and Balusamy, B. (2020). Securing e-health Records Using Keyless Signature Infrastructure Blockchain Technology in the Cloud. *Neural Computing and Applications*, 32, 639–647. doi:10.1007/s00521-018-3915-1

6

Application of Blockchain Technology in Patient Medical Records

A. Averin and K. Nikolskaia

CONTENTS

6.1 Introduction: Background and Driving Forces

In recent years the medical sector has been facing the problem of document authenticity, which includes the availability and integrity of the patient's medical record. This chapter describes the model of keeping medical records with the help of blockchain technology. It facilitates the chronological structure of all the entries in the medical record and ensures high availability of this information, with the data being saved from changes at the same time. This technology can reduce to zero the possibility of chronological distortion of the input information and can also help to detect and correct medical errors immediately. In future, to achieve higher performance, it will be possible to join blockchain systems and artificial intelligence algorithms.

6.2 Architecture Monitoring System for Patient Medical Records

A typical blockchain stores information in a chain of blocks. Every block includes a cryptographic hash of the previous block in the blockchain to link two neighboring blocks. The linkages of blocks are "chains." Blockchain, as a new computing paradigm and model of cooperation in untrustworthy competitive surroundings, changes application scenarios and canons of work in many industries due to its unique mechanism for creating a trust-building mechanism [1][3][6]. The model under study is based on the classical public blockchain using hashing algorithm SHA-256 [4]. Some changes have been made though. New meanings in the classical blockchain architecture were created. The improved model was presented as a private blockchain. The key elements of the system are listed below:

DOI: 10.1201/9781003133179-6

A. "Recipient" address—a new patient being registered, s/he is granted a unique "recipient" address, which means a unique identification of a patient. It is a hash generated from the patient's data with the help of hashing algorithm SHA-256 [4]. It includes the following information: A patient's full name, date of birth, passport (or insurance certificate) number, date of entry. Example: Andrey Averin 15.12.1989, XXXX XXXXXX. Then recipient address generated by SHA-256 will look like this: 6533883a4fcae44dad89c7691c3bfc318e77845678175215e7d074358b9afb00.

B. "Sender's" address—is an identifier of a digital service of the medical establishment. It sends the data of the diagnoses, medical procedures, medical services and a patient's condition, etc. It consists of: Name of the medical establishment, ID of the department, ID of the doctor, ID of the service through which the work has been performed, supplementary information. For example, a sender's name will look like this: MGKB №1 002 23 123132. A sender is always a privileged user. A sender may be a consulting doctor or software which can provide automated service. Every sender, as well as recipient, has its own unique address.

C. "Data"—are results added to the blocks by the electronic service of the medical establishment which provides data of the medical procedures performed to a certain patient by a certain doctor. They include the date of the action toward a patient, time of the action toward a patient, code of the action (0—consultation, 1—diagnosis, 2—operation), code of the medical service (if there is not any, then put 0), code of the diagnosis (if there is not any, then put 0). Example: 01.12.2021 15:40 2 A11.01.001 0.

D. "Transactions"—are a partition of information that is transmitted over the blockchain network and collected in blocks. The structure of the transaction is demonstrated in Figure 6.1. All transactions joined in a chain of blocks can be found and checked, all transactions within the blockchain can be tracked. Transactions in their turn include sender address, data, recipient address.

E. "Blocks"—each block of the described model contains: Hash of the current block, hash of the previous block, date and time of block creation, nonce parameter, list of transactions. A nonce parameter is used to confirm the solution of a mathematic problem solved by miners as a part of a consensus algorithm Proof of Work (PoW) [5]. The number of inputs in every block corresponds to the number of senders' addresses, and the number of outputs corresponds to the number of recipients' addresses. The structure can be seen in Figure 6.2.

F. "Creating blocks"—all the information about medical actions concerning every patient is created by the doctor in charge or by software capable of assessing patients' conditions. After this, all the transactions are placed in the transaction pool [2], which is the place containing all the unverified transactions. A transaction pool is stored on a special device and its contents can be accessed and observed

TRANSACTIONS

SENDER ADDRESS	DATA	RECIPIENT ADDRESS
MGKB №1 002 23 123132	01.12.2021 15:40 0 A11.01.001 0	6533883a4fcae44dad89c7691c3bfc318e77845678175215e7d074358b9afb00

FIGURE 6.1
Transaction structure.

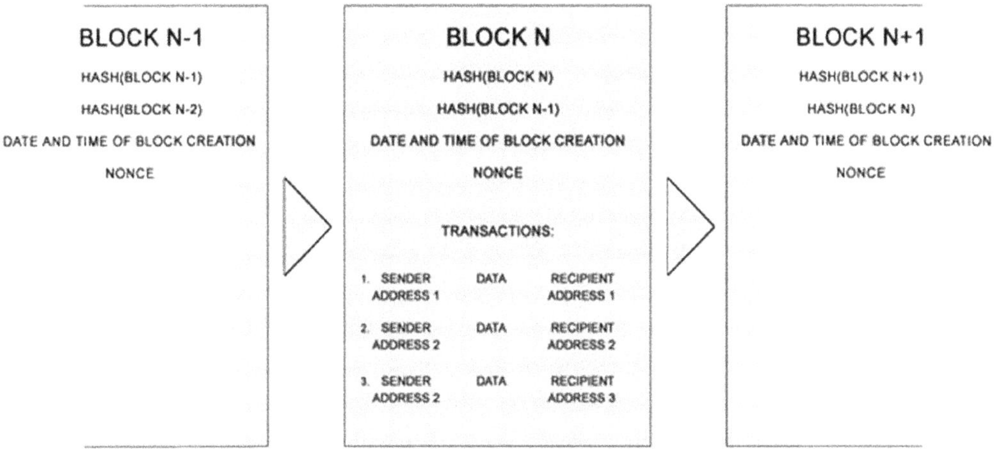

FIGURE 6.2
Block structure.

in real time. After miners get these transactions from the transaction pool and include them in blocks, and also add blocks into the blockchain, the transactions will be confirmed. For a transaction to become completed, it needs to be verified/ confirmed. To check transaction, there needs to be at least one miner. Miners are people who employ their computers to cultivate and confirm transactions. In this model medical establishments or third parties act as miners. Adding blocks is performed by the consensus algorithm PoW or future solutions in the field which are more efficient and cost-efficient.

6.3 Formation of a Medical Record and Monitoring of the Patient's Condition

Knowing a recipient's address in the system, one can form a chronological medical record by blockchain parsing.

A. Medical record formation: One can perform parsing of a blockchain, after this the system uploads received information into the graphic pattern, signs the medical record by the recipient's address and finally signs all the records with the hash received from all the input data. Thus, at any time it is possible to check the history of medical records and the patient's present status in chronological order. Figure 6.3 graphically shows the process of medical record formation.

B. Patient condition monitoring (in the global model): Using this model locally or at even higher levels gives the opportunity to monitor a patient's status regardless of his/her location. Monitoring a patient's conditions is also performed by blockchain parsing, after which the doctor in charge of the patient may receive information of the patient's treatment in another city or abroad. Monitoring a patient's status may be implemented as a secure web application.

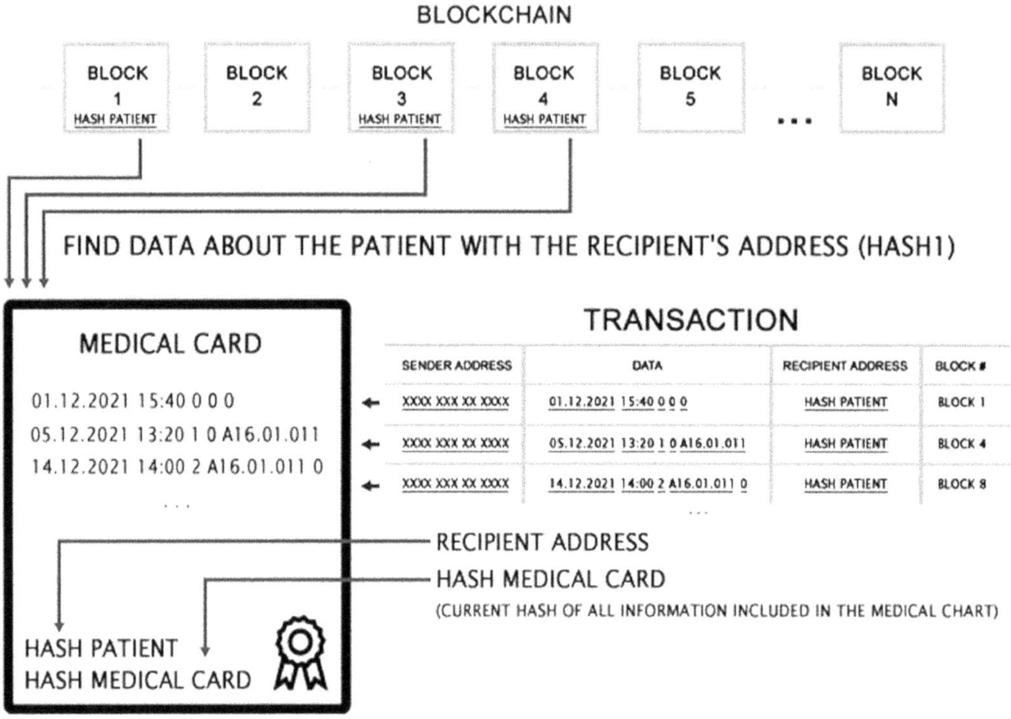

FIGURE 6.3
Formation of a medical card.

6.4 Conclusion

The work describes the model for keeping medical records and monitoring patient status, its elements and structure. The model gives the algorithm of medical record formation and the possibility of further monitoring of a patient's condition regardless of the medical establishment where they are treated. The given model is capable of solving problems in the medical field connected with the necessity to structure chronologically all the entries of the medical record and provide high availability for this information, with the data being protected from changes at the same time. The model also allows for the detection and correction of medical errors. Safety and decentralization of the system creates trust, which is necessary for mass adoption. In future, the model may be implemented in any medical establishment.

References

1. Satoshi, N. (2008). Bitcoin: A peer-to-peer electronic cash system. Available at: https://bitcoin.org/bitcoin.pdf (accessed 12 September 2020).
2. Manh Phan, Transaction pool in Blockchain. Available at: https://ducmanhphan.github.io/2018-12-18-Transaction-pool-in-blockchain (accessed 18 September 2020).

3. Desjardins, J. (2015). Its official: Bitcoin was the top performing currency of 2015. Available at: http://money.visualcapitalist.com/its-official-bitcoin-was-the-top-performing-currency-of-2015/ (accessed 22 September 2020).
4. Zhu, S, Zhu, C and Wang, W. (2018). A new image encryption algorithm based on chaos and Secure Hash SHA-256. *Entropy* 20(9), 716, https://doi.org/10.3390/e20090716.
5. Wikimedia Foundation, Inc., October 2021. Proof-of-work. Available at: https://ru.wikipedia.org/wiki/Proof-of-work (accessed 16 September 2020).
6. Shamsutdinova, TM. (2018). Application of the blockchain technology for digital diplomas: problems and prospects. *Open Education* 22(6), 51–58. https://doi.org/10.21686/1818-4243-2018-6-51-58.

7

IoT and Blockchain Technology-Based Healthcare Monitoring

Mohammad Wazid, Basudeb Bera, Ashok Kumar Das and Devesh Pratap Singh

CONTENTS

7.1 Introduction

The Internet of Things (IoT) characterizes the network of virtual or physical objects or things, also called smart devices that are integrated with sensors, software and other technologies to connect and exchange the information with other devices, systems and people over the wired or wireless network via the internet. These smart IoT devices range from

DOI: 10.1201/9781003133179-7

common home objects to complex industrial instruments. Today more than 10 billion IoT devices are connected via the internet and it is predicted by experts this number will grow to 22 billion by 2025. There are several fields that have adopted IoT technology such as smart manufacturing, wildlife monitoring, preventive and predictive maintenance, the food industry, smart power grids, the military, smart cities, connected and smart logistics, smart farming, smart digital supply chains and so on [35].

Though there are several effective applications for IoT technology, recently, in e- healthcare the IoT has been accepted to monitor patient information by wearable IoT devices and the application also called Healthcare IoT (H-IoT). H-IoT can be generally categorized into two subclasses: 1) personal and 2) clinical. The personal H-IoT can be used for self-monitoring and such smart devices are activity/heart-rate trackers, smart clothes and smartwatches (for example, Fitbit and Apple Watch). These smart devices are installed on a human body without guidance from a physician, to supervise their health condition. On the other hand, the clinical H-IoT smart devices are reinforced particularly for health monitoring of a patient under the guidance/care of a physician. Examples of clinical H-IoT devices are remote temperature monitoring devices for vaccines, air quality sensors, drug effectiveness tracking devices, sleep monitors, medication refill reminder devices and remote care biometrics scanners [21].

H-IoT technology produces a huge amount of data for a patient. The data of the healthcare application are private and confidential, therefore, to securely collect the data and store it on a secure database faces a security threat. As the H-IoT devices communicate over the public network (insecure channel), data hijacking, data leakage (eavesdropping) or malicious data injection can be possible by an unauthorized party (also known as an adversary). Several active and passive attacks have been reported during message communication or data access by researchers such as a man-in-the-middle attack, replay attack, physical devices capture attack, impersonation attack, privileged-insider attack, ephemeral secret leakage (ESL) attack and so on. Therefore, security is needed for information sharing such as authentication, access control, key agreement and identity management. Once the data are gathered securely form the H-IoT devices, the data can be stored in secure storage for future access or evaluation. Instead of storing the data into a single server due to the single server failure, the data can be stored into a distributed server such as blockchain. Blockchain technology is defined as a decentralized, distributed ledger which holds the records of a digital asset. It was introduced by Satoshi Nakamoto, whose real identity is still unknown, and it was released in 2008 in a white paper called "Bitcoin: A Peer-to-Peer Electronic Cash System" [32]. Moreover, blockchain is a digital ledger of transactions that are stored into a block which is replicated and distributed across the entire peer-to-peer (P2P) network. In the blockchain, each block holds a certain number of transactions, and when a new transaction occurs on the blockchain, that transaction is added to every participant's ledger. This decentralized blockchain database controlled by multiple participants in the P2P network is called Distributed Ledger Technology (DLT). The blockchain provides immutability, transparency and decentralized services. There are various ways to construct a blockchain network. Based on the access policy, they can be public, private, permissioned-based or permission-less and consortium.

Public blockchain networks: In a public blockchain network, anyone can access the network (for instance, join in the network, verify the transactions, add a new transaction and participate in mining), such as bitcoin or litecoin. The drawbacks of the public blockchain are that it requires substantial computational power, has weak security and there is no confidentiality for transactions.

Private blockchain networks: In a private blockchain, similar concepts have been used as in public blockchain, and it is a decentralized distributed P2P ledger. The only difference is that one organization governs the entire network, that is the access to the transactions, verification of the block and additions the block into blockchain are restricted. Therefore, the organization can control who is allowed to participate in the mining process, such as executing the consensus algorithm and holding the shared ledger. Hence, this kind of blockchain maintains the confidentiality of transactions between the peers and it significantly holds the privacy. In addition, it can be executed behind a corporate firewall and even be hosted on-premises. These types of blockchain are Multichain and Hyperledger projects (Fabric, Sawtooth). In a private blockchain, a single organization controls an entire network.

Permissioned blockchain networks: This blockchain network restricts who is permitted to be involved in the network, and only in certain transactions. In this blockchain, participants are required to get an invitation or permission to join the network. In these types of blockchain, a control layer executes on top of the blockchain that regulates the activities conducted by the allowed participants. The permissioned blockchain frameworks include Hyperledger, Quorum, Corda and others.

Consortium blockchains: A consortium blockchain is a semi-decentralized type where multiple organizations can share the duties of holding a blockchain. These preselected organizations decide who may add the transactions or access the data from the block. Since in this blockchain more than one authority controls it, therefore more than one authority can behave like a peer node in this network and share data or execute the consensus mechanism for block mining. Energy Web Foundation and R3 are examples of consortium-type blockchains. The detailed structure of a block for several blockchains is provided in Figure 7.3.

The blockchain-enabled IoT-based healthcare monitoring system (BIoT-HMS) has emerged with potential applications in the field of healthcare. An IoT-based healthcare monitoring system is a unique version of the IoT which consists of uniquely identifiable smart healthcare devices (like smartwatches, smart pacemakers) connected to the internet. These features help to localize and gather real-time information. It facilitates the automatic remote management of the resources. The internet-connected smart healthcare devices collect crucial health-related data which provides the physiological symptoms of the patient. The remote care facility of the system provides extra care and control of the disease of the patients (Figure 7.1).

The BIoT-HMS communication environment is applicable in various types of health-related applications. Some of the potential applications of BIoT-HMS are provided below [3], [11], [22], [30], [33], [59].

Remote health monitoring: Sometimes there is the possibility of the readmission of a patient into the hospital after completion of medical treatment. That happens because of a lack of monitoring [41]. Medical cases in an emergency situation are also challenging. The remote health monitoring of patients is possible through the use of smart healthcare devices and associated tools and technologies. Smart healthcare devices monitor the health of the patients 24/7 then send the notification to the concerned doctor according to the critical condition of the patients. It is very helpful to the people living in rural areas and who do not have access to expert doctors. Furthermore, due to remote check-ups and the

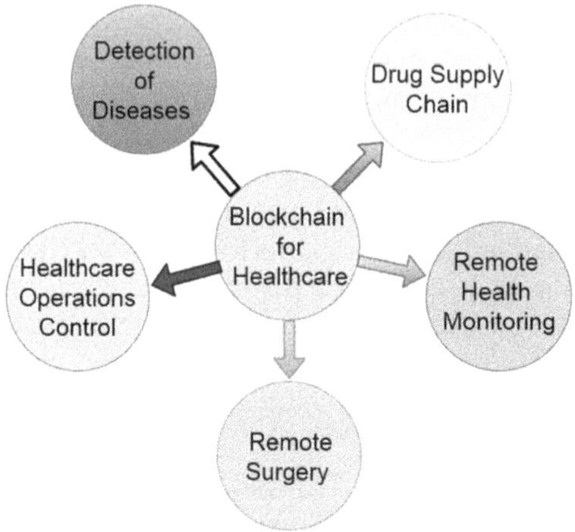

FIGURE 7.1
Various applications related to IoT and healthcare systems in blockchain technology.

guidance of expert doctors, the overall death rate in rural areas can also be reduced. Apart from that there are reductions in the expenditure related to traveling and hospitalization.

Remote surgery: BIoT-HMS-based applications are also useful in performing remote surgery. Such types of surgery can be done through robots/robotic arms employed with sensors and actuators [50]. The robot/robotic arm performs the surgery inside the body of the patient under the supervision of the surgeon(s) situated remotely. The deployed mechanism of BIoT-MS helps the surgeon(s) to perform the surgery remotely with more precision and control. This procedure is very helpful in saving the lives of people living in rural areas or at times of war or natural disaster [50].

- **Management of healthcare operations:** Sometimes it becomes very difficult for doctors to inspect multiple patients at the same time. It is very difficult to do the check-ups of multiple patients at the same time, especially in countries where the population is very high. BIoT-HMS is helpful in providing a quick response to the patients from a medical expert. The regular cost of medical equipment can be reduced by monitoring their conditions regularly, which is also facilitated through the mechanism of BIoT-HMS. This mechanism can also check the expiry of the equipment deployed in the hospital and can notify the concerned authority in case of expiry. Therefore, hospital authorities can get the notification cases of outdated equipment. Even the healthcare staff also have the information of current locations of the required equipment. Hence, BIoT-HMS is helpful in the overall management of hospital operations.
- **Detection and prevention of diseases:** BIoT-HMS can also be used for the early detection of various types of diseases, like heart attack, diabetes, asthma attack, cancer and many more. The inbuilt sensing units in the smart healthcare devices monitor the health condition of the people and send warning signals in advance. For example, the smart healthcare devices continuously monitor the level of blood sugar and send alerts in cases of increased levels. This further reduces the risk of problems like hyperglycemia. In the same way, the BIoT-HMS mechanism helps to reduce cases of asthma attacks. Asthma can be controlled by the use of inhalers. A patient can realize the symptoms of asthma attack half an hour to eight hours before it occurs. The sensing unit in the patient's smart healthcare device alerts the patient

in cases of increments in some environmental factors, like air pollution. This is further helpful to prevent the patient from suffering an asthma attack [11], [55].

- **Drug supply chain management:** The supply chain of the drugs from their production to their consumption by patients can be compromised in many ways through illegal medicine counterfeiting. The drug supply chain management can also be performed securely through the blockchain-based mechanism of BIoT-HMS [28], [14], [39]. In such mechanisms "smart tags" can be applied to the drug (i.e., tablets, vaccines) packaging. These devices help in the proper distribution and monitoring of the drugs, especially providing protection against the counterfeiting of the medicines [47]. Radio frequency identification (RFID) tags can be used to protect the drug packaging against counterfeiting. The entire data of the drug supply chain from the factory to the consumer can be maintained in the form of blockchain. If somebody tries to duplicate or counterfeit a package, such an incident can be detected with the help of a deployed "blockchain-based anti-counterfeiting technique." And thus, patients get a quality medicine which further helps to cure their disease quickly.

The remaining part of the chapter is organized as follows. The architecture of BIoT-HMS is provided in Section 7.3. The threat model, security and privacy requirements and possible attacks of BIoT-HMS are provided in Section 7.4. A summary of various security protocols related to BIoT-HMS is provided in Section 7.5. A comparative analysis of security protocols related to BIoT-HMS communication is also provided in Section 7.6. Finally, the chapter is concluded in Section 7.7.

7.2 Blockchain Evolution and its Use in Healthcare Systems

Blockchain technology can be defined as a decentralized, distributed ledger which records the provenance of a digital asset (i.e., bitcoin). It records the information in a way that makes it difficult or impossible to modify or hack the system. A blockchain is a digital ledger of transactions which is duplicated and distributed across the entire network of computer systems (i.e., a P2P cloud server network) on the blockchain. Every block in the blockchain contains a number of transactions, and every time a new transaction occurs on the blockchain, a record of that transaction is added to the ledger of participants. The decentralized database which is managed by multiple participants is called the distributed ledger. In the blockchain when the new data comes in, it is entered into a fresh block. When the block is filled with data it is chained onto the previous block and the data is chained together in a chronological way. Blockchain can be used for the storing of various types of information (like bitcoin transactions, health records, land records, digital identities, etc.). Bockchain is used in a decentralized way so that no single person or group has control over it. Rather, all users collectively have control. A typical structure of a block in a blockchain is provided in Figure 7.2. It contains information like "identity of the block," "hash of previous block," "Merkle tree root," "timestamp," "owner of the block," "public key of the owner," "encrypted transactions," "current block hash," "signature on block through a digital signature algorithm (i.e., elliptic curve digital signature algorithm (ECDSA))." All these different fields of a block are helpful to achieve the security and privacy properties (like protection against data leakage, protection against data modification, etc.) during the data exchange and storage.

Block Header	
Identity of block	*BID*
Hash value of previous block	H_{PB}
Merkle tree root value	*MTR*
Timestamp value	*TS*
Owner of block	*OB*
Public Key of owner	X_{OB}
Payload of the block (transactions in encrypted form)	
Transactions in encrypted form #1 Transactions in encrypted form #2 . Transactions in encrypted form #n_t	$E_{X_{OB}}(Tx_1)$ $E_{X_{OB}}(Tx_2)$. $E_{X_{OB}}(Tx_{n_t})$
Current block's hash value Signature on block via ECDSA procedure	H_{CB} sig_{BK}

FIGURE 7.2
Block structure.

7.2.1 Blockchain Evolution in Healthcare Systems

Blockchain was introduced by Satoshi Nakamoto for a cryptocurrency called bitcoin, and it was released in 2008 in a white paper entitled "Bitcoin: A Peer-to-Peer Electronic Cash System" [32]. After that it was used in Ethereum, also a cryptocurrency, for a long time. The blockchain has spread over the business network known as Hyperledger and DLT. In 2018, blockchain technology was utilized for the IoT system such as industrial IoT (IIoT), agricultural application, smart home application, supply chain and so on. E-healthcare systems also adopted blockchain technology for its immutability, decentralized structure and cryptographic protection of data as the healthcare data are private and confidential. The detailed evaluation process of blockchain in the healthcare application is shown in Figure 7.3.

The healthcare industry is growing rapidly. According to a report, it was worth US$60 billion in 2010, US$104 billion in 2015, US$280 billion in 2020 and it will be worth US$372 billion in 2022. Due to lifestyles and other environmental factors the number of chronic diseases is increasing day by day. However, the use of technology (like blockchain-enabled IoT- based healthcare monitoring systems) cannot stop people from aging or getting affected by various chronic diseases. Accordingly, it should be accessible and cheaper to the people. The expenses of health diagnosis are the biggest share of the hospital bills. Due to the use of technology, we

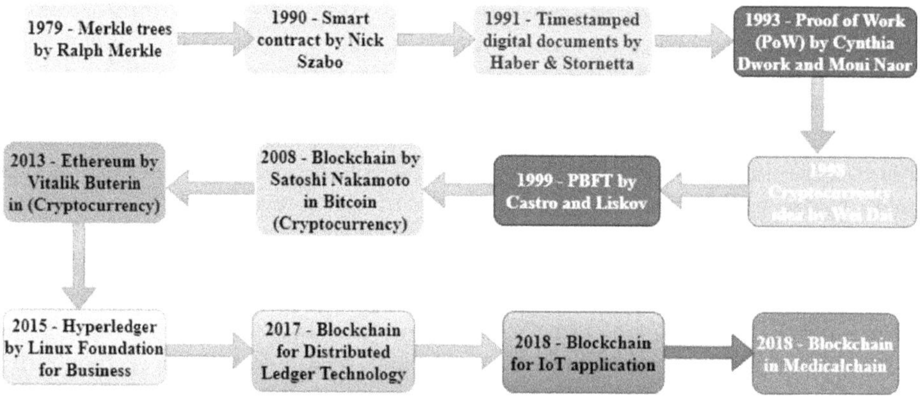

FIGURE 7.3
Blockchain evolution in healthcare systems (adopted from [6]).

have shifted from hospital-centric treatment to the home treatment approach. There are lots of benefits of using this system as it improves the quality of treatment and can also improve the health of the patient quickly [33]. Some of the advantages of using blockchain-enabled IoT-based healthcare monitoring systems are provided below (Figures 7.2 and 7.3).

7.2.3 Advantages of Blockchain-Enabled IoT-Based Healthcare Monitoring Systems

Traditional healthcare practice suffers from different types of problems and issues (like lack of real-time health monitoring, absence of remote healthcare facilities, etc.). However, BIoT-HMS provides lots of advantages; some of them are discussed below [3], [18], [30], [33]:

- **Remote healthcare support:** In BIoT-HMS, a remote doctor can provide remote healthcare support to patients where medical facilities are not available, which is very helpful in emergency situations. With the help of such a facility a doctor (or other medical staff) can get the information of patient's health to learn about his/her illness. Moreover, the doctor can prescribe the required medicines to the patients according to their illnesses, which can be further delivered to them by the associated medicine delivery firm. It reduces the number of patient visits to the hospitals as well as decreasing their healthcare expenditure.
- **Real-time health monitoring of patients:** BIoT-HMS provides the real-time health monitoring of patients through connected smart healthcare devices, which is further helpful in medical emergency cases like heart attacks. In BIoT-HMS, the connected smart healthcare devices monitor the health data of the patients which is also available to legitimate users (i.e., doctors, nursing staff) through their smartphone applications anytime from anywhere. Thus, the healthcare experts get real-time patient health information , which is essential in cases of critical medical illness.
- **Healthcare data storage and analysis:** BIoT-HMS smart healthcare devices produce an enormous amount of data. This can also be called big healthcare data, which is stored in the form of blockchain over the peer-to-peer cloud server (P2PCS) network. The healthcare data can be made available to legitimate users at anytime from anywhere. As the P2PCS network is distributed, therefore there is no single point of failure, which further improves the reliability of the system. Moreover, in the fog server-based architecture, the use of a fog server provides an efficient service to the users, which is another advantage over the traditional system (Figure 7.4) [49]. Healthcare data which is stored over the P2PCS network can be used in big data analytics to draw some useful conclusions (i.e., chances of severe heart attack). Thus, this process is very helpful in case of critical health conditions. Apart from that, the system can also alert the healthcare staff in case of any life-threatening situation.
- **End-to-end connectivity:** BIoT-HMS provides the automation of the entire healthcare process by "healthcare mobile methods" and "other use of advanced technologies." It permits "machine-to-machine communication," "interoperability," "information exchange" and "data transfer." Thus, the delivery of healthcare services becomes effective. In BIoT-HMS, different mechanisms like "Bluetooth," "Wi-Fi" and "ZigBee" are utilized, which change the way medical experts discover the presence of different diseases in patients. Thus, the use of smart tools and technologies reduces the overall treatment costs as well as the number of clinical visits. Moreover, the available system resources are utilized in a better way.

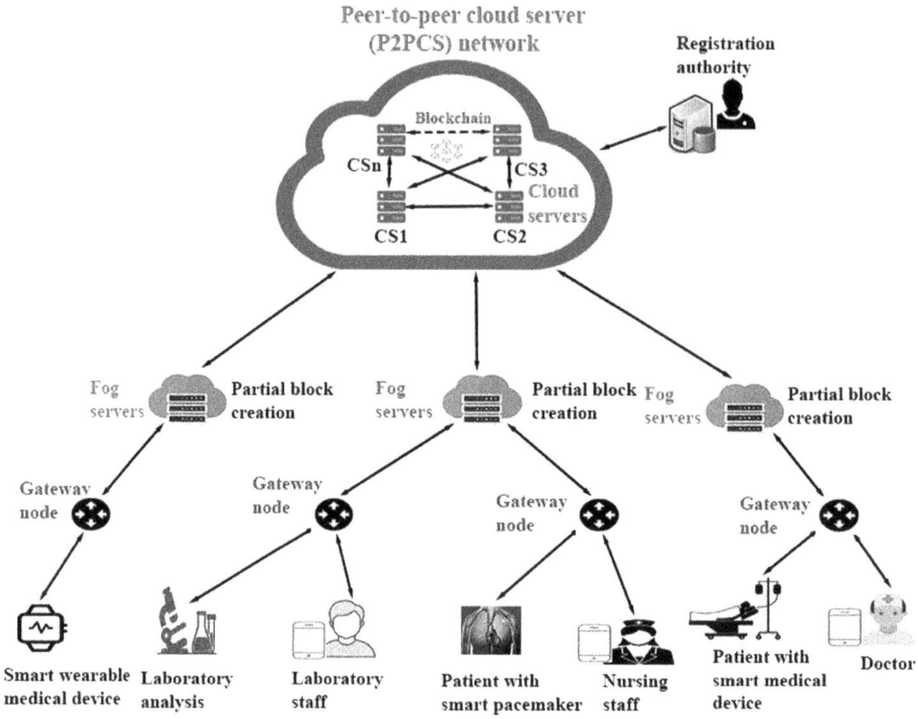

FIGURE 7.4
Architecture of blockchain-enabled fog-based IoT for healthcare monitoring systems (adapted from [49], [52]).

- **Blockchain-enabled security for healthcare data:** In BIoT-HMS, the entire healthcare data are stored in the form of a blockchain over the P2PCS network. The use of the blockchain mechanism provides various types of advantages over the traditional architecture, such as, the decentralized approach, security and privacy features of blockchain. That further mitigates the single point of failure problem, provides better and efficient delivery of information. Furthermore, it provides protection against various types of attacks like replay, man-in-the-middle (MiTM), impersonation, denial of service, credentials leakage and unauthorized disclosure of healthcare data.

Though an IoT-based healthcare monitoring system has lots of advantages, at the same time it also suffers from various security and privacy issues, which are discussed below.

7.2.3 Security and Privacy Issues in IoT-Based Healthcare Monitoring Systems and Their Mitigation through Blockchain Mechanism

In an IoT-based healthcare monitoring system, smart healthcare devices are connected to the public channel. That gives a chance for attackers to hijack them or to launch other kinds of attacks on these devices or on the related healthcare data. Therefore, the communication which happens in an IoT-based healthcare monitoring system is vulnerable to various types of attacks. However, these issues can be resolved by involving the blockchain mechanism. Some of the security and privacy issues of an IoT-based healthcare monitoring system along with their mitigation are provided below [17], [18], [19], [24], [37] [43], [44]:

- **Failure of data protection schemes:** In the IoT-based healthcare monitoring system, most of the data protection schemes use various types of "encryption algorithms" for the protection of healthcare data (i.e., data at rest and data in transit). However, some of the encryption algorithms are vulnerable to various attacks. The secret health-related data of the patient can be revealed to the unauthorized third parties. Thus, the secrecy of the healthcare data is at risk. However, in the security schemes by making the use of the blockchain mechanism we can secure such types of attacks up to certain extent.
- **Lack of data transparency:** In the IoT-based healthcare monitoring system, the health data are stored at the healthcare servers (i.e., cloud servers). However, in such kinds of communication, we may get issues related to data transparency like who is the owner of data. Further, there is also the chance that data may be exposed during its transmission. However, if we make the use of a blockchain-based mechanism in an IoT-based healthcare monitoring system, then such types of issues can be resolved. Because it is distributed and also in-built with other essential security features like data encryption, data owner's information, digital signature generation, verification and integrity checking.
- **Chances of unauthorized usage:** As we know, in an IoT-based healthcare monitoring system, the health-related data is stored on the healthcare servers (i.e., cloud servers), therefore, there is the possibility that the service providers could resell the patients' data to some advertising firms. Because service providers may get some money by the secondary usage of health-related data, it is essential to make a clear agreement among the customers (i.e., patients) and the service providers which includes clear guidelines like "how and where their health data can be used." However, if we make use of the blockchain-based mechanism in an IoT-based healthcare monitoring system, then such types of issues can be resolved. Because in blockchain all data is stored in the form of encrypted transactions, which can only be decrypted through the corresponding private key. Therefore, the secondary usage of health-related data is not possible for unauthorized parties.
- **Lack of skilled staff:** In an IoT-based healthcare monitoring system, the healthcare data stored are on servers (i.e., cloud servers) which are managed and administered by the concerned technical staff. Sometimes, these people are not skilled enough or lack technical knowledge. Hence, there is a requirement to conduct rigorous training and workshops for these employees to make them aware of various security attacks, privacy breaches and security mechanisms (i.e., blockchain).

As a summary, we can say that most of the issues of an IoT-based healthcare monitoring system can be resolved by making the use of blockchain technology.

7.3 Architectures of Blockchain-Enabled IoT-Based Healthcare Monitoring Systems

In this section, we provide the details of the architecture of blockchain-enabled IoT-based healthcare monitoring systems.

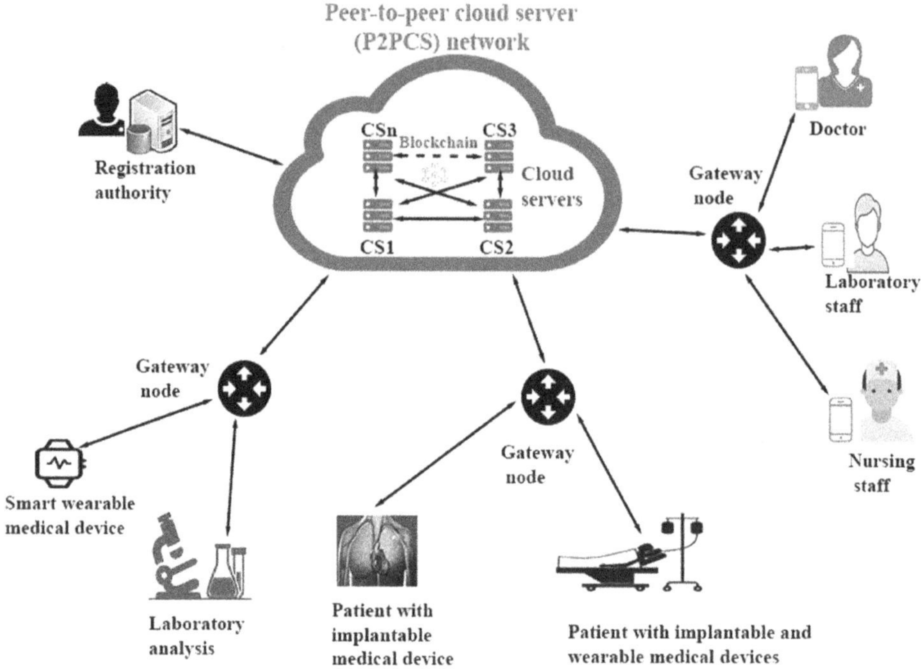

FIGURE 7.5
Generic architecture of blockchain-enabled IoT for healthcare monitoring systems (adapted from [9], [52]).

7.3.1 Generic Architecture

The generic architecture of blockchain-enabled IoT for healthcare monitoring systems is provided in Figure 7.5. The architecture consists of various types of smart implantable and wearable healthcare devices, like smartwatches and smart pacemakers, which sense and process the data related to the health conditions of a person (i.e., a patient). Further, smart healthcare devices send the health data to its nearby gateway node. After receiving the data from all nearby smart devices, the gateway node creates the transactions from the received data and encrypts them using its own public key. Then the gateway node sends the encrypted transactions to a P2PCS network in a secure way. After receiving the encrypted transactions securely from the corresponding gateway node, the cloud server, first creates a block from this transaction. A block contains fields like the block's ID, owner of the block, public key of the owner, hash of this block, hash of previous block, Merkle tree root value of the encrypted transactions, encrypted transactions and signature of this block. After the creation of the block, it is sent to the other peers (i.e., cloud servers) for its addition to the blockchain by the leader of the P2PCS network. Then the steps of the consensus algorithm are executed among the cloud servers of the P2PCS network. Here it is important to mention that a particular cloud server is elected as the leader of the P2PCS network for a certain time period [5], [18], [53]. When all peers of P2PCS network commit to the addition of this particular block in the blockchain, then that block is added to the blockchain. If a legitimate user (i.e., doctor, laboratory staff, nursing staff) is interested in accessing the data of the blockchain, then the corresponding cloud server can provide the requested data to that user in a secure way. In this particular mechanism, we need to perform the steps of authentication and session key establishment between the smart healthcare device and gateway node, between the gateway node and cloud server, between a cloud server to the other cloud server and between the cloud server and the user. All these entities exchange their data in an encrypted form through the established session keys [9], [10], [12], [25], [41], [48].

7.3.2 Fog-Based Architecture

The generic architecture of blockchain-enabled IoT for healthcare monitoring systems, which is provided in Figure 7.5, suffers from certain problems. As it has issues related to high latency, which is not preferable for efficient services [49], another architecture called "blockchain-enabled fog based IoT for healthcare monitoring system" is presented in Figure 7.5. In this architecture, there is another layer of servers called fog servers in between the smart healthcare devices and the cloud servers (P2PCS network). In this architecture, the smart healthcare devices send the health data to its nearby gateway node. After receiving the data from all nearby smart devices, the gateway node creates the transactions from the received data and encrypts them using its own public key. Then the gateway node sends the encrypted transactions to the corresponding fog server.

The server then creates a partial block from it by putting important information like, block ID, owner of the block, public key of the owner, encrypted transactions and Merkle tree root value of the encrypted transactions. Afterwards, the fog server sends the created partial block to the corresponding cloud server of the P2PCS network in a secure way. After receiving the partial block from the corresponding fog server, the cloud server first creates a full block from the partial block by adding other important values like the hash of this block, the hash of previous block and the signature of this block. After the creation of a full block, it is sent to the other peers (i.e., cloud servers) for its addition to the blockchain by the leader of the P2PCS network. Then the steps of consensus algorithm are executed among the cloud servers of the P2PCS network [5], [18], [53]. After getting the commitment from the other peers the leader adds the block to the blockchain. Similar to the generic architecture, if a legitimate user (i.e., doctor) is interested in accessing the data of the blockchain, then the corresponding cloud server can provide the requested data to that user in a secure way. However, there is a requirement to perform the steps of authentication and session key establishment among the various entities like smart healthcare devices, gateway nodes, fog servers, cloud servers and users. Then, these entities can exchange their data in the encrypted form by the help of established session keys [9], [10], [12], [25], [41], [48], [49].

7.4 Security and Privacy in Blockchain-Enabled IoT-Based Healthcare Monitoring Systems (BIoT-HMS)

In this section, we discuss the "threat model" applicable for BIoT-HMS. We also discuss various types of security and privacy needs of BIoT-HMS along with the possible attacks [45], [47].

7.4.1 Threat Model

The widely-accepted "Dolev-Yao (DY) threat model" [15] is useful for the designing of security mechanisms in BIoT-HMS. As per the guidelines of this model, the communicating parties exchange their data over a public channel. The smart healthcare devices, gateway nodes, fog servers and cloud servers cannot be treated as the trusted entities of the network, because several types of attacks can be launched using them, like data leakage, data modification, illegal smart healthcare device hijacking and control. The attacker (A) has the ability to eavesdrop, delete or update the exchanged messages due to the openness of the channel. Another important model, "Canetti and Krawczyk's adversary model," in short called the "CK-adversary model" [7], [8], which is a current *de facto* standard model for the designing and modeling of security mechanisms, such as "authentication," "access control" and "key management" can be utilized. As per the CK-adversary model, A can have the same capabilities as in the DY model. Moreover, A can also get the secret credentials along with the "session states and session keys" corresponding to a session. Another important assumption can also be made that all gateway nodes are installed under some physical locking system, where their physical stealing is not possible [51]. Apart from that there is also the capability of psychical capturing of some smart healthcare devices, and thus, some of the smart healthcare devices which can be further utilized for the unauthorized extraction of stored information from their memory through the steps of sophisticated "power analysis attack" [31], [36]. Then the extracted secret information can be used for the launching of other types of potential attacks like, "impersonation," "session key computation" and "password guessing."

7.4.2 Security and Privacy Requirements

The security and privacy requirements of blockchain-enabled IoT-based healthcare monitoring systems are provided below [17], [19], [24], [37], [42], [43], [44], [52]:

- *Confidentiality:* This property provides assurance against any kind of data disclosure attack. It is also called secrecy or privacy. In the case of IoT-based healthcare monitoring systems the secrecy of stored and transmitted data should both be achieved. We usually use a data encryption mechanism to maintain the secrecy of the stored and transmitted data.
- *Integrity:* This property provides assurance of the integrity of the stored and transmitted data. This means there should not be any unauthorized updates on the stored and transmitted healthcare data. Moreover, there should not be any unauthorized insertion or deletion of information. To maintain integrity, we use mechanisms like secure hash algorithms (i.e., SHA256, MD5, etc.).
- *Authentication*: Authentication is a process of checking the genuineness of somebody or some device. In IoT-based healthcare monitoring systems, it can be device-to-device authentication, user-to-device authentication or user-to-user authentication. For such purposes, we use mechanisms like a "two-factor user authentication protocol" or a "three-factor user authentication protocol." After the successful completion of all the steps in an "authentication protocol," the communicating entities establish session keys for their secure communication.
- *Non-repudiation:* It is another essential property. It provides the assurance that the communicating party should not refuse the validity of something like the transmitted messages. This property assures the "proof of data origin" along with its integrity. Hence it is not easy to refuse "who has sent the message" or "from where a message came." Non-repudiation can be classified as follows:
  - *Non-repudiation of origin:* This property confirms the legitimacy of the sender (i.e., the message was sent by a genuine party).

- *Non-repudiation of destination:* This property confirms the legitimacy of the receiver (i.e., the message was received by a genuine party).
- *Authorization:* Authorization assures that authentic parties, for example legitimate smart healthcare devices in the IoT-based healthcare monitoring system, provide the data to other parties (for example, the healthcare expert).
- *Freshness:* It assures the freshness of the exchanged messages to mitigate re-transmission attempts (i.e., replay attacks).
- *Availability:* This property assures that the affiliated network services should also be made available to genuine entities even in the worst situations (i.e., "Denial-of-Service (DoS)" attacks).
- *Third-party protection:* This property provides the assurance of different resources (i.e., smart healthcare devices and their data) against the damage done by third parties (i.e., service providers of IoT-based healthcare monitoring systems) [58].
- *Forward secrecy:* It assures the "forward secrecy" of the exchanged messages. It means, if a smart healthcare device leaves the IoT-based healthcare monitoring system, then it must no longer have access to the messages which will be exchanged in the future.
- *Backward secrecy:* It assures the "backward secrecy" of the exchanged messages. It means, if a smart healthcare device has recently joined the IoT-based healthcare monitoring system, then it must not have any access to the messages exchanged in the past.

7.4.3 Details of Possible Attacks in Blockchain-Enabled IoT-Based Healthcare Monitoring Systems

The following types of passive and active attacks are possible in blockchain-enabled IoT-based healthcare monitoring systems [13], [52], [18], [34]:

- *Eavesdropping:* Eavesdropping is performed through the sniffing of exchanged messages. Later on, the eavesdropped messages can be utilized to launch other types of attacks like an impersonation attack, credential guessing, etc.
- *Traffic analysis:* In this malicious act the adversary intercepts messages to find out which kind of communication is taking place on the channel. For example, the adversary can find out which party is communicating with whom and for how long.
- *Replay attack:* In this malicious act the adversary records the exchanged messages at one place and later tries to replay them to mislead the recipient party.
- *Man-in-the-middle (MiTM) attack:* In this malicious act the adversary captures the exchanged messages, and later tries to delete or update the intercepted messages before forwarding them to the intended receiver.
- *Impersonation attack:* In this attack, the adversary first tries to compute the identity of the sender through the eavesdropped messages and later tries to update or create new messages, and then sends them to the intended receiver. After receiving such messages, the receiver believes that messages come from a legitimate sender. However, in reality, messages come from the adversary.

- *Denial-of-service (DoS) attack:* In this malicious act, the adversary stops legitimate users from accessing the services of the BIoT-HMS. The adversary does this by deploying the attacker system (or the system with the malicious script) which sends fake requests or attack packets to the legitimate devices or servers of the BIoT-HMS. Therefore, the devices or servers are not able to provide the service to the legitimate users. "Distributed DoS (DDoS)" is the variant of DoS, which can be conducted with the help of multiple attacker systems like botnets. For example, if a genuine doctor is not able to access the health data of patient or not accessible to get it during the desired period of time. Due to that act, a doctor is not able to prescribe the treatment to the patient. In some of the worst cases a patient may die. Some of the examples of DoS and DDoS attacks are UDP floods, ICMP floods, HTTP floods, SYN floods, Ping of Death and Smurf DDoS [16], [20], [27].
- *Protection against 51% attack and selfish mining:* Some attacks, like 51% attacks and selfish mining are possible on the BIoT-HMS, when we do not select the consensus algorithm wisely. Such types of malicious acts may happen when an adversary has a large amount of hashing power [40]. In particular, a 51% attack demands that an adversary needs to carry more than half of the hashing power. Typically, a 51% attack is organized against cryptocurrencies in which adversary performs malicious activities, such as double spending. Apart from that, selfish mining is another well-known vulnerability in a blockchain-based environment. This can be exploited by malicious miners (adversaries) in order to steal block rewards. Recent attacks proved that "Proof-of-Work (PoW)" is vulnerable to 51% attacks. Hence, it is recommended that we should select the consensus algorithm wisely. Consensus algorithms like the "Ripple Protocol Consensus Algorithm (RPCA)," and "practical Byzantine Fault Tolerance(pBFT)" can be used.
- *Malware attack:* Remote siting adversary performs malware attacks with the help of the execution of malicious scripts in the system. Under the execution of malware attacks, malicious tasks like the stealing of information, encryption of sensitive information and hijacking the shell of a smart healthcare device can be performed [52].
- *Database attack:* In BIoT-HMS, most of the healthcare data is stored on a server, like fog servers and cloud servers. In this communication environment, database-related attacks are also possible. Sensitive healthcare data can be revealed through the application of attacks like a "Structured Query Language (SQL) injection attack" and a "Cross-Site Scripting (XSS) attack." In a SQL injection attack, the attacker tries to inject malicious code into the existing SQL statements, so that the maintained database surrenders some of the sensitive information [2]. Whereas in the XSS attack, the attacker tries to inject the malicious scripts into benign and trusted websites to extract the sensitive information (like, identity information, password information, etc.) from them [1].
- *Physical device stolen attack:* As the information provided in the "threat model" in Section 7.4.1, the physical theft of smart healthcare devices is possible by the adversary because these devices cannot be monitored for 24 hours per day, seven days per week. Then these stolen healthcare devices can be utilized to deduce sensitive information through the application of the steps of sophisticated "power analysis attacks" [31], [36]. Furthermore, the situation becomes worse if the adversary tries

to utilize the extracted information to launch further attacks like "MiTM," "illegal session key computation," "impersonation attacks," etc. [9], [29], [51]).

- *Privileged-insider attack:* In this malicious act, the privileged-insider user of the registration authority who has access to the sensitive registration information of the various users and devices may create a problem. A privileged insider user may act as an attacker and can misuse the deduced registration information of the various users and devices to launch potential attacks, like "offline password guessing attack," "impersonation attacks" and "illegal session key computation" on the system [9], [18], [48], [51].
- *Stolen verifier attack:* In this malicious act, the adversary tries to extract sensitive information (i.e., identities, secret keys) from the memory of the devices and servers to launch further attacks (i.e., "MiTM," "offline password guessing attack," "impersonation attacks" and "illegal session key computation") in BIoT-HMS. However, it is recommended that all secret values should be stored in the secured section of the database of the devices. Here it is important to mention that the same mechanism is also used in cases of RSA, ECC and AES based secure communication systems, where it is assumed that all secret information is stored in the secure section of the database (memory). This further prevents any unauthorized access to the secret information. Thus, the required information is not available to the adversary to launch other potential attacks [18], [46], [53], [54].

7.5 Analysis of Blockchain-Enabled Security Protocols for IoT-Based Applications

In this section, we discuss blockchain-enabled security protocols for IoT-based healthcare applications. Moreover, we provide a comparative study of these protocols.

7.5.1 Review of Neha et al.'s Scheme [23]

Neha et al. [18] presented a blockchain-enabled authenticated key management protocol for Internet of Medical Things (IoMT) deployment applicable in healthcare (BAKMP-IoMT). Some of the features of Neha et al.'s protocol [18] are as follows:

- In the design of BAKMP-IoMT, private blockchain was considered.
- Fast "one-way cryptographic hash function" and "bitwise XOR operations" were used in the design of their protocol.
- BAKMP-IoMT contained important phases, like the pre-deployment phase, key management phase, user registration phase, authentication and key agreement phase, password and biometric update phase, dynamic device addition phase and blockchain construction and addition phase.
- The "formal security verification" of the presented protocol through the widely known Automated Validation of Internet Security Protocols and Applications tool was done to discover its resilience against replay and MiTM attacks. Informal

security analysis of their protocol was also conducted to prove its resilience against other attacks, like "impersonation attacks," "Ephemeral Secret Leakage (ESL) attacks," "privileged-insider attacks," "physical medical devices capture attacks" and "data modification attacks." It was also proved that BAKMP-IoMT preserved the "anonymity" and "un traceability" properties.

- A comparative study among BAKMP-IoMT and other related existing methods was also conducted which proved that BAKMP-IoMT had high security and extra functionality features along with low communication and computational costs compared to the existing schemes.
- A practical demonstration of BAKMP-IoMT was also provided to measure its impact on some important performance parameters (i.e., transactions per second, computation time).

7.5.2 Review of Saha et al.'s Scheme

Saha et al. [38] presented a blockchain-based access control protocol for IoT-enabled healthcare applications. Some of the features of Saha et al.'s protocol [38] are as follows:

- An access control mechanism with inclusion of private blockchain technology was proposed.
- Their protocol could be used by a trusted group of hospitals for the secure sharing of sensitive healthcare data.
- The Elliptic Curve Cryptography (ECC)-based signature technique was used in their protocol. The security of the presented protocol was dependent on solving the Elliptic Curve Discrete Logarithm Problem (ECDLP) and "collision-resistant one-way hash function."
- Their protocol contained important phases, like the registration/enrolment phase, login and access control phase and blockchain formation phase.
- Their protocol could resist various types of known attacks such as "replay attacks," "MiTM attacks," "impersonation attacks" and "ESL attacks." Their protocol also preserved the "anonymity" and "untraceability" properties.

7.5.3 Review of Xiang et al.'s Scheme

Xiang et al. [56] presented a permissioned blockchain-enabled identity management and user authentication protocol for e-health systems. Some of Xiang et al.'s features [56] are as follows:

- They presented a permissioned blockchain-enabled identity management and user authentication (PBBIMUA) protocol for e-health applications.
- Their protocol satisfied the extensive security requirements of health-related data.
- Their protocol contained important phases, like the installation phase, enrolment phase, login phase, authentication and key agreement phase, password update phase. However, important phases like dynamic device addition and key revocation are missing in their protocol.
- The provided security analysis proved the security of their protocol against the various types of possible attacks.

- The experimental results proved that the protocol was efficient compared to other protocols.

7.5.4 Review of Xu et al.'s Scheme

Xu et al. [57] presented a blockchain-enabled smart healthcare system (healthchain) for large-scale health data privacy. Some of Xu et al.'s features of [57] are as follows:

- A blockchain-enabled smart healthcare system (healthchain) for large-scale health data privacy preserving was presented.
- In the presented scheme, the users were enabled to upload IoT data and read doctors' diagnoses. Moreover, doctors had the facility to read users' data and could upload the diagnoses.
- The presented model separated the transactions to publish the data from the available trans actions to achieve the access control. The healthcare data is encrypted and stored in an "interplanetary file system (IPFS)."
- The presented model reduced the communication and computation costs along with the privacy preservation.
- In healthchain, the key revocation facility was also provided. Using this key revocation mechanism, the keys of various entities like doctors could be revoked.

7.5.5 Review of Aujla et al.'s Scheme

Aujla et al.'s scheme [4] presented a blockchain-enabled protocol for the security of the healthcare data. Some of the features of Aujla et al.'s scheme [4] are as follows:

- They presented a technique for the secure transmission of the health-related information to the cloud servers with the help of edge nodes.
- They used the blockchain mechanism for the data security to preserve the privacy of healthcare data.
- Furthermore, an incremental "tensor train decomposition model" was provided for the storage of health-related information over the cloud servers to prevent the information duplication.
- Their protocols were designed with important phases like registration, block creation along with validation, data generation and block updates.

7.5.6 Review of Islam and Shin's Scheme

Islam and Shin [26] presented a blockchain-enabled protocol for the security of healthcare data with the assistance of an unmanned aerial vehicle (UAV) in the IoT domain. Some of the features of Islam and Shin's scheme [26] are as follows:

- In their protocol they presented the system model for health-related data collection with the help of UAVs and blockchain-enabled mechanisms.
- A procedure for health-related data collection was given.
- A "two-phase authentication procedure" was also discussed for the considered system.

- They provided a threat model along with the security analysis of their protocol to prove its resilience against various possible attacks.
- Their protocols are designed with important phases like the device registration phase, body sensor hive synchronization phase, data acquisition phase and data storage phase.
- Furthermore, a consortium network of blockchains was built through the Ethereum platform. They also computed and analyzed the network performance parameters like throughput, latency and block size for their presented protocol.

7.6 Comparative Study of Blockchain-Enabled Security Protocols for IoT-Based Healthcare Applications

In this section, we provide a comparative study of various blockchain-enabled security protocols for IoT-based healthcare applications. Various protocols like Neha et al.'s scheme [18], Saha et al.'s scheme [38], Xiang et al.'s scheme [56], Xu et al.'s scheme [57], Aujla et al.'s scheme [4] and Islam and Shin's scheme [26] are analyzed and compared. The comparison is provided in Table 7.1.

TABLE 7.1

Comparison of Security and Functionality Features

Feature	Neha et al. [18]	Saha et al. [38]	Xiang et al. [56]	Xu et al. [57]	Aujla et al. [4]	Islam and Shin [26]
SFF_1	C	C	C	C	C	C
SFF_2	C	C	C	C	C	C
SFF_3	C	C	C	C	C	C
SFF_4	C	C	C	×	C	×
SFF_5	C	C	×	×	×	×
SFF_6	C	C	C	C	C	C
SFF_7	C	C	C	C	C	C
SFF_8	C	C	C	C	C	C
SFF_9	C	C	C	C	C	C
SFF_{10}	C	*NA*	C	*NA*	×	*NA*
SFF_{11}	C	*NA*	C	*NA*	×	*NA*
SFF_{12}	C	*NA*	×	*NA*	×	*NA*
SFF_{13}	C	×	×	×	×	×
SFF_{14}	C	×	×	×	×	×
SFF_{15}	C	*NA*	C	*NA*	*NA*	*NA*
SFF_{16}	C	C	C	C	C	C
SFF_{17}	C	×	C	×	×	×
SFF_{18}	×	×	×	×	×	×
SFF_{19}	C	×	C	C	C	C

Note—x: "a scheme does not protect from a specific attack, nor it does support a particular feature;" C: "a scheme protects against a specific attack, or it supports a particular feature;" *NA*: "not applicable in a scheme."

The following features have been considered in the comparative study:

- SFF_1: "provides mutual authentication/access control."
- SFF_2: "supports anonymity property."
- SFF_3: "supports untraceability property."
- SFF_4: "provides session-key agreement."
- SFF_5: "provides session key security under CK adversary model."
- SFF_6: "provides data confidentiality."
- SFF_7: "provides data integrity."
- SFF_8: "protection against strong replay attack."
- SFF_9: "protection against man-in-the-middle attack."
- SFF_{10}: "availability of efficient login phase."
- SFF_{11}: "availability of password update phase."
- SFF_{12}: "availability of biometric update phase."
- SFF_{13}: "availability of dynamic controller node (personal server) addition phase."
- SFF_{14}: "availability of dynamic smart healthcare device addition."
- SFF_{15}: "protection against stolen mobile device/programmer attack."
- SFF_{16}: "protection against impersonation attack."
- SFF_{17}: "provides formal security verification using AVISPA/SCYTHER tool."
- SFF_{18}: "provides formal security analysis under Real-or-Random (RoR) model."
- SFF_{19}: "provides practical implementation."

From Table 7.1, it is clear that schemes of Saha et al. [38], Xiang et al. [56], Xu et al. [57], Aujla et al. [4] and Islam and Shin [26] lack most of desired security and functionality features like, "provides session-key agreement," "provides session key security under CK adversary model," "availability of password update phase," "availability of biometric update phase," "availability of dynamic controller node (personal server) addition phase," "availability of dynamic smart healthcare device addition," "provide formal security verification using AVISPA/SCYTHER tool" and "provides formal security analysis under Real-or-Random (RoR) model." However, of Neha et al.'s [18] scheme achieved most of the required "security and functionality features." Therefore, of Neha et al.'s [18] scheme seems suitable for the security of a blockchain-enabled IoT-based healthcare monitoring system.

7.7 Concluding Remarks

The blockchain mechanism helps to improve the security of IoT-based healthcare monitoring systems, which can be further considered as the blockchain-enabled IoT-based healthcare monitoring system (BIoT-HMS) in which the blockchain mechanism helps to protect the data against various types of possible attacks, as discussed earlier. We provided details of different architectures of BIoT-HMS. We also discussed the security and privacy requirements of BIoT-HMS. Some of the possible attacks on BIoT-HMS were also highlighted. A threat model for BIoT-HMS was provided, which would be further helpful to researchers in the designing of security protocols for BIoT-HMS. Furthermore, we provided the summary of various existing security protocols related to BIoT-HMS. A comparative study of various existing security protocols related to BIoT-HMS was provided. The scheme of Neha et al. [18] achieved most of the required security and functionality features like "supports anonymity property," "supports untraceability property," "provides session key security under CK adversary model," "provides data confidentiality," "provides data integrity," "protection against strong replay attack," "protection against man-in-the-middle attack," "protection against impersonation attack," "protection against stolen mobile device attack" and many more.

References

1. S Kirsten. (2020). Cross Site Scripting (XSS). OWASP. https://owasp.org/www-community/attacks/xss/. Accessed in March 2020.
2. What is an SQL Injection Attack? (2020). https://sucuri.net/guides/what-is-sql-injection/. Accessed in March 2020.
3. M Asif-Ur-Rahman, F Afsana, M Mahmud, MS Kaiser, MR Ahmed, O Kaiwartya and A James-Taylor. (2019). Toward a Heterogeneous Mist, Fog, and Cloud-Based Framework for the Internet of Healthcare Things. *IEEE Internet of Things Journal*, 6(3), 4049–4062.
4. GS Aujla and A Jindal. (2020). A Decoupled Blockchain Approach for Edge-envisioned IoT-based Healthcare Monitoring. *IEEE Journal on Selected Areas in Communications*, 39(2), 491–499.
5. B Bera, D Chattaraj and AK Das. (2020). Designing Secure Blockchain-based Access Control Scheme in IoT-enabled Internet of Drones Deployment. *Computer Communications*, 153, 229–249.
6. B Bera, AK Das, M Obaidat, P Vijayakumar, KF Hsiao and Y Park. (2020). AI-Enabled Blockchain- Based Access Control for Malicious Attacks Detection and Mitigation in IoE. *IEEE Consumer Electronics Magazine*, 1–1.
7. R Canetti and H Krawczyk. Analysis of Key-exchange Protocols and Their Use for Building Secure channels. In *International Conference on the Theory and Applications of Cryptographic Techniques– Advances in Cryptology (EUROCRYPT'01)*, pages 453–474. Springer, Innsbruck (Tyrol), Austria, 2001.
8. R Canetti and H Krawczyk. (2002). Universally Composable Notions of Key Exchange and Secure Channels. In *International Conference on the Theory and Applications of Cryptographic Techniques– Advances in Cryptology (EUROCRYPT'02)*, 337–351, Amsterdam, The Netherlands
9. S Challa, M Wazid, AK Das, N Kumar, AG Reddy, E Yoon and K Yoo. Secure Signature-Based Authenticated Key Establishment Scheme for Future IoT Applications. *IEEE Access*, 5:3028–3043, 2017.
10. S Chatterjee, AK Das and JK Sing. (2014). A Novel and Efficient User Access Control Scheme for Wireless Body Area Sensor Networks. *Journal of King Saud University - Computer and Information Sciences*, 26(2), 181–201.
11. R Chowdhury. (2019). IoT in Healthcare: 20 Examples That'll Make You Feel Better. https://www.ubuntupit.com/ iot-in-healthcare-20-examples-thatll-make-you-feel-better/. Accessed in March 2020.
12. AK Das, M Wazid, N Kumar, MK Khan, KR Choo and Y Park. (2018). Design of Secure and Lightweight Authentication Protocol for Wearable Devices Environment. *IEEE Journal of Biomedical and Health Informatics*, 22(4), 1310–1322.
13. AK Das and S Zeadally. (2019). Chapter 13 - Data Security in the Smart Grid Environment. In A Tascikaraoglu and O Erdinc, editors, *Pathways to a Smarter Power System*, 371–395. Cambridge, MA: Academic Press, Elsevier,

14. M Debe, K Salah, R Jayaraman and J Arshad. (2020). Blockchain-Based Verifiable Tracking of Resellable Returned Drugs. *IEEE Access*, 8, 205848–205862.
15. D Dolev and AC Yao. (1983). On the Security of Public Key Protocols. *IEEE Transactions on Information Theory*, 29(2), 198–208.
16. W Eddy. TCP SYN Flooding Attacks and Common Mitigations. https://tools.ietf.org/html/rfc4987. Accessed in March 2020.
17. F Fernandez and GC Pallis. (2014). Opportunities and Challenges of the Internet of Things for Healthcare: Systems Engineering Perspective. In *4th International Conference on Wireless Mobile Communication and Healthcare - Transforming Healthcare Through Innovations in Mobile and Wireless Technologies (MOBIHEALTH)*, 263–266, Athens, Greece,
18. N Garg, M Wazid, AK Das, DP Singh, JJPC Rodrigues and Y Park. (2020). BAKMP-IoMT: Design of Blockchain Enabled Authenticated Key Management Protocol for Internet of Medical Things Deployment. *IEEE Access*, 8, 95956–95977. doi:10.1109/ ACCESS.2020.2995917.
19. D Goad, AT Collins and U Gal. (2021). Privacy and the Internet of Things–An experiment in discrete choice. *Information & Management*, 58(2), 103292. doi:10.1016/j.im.2020.103292.
20. H Wang, D Zhang and KG Shin. (2004). Change-point Monitoring for the Detection of DoS Attacks. *IEEE Transactions on Dependable and Secure Computing*, 1(4), 193–208.
21. H Habibzadeh, K Dinesh, O Rajabi Shishvan, A Boggio-Dandry, G Sharma and T Soyata. (2020). A Survey of Healthcare Internet of Things (HIoT): A Clinical Perspective. *IEEE Internet of Things Journal*, 7(1), 53–71.
22. H Habibzadeh, K Dinesh, O Rajabi Shishvan, A Boggio-Dandry, G Sharma and T Soyata. (2020). A Survey of Healthcare Internet of Things (HIoT): A Clinical Perspective. *IEEE Internet of Things Journal*, 7(1), 53–71.
23. R Hamza, Z Yan, K Muhammad, P Bellavista and F Titouna. (2020). A Privacy-preserving Cryptosystem for IoT E-healthcare. *Information Sciences*, 527, 493–510. http://www.sciencedirect.com/science/article/pii/S002002551930088X.
24. JJ Hathaliya and S Tanwar. (2020). An Exhaustive Survey on Security and Privacy Issues in Healthcare 4.0. *Computer Communications*, 153, 311–335.
25. MH Ibrahim, S Kumari, AK Das, M Wazid and V Odelu. (2016). Secure Anonymous Mutual Authentication for Star Two-tier Wireless Body Area Networks. *Computer Methods and Programs in Biomedicine*, 135, 37–50.
26. A Islam and SY Shin. A Blockchain-based Secure Healthcare Scheme with the Assistance of Unmanned Aerial Vehicle in Internet of Things. *Computers & Electrical Engineering*, 84:106627, 2020.
27. GA Jaafar, SM Abdullah and S Ismail. (2019). Review of Recent Detection Methods for HTTP DDoS Attack. *Journal of Computer Networks and Communications*, 2019, 1–10, Article ID 1283472.
28. S Jangirala, AK Das and AV Vasilakos. (2019). Designing Secure Lightweight Blockchain-Enabled RFID- Based Authentication Protocol for Supply Chains in 5G Mobile Edge Computing Environment. *IEEE Transactions on Industrial Informatics*, doi:10.1109/TII.2019.2942389.
29. R Kumar, X Zhang, W Wang, RU Khan, J Kumar and A Sharif. (2019). A Multimodal Malware Detection Technique for Android IoT Devices Using Various Features. *IEEE Access*, 7, 64411–64430,
30. PA Laplante and N Laplante. (2016). The Internet of Things in Healthcare: Potential Applications and Challenges. *IT Professional*, 18(3), 2–4.
31. TS Messerges, EA Dabbish and R H. Sloan. (2002). Examining Smart-card Security Under the Threat of Power Analysis Attacks. *IEEE Transactions on Computers*, 51(5), 541–552.
32. S Nakamoto. (2008). Bitcoin: A Peer-to-peer Electronic Cash System, http://bitcoin.org/bitcoin.pdf.
33. P Nasrullah. (2020). Internet of Things in Healthcare: Applications, Benefits, and Challenges. https://www.peerbits.com/blog/internet-of-things-healthcare-applications-benefits-and-challenges.html. Accessed in March 2020.
34. S Pundir, M Wazid, DP Singh, AK Das, JJPC Rodrigues and Y Park. (2020). Intrusion Detection Protocols in Wireless Sensor Networks Integrated to Internet of Things Deployment: Survey and Future Challenges. *IEEE Access*, 8, 3343–3363.

35. YA Qadri, A Nauman, YB. Zikria, AV Vasilakos and SW Kim. (2020). The Future of Healthcare Internet of Things: A Survey of Emerging Technologies. *IEEE Communications Surveys & Tutorials*, 22(2), 1121–1167.
36. J Ryoo, D Han, S Kim and S Lee. (2008). Performance Enhancement of Differential Power Analysis Attacks with Signal Companding Methods. *IEEE Signal Processing Letters*, 15, 625–628.
37. R Saha, G Kumar, MK Rai, R Thomas and S Lim. (2019). Privacy Ensured *e*-Healthcare for Fog-Enhanced IoT Based Applications. *IEEE Access*, 7, 44536.
38. S Saha, AK Sutrala, AK Das, N Kumar and JJPC Rodrigues. (2020). On the Design of Blockchain-Based Access Control Protocol for IoT-Enabled Healthcare Applications. In *ICC 2020– 2020 IEEE International Conference on Communications (ICC)*, 1–6, Dublin, Ireland,
39. N Saxena, I Thomas, P Gope, P Burnapand N Kumar. (2020). PharmaCrypt: Blockchain for Critical Pharmaceutical Industry to Counterfeit Drugs. *Computer*, 53(7), 29–44.
40. S Sayeed and H Marco-Gisbert. (2019). Assessing Blockchain Consensus and Security Mechanisms against the 51% Attack. *Applied Sciences*, 9(9), 1–17.
41. J Srinivas, AK Das, N Kumar, and JJPC Rodrigues. (2019). Cloud Centric Authentication for Wearable Healthcare Monitoring System. *IEEE Transactions on Dependable and Secure Computing*, doi:10.1109/TDSC.2018.2828306.
42. W Stallings. (2010). *Cryptography and Network Security: Principles and Practice*. Prentice Hall Press: Upper Saddle River, NJ, 5th edition,
43. Y Sun, FP Lo and B Lo (2019). Security and Privacy for the Internet of Medical Things Enabled Healthcare Systems: A Survey. *IEEE Access*, 7, 183339–183355.
44. Q Wang, D Zhou, S Yang, P Li, C Wang and Q Guan. (2019). Privacy Preserving Computations over Healthcare Data. In *International Conference on Internet of Things (iThings) and IEEE Green Computing and Communications (GreenCom) and IEEE Cyber, Physical and Social Computing (CPSCom) and IEEE Smart Data (SmartData)*, 635–640, Atlanta, USA,
45. M Wazid, P Bagga, AK Das, S Shetty, JJPC Rodrigues and Y Park. (2019). AKM-IoV: Authenticated Key Management Protocol in Fog Computing-Based Internet of Vehicles Deployment. *IEEE Internet of Things Journal*, 6(5), 8804–8817.
46. M Wazid, B Bera, A Mitra, AK Dasand R Ali. (2020). Private Blockchain-Envisioned Security Frame- work for AI-Enabled IoT-Based Drone-Aided Healthcare Services. In *Proceedings of the 2nd ACM MobiCom Workshop on Drone Assisted Wireless Communications for 5G and Beyond, DroneCom '20*, 37–42, London, United Kingdom,
47. M Wazid, AK Das, MK Khan, AA Al-Ghaiheb, N Kumar and AV Vasilakos. (2017). Secure Authentication Scheme for Medicine Anti-Counterfeiting System in IoT Environment. *IEEE Internet of Things Journal*, 4(5), 1634–1646.
48. M Wazid, AK Das, N Kumar, M Conti and AV Vasilakos. (2018). A Novel Authentication and Key Agreement Scheme for Implantable Medical Devices Deployment. *IEEE Journal of Biomedical and Health Informatics*, 22(4), 1299–1309.
49. M Wazid, AK Das, N Kumar and AV Vasilakos. (2019). Design of Secure Key Management and User Authentication Scheme for Fog Computing Services. *Future Generation Computer Systems*, 91, 475–492.
50. M Wazid, AK Das and J-H Lee. (2019). User Authentication in a Tactile Internet Based Remote Surgery Environment: Security Issues, Challenges, and Future Research Directions. *Pervasive and Mobile Computing*, 54, 71–85.
51. M Wazid, AK Das, V Odelu, N Kumar and W Susilo. (2020). Secure Remote User Authenticated Key Establishment Protocol for Smart Home Environment. *IEEE Transactions on Dependable and Secure Computing*, 17(2), 391–406.
52. M Wazid, AK Das, JJPC Rodrigues, S Shetty and Y Park. (2019). IoMT Malware Detection Approaches: Analysis and Research Challenges. *IEEE Access*, 7, 182459–182476.
53. M Wazid, AK Das, S Shetty and M Jo. (2020). A Tutorial and Future Research for Building a Blockchain- Secure Communication Scheme for Internet of Intelligent Things. *IEEE Access*, 8, 88700–88716.

54. M Wazid, AK Das, S Shetty and JJPC Rodrigues. (2020). On the Design of Secure Communication Framework for Blockchain-Based Internet of Intelligent Battlefield Things Environment. In *IEEE IN- FOCOM 2020 - IEEE Conference on Computer Communications Workshops (INFOCOM WKSHPS),* 888–893, Toronto, ON, Canada.
55. M Wazid, S Zeadally, AK Das and V Odelu. (2016). Analysis of Security Protocols for Mobile Healthcare. *Journal of Medical Systems,* 40(11), 1–10.
56. X Xiang, M Wang and W Fan. (2020). A Permissioned Blockchain-Based Identity Management and User Authentication Scheme for E-Health Systems. *IEEE Access,* 8, 171771–171783.
57. J Xu, K Xue, S Li, H Tian, J Hong, P Hong and N Yu. (2019). Healthchain: A Blockchain-Based Privacy Preserving Scheme for Large-Scale Health Data. *IEEE Internet of Things Journal,* 6(5), 8770–8781.
58. Y Yan, Y Qian, H Sharif and D Tipper. (2012). A Survey on Cyber Security for Smart Grid Communications. *IEEE Communications Surveys and Tutorials,* 14(4), 998–1010.
59. H Zhu, CK Wu, CH Koo, YT Tsang, Y Liu, HR Chi and K Tsang. (2019). Smart Healthcare in the Era of Internet-of-Things. *IEEE Consumer Electronics Magazine,* 8(5), 26–30.

8

Connecting Patient-Centric Blockchains with Multilayer P2P Networks and Digital Platforms

Roberto Moro-Visconti

CONTENTS

8.1 Introduction

Healthcare represents a data-sensitive industry, and blockchain validation is a disrupting innovation that reshapes the patient-centric supply and value chains.

A blockchain is a distributed ledger that shares data among a network of peers (Holbl et al., 2018). It can be defined as a chain of blocks that are timestamped and linked using cryptographic hashes. These blocks are sealed in a secure and immutable manner (Rohers et al., 2017). The chain is constantly growing, and new blocks are being appended to the end, whereby each new block holds a reference (i.e., a hash value) to the content of the previous block (Sleiman et al., 2015). The shareholders represent the nodes of the blockchain and are organized in a decentralized peer-to-peer (P2P) network. Each node holds two keys (Aumasson, 2017): A public key for encrypting the messages sent to a node and a private key to decrypt and read the messages. Thus, the public key encryption mechanism is used to ensure the consistency, irreversibility, and non-repudiability of a blockchain (Zheng et al., 2017). Only the proper private key can decrypt the messages encrypted with the corresponding public key.

Blockchain is a consequential list (chain) of blocks (records) that are linked using cryptography. Each block contains a cryptographic hash of the previous block, a timestamp and transaction data (Economist, 2015).

Blockchain could be regarded as a public ledger technology in which all committed transactions are stored in a chain of blocks. This chain continuously grows when new blocks are added to it. Blockchain technology has characteristics such as decentralization,

DOI: 10.1201/9781003133179-8

persistence, anonymity, verifiability and auditability. It can then be used to ensure the authenticity, reliability and integrity of data and business activities. Blockchain can work in a decentralized environment thanks to the integration of technologies such as cryptographic hash, digital signature (based on asymmetric cryptography) and distributed consensus mechanisms. With blockchain technology, a transaction can take place in a decentralized manner. As a result, blockchain can produce notable cost savings and efficiency gains (Zheng et al., 2018).

Blockchains are becoming increasingly popular thanks to the success of controversial cryptocurrencies. Bitcoins and their "relatives" represent a powerful instrument of financial disintermediation that refreshes a barter economy, bypassing central authorities. Whereas the author of this chapter shares the growing skepticism towards an instrument that favors tax evasion, money laundering and boundless speculation, other less-known blockchain applications deserve more attention. This is, for instance, the case of healthcare blockchains that validate data-sharing in an extremely sensitive industry, producing efficiency gains and tangible savings.

In summary, a blockchain has the following key characteristics (Zheng et al., 2018):

1. Decentralization: In conventional centralized transaction systems, each transaction needs to be validated through the central trusted agency (e.g., the central bank) with fixed cost and performance bottlenecks at the primary servers. A transaction in the blockchain network can instead be conducted between any two peers (P2P) without authentication by the central agency. In this manner, blockchain significantly reduces server costs (including the development and the operation costs) and mitigates the performance bottlenecks at the central server.
2. Persistency: Since each of the transactions spreading across the network needs to be confirmed and recorded in blocks distributed in the whole network, it is nearly impossible to tamper with. Furthermore, each broadcasted block would need to be validated by other nodes, and transactions would be checked. In this way, any falsification could be easily detected.
3. Anonymity: Each user can interact with the blockchain network with a generated address. In addition to this, a user could create many addresses to avoid identity exposure. There is no longer a central party recording users' private information. This mechanism preserves privacy on the transactions in the blockchain.
4. Auditability: Since each of the transactions on the blockchain is validated and recorded with a timestamp, users can easily verify and trace the previous records by accessing any node in the distributed network. In a bitcoin blockchain, each transaction could be traced to previous transactions iteratively. This improves the traceability and transparency of the data stored in the blockchain.
5. Trust: Confidence is shifted away from human actors towards a cryptographic system, with incentives for participating actors (Figure 8.1).

Figure 8.2 shows the blockchain formation. The main chain (black) consists of the longest series of blocks from the genesis block (red) to the current block. Orphan blocks (blue) exist outside of the main chain.

The importance of the topic is confirmed by a growing literature, as can be shown, for instance, by recent surveys concerning healthcare applications (see for example Agbo et al., 2019; Hasselgren et al., 2020; Hölbl et al., 2018; Hussien et al., 2019; Kuo et al., 2019; Xu et al., 2019; Prokofieva & Miah, 2019; Khezr et al., 2019; Mazlan et al., 2020).

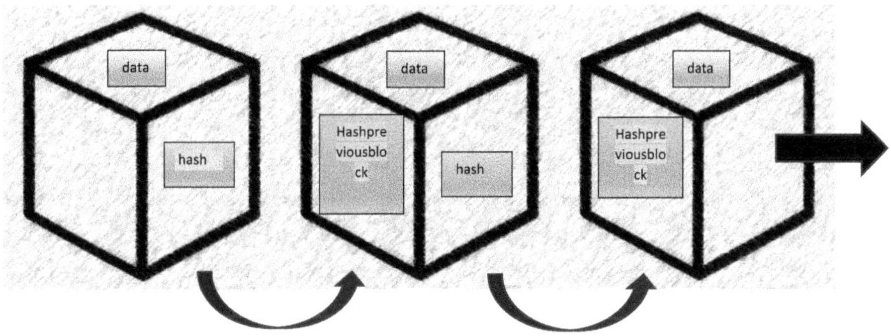

FIGURE 8.1
Blockchain as a sequential chain of data.

One significant advantage of using blockchain technology in the healthcare industry is that it can reform the interoperability of healthcare databases, providing increased access to patient medical records, device tracking, prescription databases and hospital assets, including the complete life cycle of a device within the blockchain infrastructure (Tanwar et al., 2020). There are, however, some aspects that are still neglected but may deserve further investigation.

Blockchains represent a peculiar P2P decentralized and distributed digital ledger and network, as it can be seen at first sight even considering their supply and value chain, represented in graphical terms. It may so be worth examining their networking properties and some possible practical applications.

The (trivial) consideration that blockchains process and validate IT data can be linked to the digitalization trend. Data are increasingly digitized, so becoming suitable for IT manipulation and consequent blockchain use. It will be shown that digital platforms can act as a powerful catalyzer of information and transactions, connecting patients and other

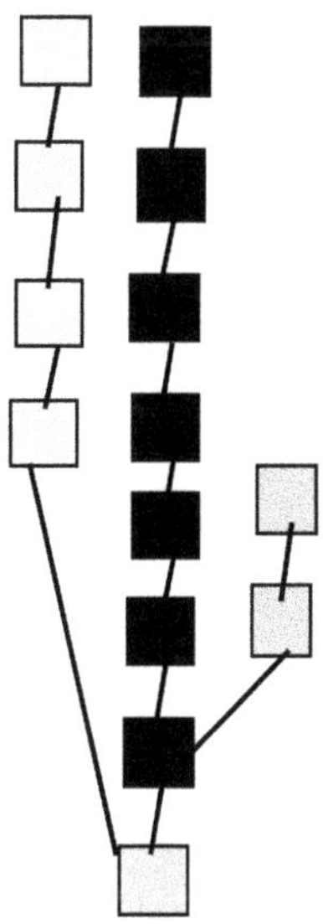

FIGURE 8.2
Blockchain formation.

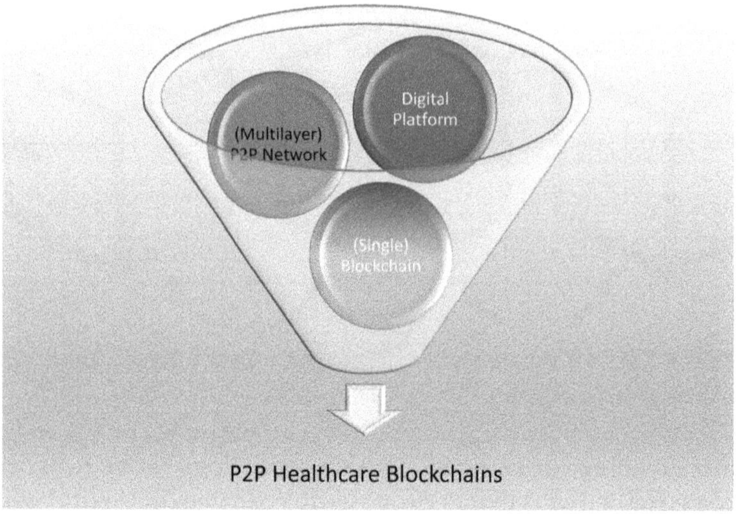

FIGURE 8.3
Interacting digital platforms and P2P networks for the connection of blockchains.

key stakeholders to validating blockchains. Scattered data can be coalesced through platforms, becoming big, and so improving their value. Blockchains add further value.

The final aim of this chapter is to show that the networking features of the blockchains, linked to the intermediating function of bridging platforms, add value to the whole healthcare ecosystem, improving its sustainability.

Figure 8.3 shows which are the interacting variables that can foster patient-centric P2P healthcare blockchains: Digital platforms applied to P2P networks and to single blockchains that become digitally connected.

This contribution is structured as follows: After this introductory framework, the strategic impact of blockchains on different industries is synthesized in Section 8.2. A short introduction to healthcare blockchains and the related literature is contained in Section 8.3. The rationale of the public versus private blockchain model in the healthcare industry is synthetically described in Section 8.4. Section 8.5 is inspired by the (trivial) consideration that blockchains are a (peculiar) network that hosts P2P interactions. Network theory can so be adapted to this relevant case. Section 8.6 considers a patient-centric application of IT networks that are connected to blockchains through digital platforms. Section 8.7 extends these considerations to a multilayer network ecosystem, where complementary healthcare blockchains interact, again thanks to bridging digital platforms. Section 8.8 is dedicated to some concluding remarks.

8.2 Disrupting Traditional Business Models

Numerous industries are implementing blockchain as part of their business processes. Valuation patterns may therefore be concerned not only with public or private blockchains but also with their impact on traditional businesses.

Blockchain technology was used at first for controversial cryptocurrencies like bitcoins and FinTech applications and later in many other industries as:

- Energy (Fan et al., 2017) IoT electric business model (Veuger, 2018).
- Property transfer (intangibles, real estate property, registered movable property ...).
- Industry/manufacturing.
- Logistics and transport (tracking of goods, etc.).
- Automotive (shipment of vehicles with frictionless information among connected systems; tracking of original spare parts; car-sharing; fidelization of the clients, etc.).
- Food supply chain (Mao et al., 2018).
- e-commerce.
- Stock markets (asset pricing; appraisal of shareholders, etc.).
- Healthcare (for track-record; clinical trials; personalized medicine; pharmaceutical supply chains; prescription drug management; health records management, etc.); see Shing et al., 2016.
- Contemporary art (Lotti, 2016).
- Insurance (InsurTech).
- FinTech (validation of payments; P2P lending and crowdfunding, etc.).
- Microfinance (assisting with smart contracts between several microfinancing bodies without the need for mediators or central authorities).
- E-governance (transparency and accessibility of government information; information sharing, etc.).
- Crowdsourcing (decentralized and secured petition systems).

This list is far from being exhaustive and just represents an example of some possible applications of this versatile technology.

Since it allows payments to be finished without any bank or any intermediary, a blockchain can be used in various financial services such as digital assets, remittances and online payments. Additionally, blockchain is becoming one of the most promising technologies for the next generation of internet interaction systems, such as smart contracts, public services, the Internet of Things (IoT), reputation systems and security services.

Blockchains so go well beyond the cryptocurrencies (like bitcoin) that made them famous. It is my firm opinion that cryptocurrencies may fuel money laundering and other malpractices and that their market is opaque, irrespective of any regulation, and subject to speculative bubbles. For these very reasons I think that cryptocurrencies should be regulated or, if this is not possible, prohibited. This, however, does not interfere with other potential applications of blockchain technology.

These applications contribute to the evaluation patterns: The wider, the higher the potential value of a blockchain that can enable and forge new products, processes, and business models.

Technological evolution ignites an extension to many other sectors. Synergies among complementary industries are also possible.

8.3 Healthcare Blockchains

The characteristics of the blockchain (its decentralized nature, openness and permissionlessness) may offer a unique solution for healthcare (Dhillon et al., 2021; Sharma et al., 2021; Gupta et al., 2021; Bittins et al., 2021; Ciampi et al., 2021; Saharan & Prasad, 2021). Wider applicability of the technology paves its way into different aspects of healthcare, including wearables and the progress of medical research. The healthcare sector has growing demands for blockchain developments (Deloitte, 2018).

The immutability of the blockchain is a vital option for healthcare data. It can secure health records, the results of clinical trials and ensure regulatory compliance. The employment of smart contracts demonstrates how blockchain can be used to support real-time patient monitoring and medical interventions (Griggs et al., 2018). Further application of blockchain relates to the supply chain in pharma and developing measures against counterfeit drugs. Blockchain technology has the potential to transform healthcare, placing the patient at the center of the healthcare ecosystem and increasing the security, privacy and interoperability of sensitive health data. Healthcare records that contain confidential patient data make this system extremely complicated because there is a risk of a privacy breach (De Aguiar et al., 2020).

Hölbl et al. (2018) accordingly say that "one field where blockchain technology has tremendous potential is healthcare, due to the need for a more patient-centric approach to healthcare systems and to connect disparate systems and increase the accuracy of electronic healthcare records (EHRs)."

Blockchain will prove to be indispensable in building a global precision-medicine ecosystem that optimally connects patients, clinicians, researchers, insurers and clinical laboratories to one another. Blockchain will improve data security, data sharing, interoperability, patient engagement, big data analytics (Muneeswaran et al., 2021), health information exchange, fighting counterfeit drugs, R&D processes, AI-based diagnostics and fostering vertical business models (Schumacher, 2017).

Healthcare blockchain technology can be used to support (Angraal et al., 2017):

- Interoperability to facilitate the exchange of health-related information.
- Drug prescriptions.
- Supply and value chain management.
- Pregnancy and any risk data management.
- Access control to (sensitive) health data.
- Data sharing and managing of an audit trail of medical activities.
- Precision medicine and care / orphan pathologies.
- Provider credentials.
- Medical billing.
- Contracting.
- Medical record exchange.
- Clinical trials.
- Validation of client identities.
- Automated validation of claims.
- Anti-counterfeiting drugs.
- Internet of Medical Things.

- A decentralized approach to managing permissions, authorization, and data sharing between healthcare systems.
- Safe storing of medical data.

8.4 Public or Private Healthcare Blockchains?

The Hamletic dilemma between private or public blockchains, mitigated by consortial variants, is particularly meaningful in the sensitive healthcare industry, where privacy concerns peak and quality (of care) often becomes a question of survival.

A blockchain does not represent a firm but a semi-public good (being a public or private blockchain) that is shared among different stakeholders that co-create value participating in the construction and implementation of a sequential pattern of codes. The evaluation of a blockchain is so vastly different from that of a firm or an asset.

There are different types of blockchains depending on the managed data, on their availability and on what actions can be performed by the user. These include:

- Public permissionless (Norman et al., 2018).
- Consortium (public permissioned).
- Private.

Public blockchains are non-marketable, and so it is difficult to assess their potential value; they may have a figurative value that emerges from the public savings that they make possible.

A private blockchain may be owned by a firm, and valuation patterns may follow its innovative revenue model. Revenues deriving from new businesses are hard to assess since they lack a historical background and are not clear-cut. Profit streams may derive from subscriptions, pay-per-use income, performance-based fees (cashing in part of the savings of the blockchain users), or extraction of validated big data (sold outside for vertical advertising; e-commerce applications, etc.).

Public blockchains lack ultimate private ownership and may be harder to evaluate. They represent the only fully decentralized model.

Semi-public blockchains may somewhat resemble consortia. A consortium is an association of two or more individuals, companies, organizations or governments (or any combination of these entities) to participate in a common activity or pooling their resources for achieving a common goal. This may be consistent with blockchains, joint ventures, company networks and value co-creation paradigms, so representing an innovative business model. Different stakeholders may join in setting up "co-opetition," merging cooperation and competition. It is used when companies which are otherwise competitors collaborate in a consortium to cooperate on areas which are non-strategic for their core businesses. They prefer to reduce their costs in these non-strategic areas and compete in other areas where they can differentiate better. The value of consortium membership is typically represented by the private rents that any participants can extract from it since the consortium is a non-profit alliance.

The business model of the blockchain influences its peculiar corporate governance issues (Yermack, 2017). Stakeholders may be linked by their P2P interactions and in general, are not represented by the ordinary stakeholders that rotate around a firm (shareholders, debtholders, employees, managers, suppliers, clients, etc.). Whereas value co-creation is typical of digital businesses, sharing of co-created value may not follow a similar pattern. For example, social networks are based on shared information (personal data) that platforms can monetize unilaterally, with the tacit and unaware consent of the participants. Blockchains work differently, and their decentralization prevents the abuses of a pivoting platform and minimizes information asymmetries.

> Consortium blockchains differ from their public counterpart in that they are permissioned, thus, not just anyone with an Internet connection could gain access to a consortium blockchain. These types of blockchains could also be described as semi-decentralized. Control over a consortium blockchain is not granted to a single entity, but rather a group of approved individuals. With a consortium blockchain, the consensus process is likely to differ from that of a public blockchain. Instead of anyone being able to partake in the procedure, consensus participants of a consortium blockchain are likely to be a group of pre-approved nodes on the network. Thus, consortium blockchains possess the security features that are inherent in public blockchains whilst also allowing for a greater degree of control over the network (https://www.mycryptopedia.com/consortium-blockchain-explained/).

8.4.1 The Blockchain Flow

Due to their intrinsic nature, blockchains follow a peculiar consequential flow that shapes their supply chain features. Figure 8.4 depicts a typical process that can be consequently customized for healthcare applications.

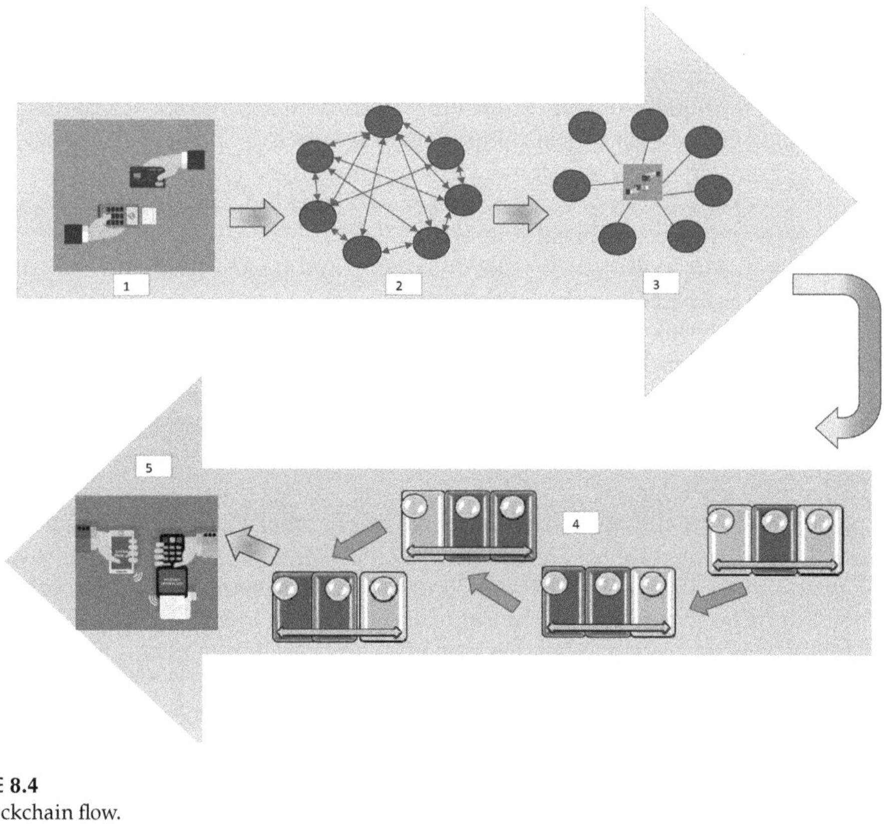

FIGURE 8.4
The blockchain flow.

The blockchain supply chain (Blossey et al., 2019; Dujak & Sajter, 2019; Saberi et al., 2018) can be described with the following patterns:

1. One party (e.g., a patient) requests a transaction.
2. Each requested transaction is funneled into a decentralized P2P network, reaching each (computer) node.
3. Each peer node (being the blockchain a P2P network) validates the transaction through an algorithm.
4. Any approved transaction forms a block and is added to a distributed public ledger (blockchain).
5. Once a new block is added to an existing blockchain, the transaction embodied in that block is permanently validated.

The features of the networked chains will be shortly described in Section 8.5.

Supply and value chain management concerns all the stakeholders of the healthcare ecosystem that interact around the networked chain:

- The patients.
- The public authorities.
- Private players from MedTech to other suppliers, etc.

Supply and value chain management so interacts with digital processes, ranging from e-Health/m-Health applications to digital identity management. Figure 8.5 shows an example of these possible interactions that may well be extended to accommodate further products and services.

The interaction between the stakeholders, the healthcare applications, and the blockchain is exemplified in Figure 8.6.

8.5 Adaptation of Network Theory to P2P Interactions and Blockchains

Network (graph) theory describes the interaction between nodes connected by edges. Blockchains can be interpreted as a peculiar network where blocks (nodes or vertices, using standard network terminology) are connected through hashes (edges) that ensure anonymity, immutability and compactness of the block. These characteristics (evident in the blockchain flow represented in Figure 8.4) are crucial in the sensitive healthcare industry.

The blockchain network is a P2P platform where interacting peer nodes cooperate. Nodes are digitally represented by connected computers with blockchain clients (stakeholding nodes) behind them. "Democratic" P2P features are consistent with the decentralized nature of blockchains.

P2P architecture is typical of crowdfunding, a networking structure where equity-holders interact to raise capital.

The networking features of the blockchains are peculiar, since they are incremental (each block adds up to the previous ones) and unidirectional (data embedded in certified blocks are immutable and the validating system is forward-looking).

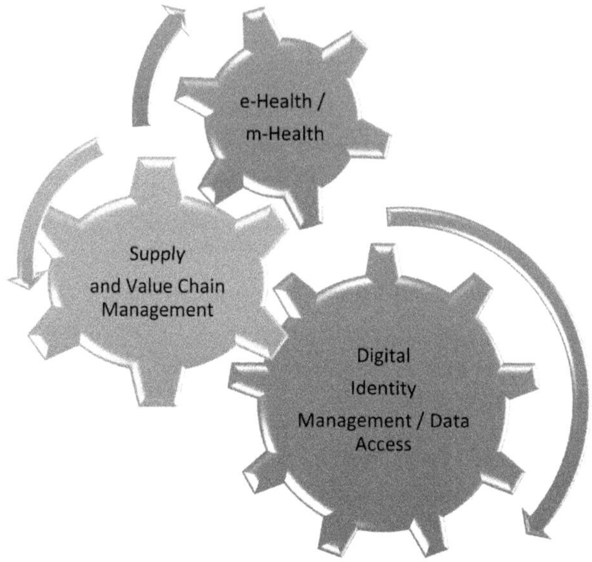

FIGURE 8.5
Digital interaction of healthcare components.

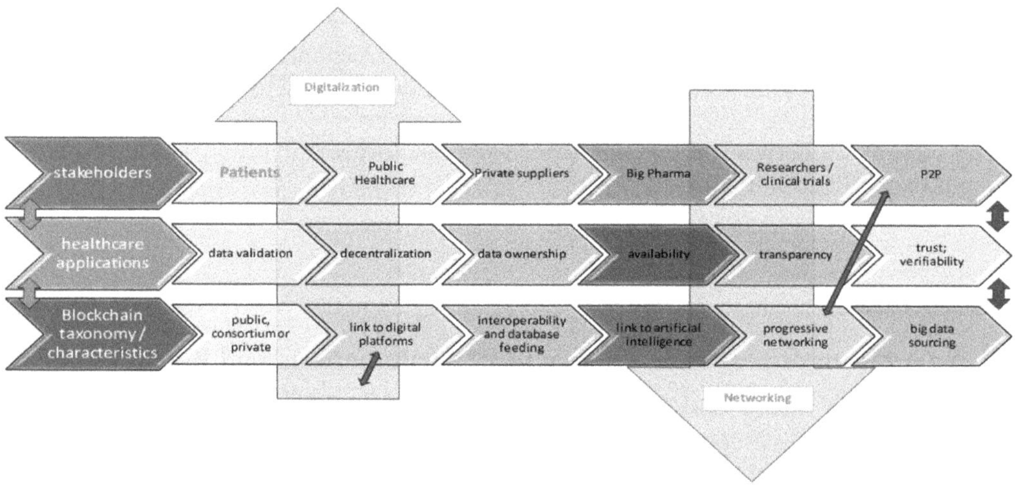

FIGURE 8.6
Interaction between the stakeholders, the healthcare applications and the blockchain.

Network (graph) theory is based on its widely investigated mathematical properties (Bapat, 2011; Barabási, 2016, Caldarelli & Catanzaro, 2011; Erdős & Rényi, 1959; Estrada & Knight, 2015; Jackson, 2008; Van Steen, 2010) that are not considered in this chapter. What matters here—and may represent a tip for fruitful research—is the mathematical comparison between traditional networks and blockchains (see, for instance, Ferretti & D'Angelo, 2019). Research may well be extended to include multilayer networks (Bianconi, 2018; Kennet, 2015; Lee, 2015; Tomasini, 2015).

The mathematical analysis is the founding element for the interpretation of the workings of the blockchain ecosystem. Blockchains are validated with mathematical/IT consensus rather than by humans. The structure (design outlay) of the blockchain and its effective functioning is described by mathematical properties that are also the basis for any economic valuation. In other terms, whenever it becomes important to assess the economic value of the blockchain (see Moro-Visconti, 2020), the appraisal process should conveniently start from adjacent matrix algebra.

Corporate and digital networks are particularly relevant for blockchains and their fueling (big) data. Blockchains have an intrinsic reticular structure where protocols of distributed ledgers follow sequential and incremental patterns where each ring of the chain is linked to the previous one. This pattern shows analogies with network architecture.

The graphical representation of a social network is depicted in Figure 8.7.

From the graph, it can be intuitively guessed that the differences between digital networks and blockchains are relevant. (Social) networks are typically not sequential and blockchains do not have a pivoting hub and are not bi-directional (since they can only move forward). But there are also intersections, especially if a (social) network of individuals (e.g., patients) uses a blockchain for securing its transactions.

Networks try to explain how a system of isolated elements can be transformed through their interaction (using, for instance, digital platforms) into groups and communities. The implications may be relevant, even if largely unexplored. The value of a network can be estimated as the incremental value of the intangibles related to that network.

There are special nodes in a blockchain network that are responsible for running the consensus algorithms (i.e., for validating transactions and determining the order in which transaction blocks are added to the blockchain). These special nodes are called miners, and the process of validating transactions and ordering them in the blockchain is referred to as mining. Once a transaction proposal is received by a miner, the miner proceeds to check if the transaction is valid. Validated transactions are included in a block. After a period (or block) of time, the new block of validated transactions is linked (or chained) to the previous blocks, creating a chain of blocks, known as a blockchain. The blockchain is replicated among all the nodes in the network, such that every node has an identical database or ledger of all the transactions in the network (Agbo et al., 2019).

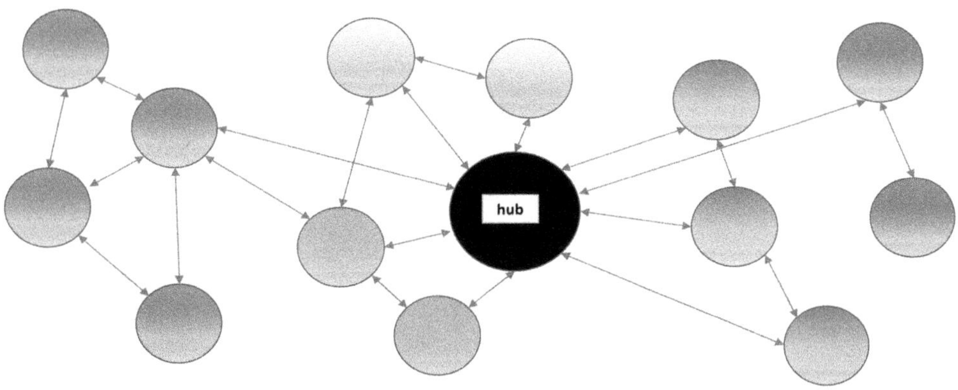

FIGURE 8.7
Social networks.

P2P computing or networking is a distributed application architecture that partitions tasks or workloads between peers. Peers are equally privileged, equipotent participants in the application. They are said to form a P2P network of nodes.

8.6 Patient-Centric Networks Connected to Blockchains through Digital Platforms

Networked blockchains do not have pivoting (bridging) nodes due to their decentralized nature. They are, however, increasingly patient-centric, patients being the most prominent stakeholder (Moro-Visconti & Martiniello, 2019). This consideration—which may seem evident—does not always have the application it deserves, and it raises corporate governance concerns when public-private conflicts of interest prevail over ethical targets.

Patients are anyway a crucial node that is connected to the blocks of the chain through IT devices (PC, smartphones and more generally, digital platforms). Digital platforms are facilitators that catalyze information and transactions, fueling the blocks and receiving precious validating feedbacks. Platforms may be considered "virtual" stakeholders or, from a network perspective, bridging nodes since they connect stakeholding nodes to each block node.

Figure 8.8 shows how the blockchain functional workings are linked to centric nodes (patients). It has already been shown, for instance, in Section 8.2, that blockchain applications to healthcare are many (and growing). Figure 8.8 accordingly describes two complementary functions that are both accessed by patients. Should these functions show

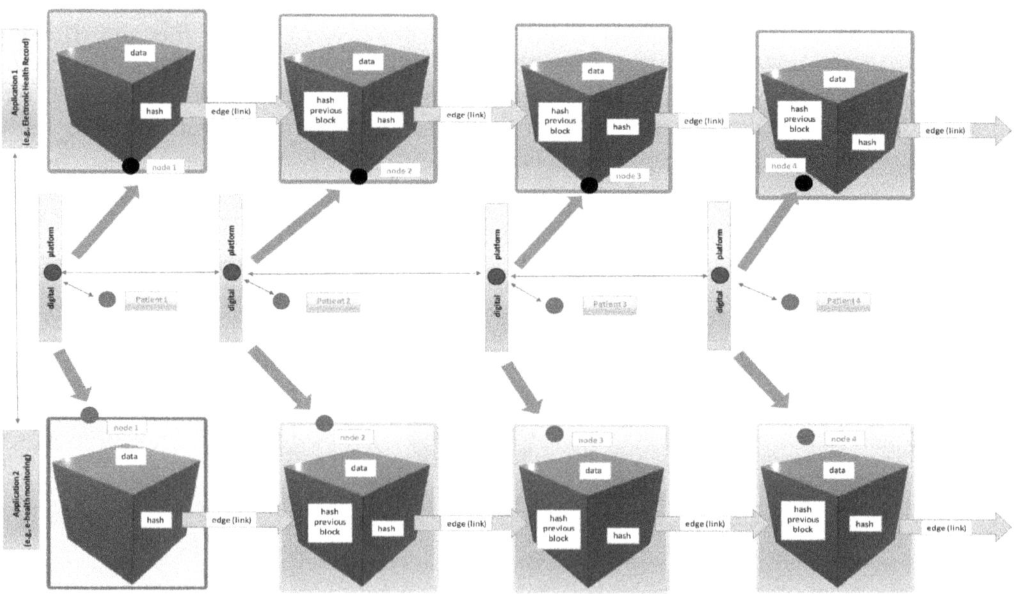

FIGURE 8.8
Digital platforms connecting patients to blockchains.

much-wanted complementarity, then they may be studied following multilayer network analysis, as it will be seen in Section 8.7.

A crucial consideration is that platform-based solutions leverage the data amassed by the network. This statement is consistent with the research question of this chapter. Platforms act as a catalyzer of data, for many complementary reasons, such as:

- Their digital nature receives (from external sources deriving from composite stakeholders) data that are only expressed in a digital format.
- The functional process of collected information that gathers in interoperable cloud databases that fuel blocks; healthcare big data (Moro-Visconti & Morea, 2019), made anonymous by cryptography, encourage value co-creation patterns, and blockchains contribute with validation to this virtuous process.
- Due to their digital nature, platforms are intrinsically fit to ease synergies with other intangible processes, such as artificial intelligence and machine learning. Whereas these applications are mostly futuristic, the potential seems dreamy and worth investigating.

8.7 Extending the Model to Multilayer Networks

Network properties are traditionally investigated as single entities in most textbooks (Bapat, 2011; Barabási, 2016, Caldarelli & Catanzaro, 2011; Estrada & Knight, 2015; Jackson, 2008; Van Steen, 2010). Recent evidence and pioneering research, however, show that reality is too complex and multiform to be represented by single layers, unrelated to other networks.

Multilayer networks (Bianconi, 2018; Kennet, 2015; Lee, 2015; Tomasini, 2015) emerge as a natural need for a correct interpretation of real ecosystems. Healthcare makes no exception. It may, for instance, be evidenced that pivoting patients simultaneously fuel more than one blockchain (and probably even more in the future, should this technology expand as expected).

Whereas this consideration adds complexity to the investigation, it may also have positive side effects, especially if considering the potential synergies embedded in the simultaneous use of healthcare blockchains.

Figure 8.9 gives a simplified representation of how four ideal blockchains may interact. The pivoting (bridging) node is unsurprisingly represented by a digital platform strictly linked to end-users (patients).

Patients and digital platforms behave as replica nodes that are simultaneously present in several layers. In this function, patients may act singularly or in clusters, especially if they are interacting through social networks, somewhat bypassing privacy concerns.

The information contents embedded in each blockchain can be easily enriched through their synergistic interaction. Coordination within a coherent healthcare ecosystem depends on the architectural design of the framework, which should ease interconnections and interoperability.

Artificial intelligence may represent the ideal engine behind this dynamic coordination.

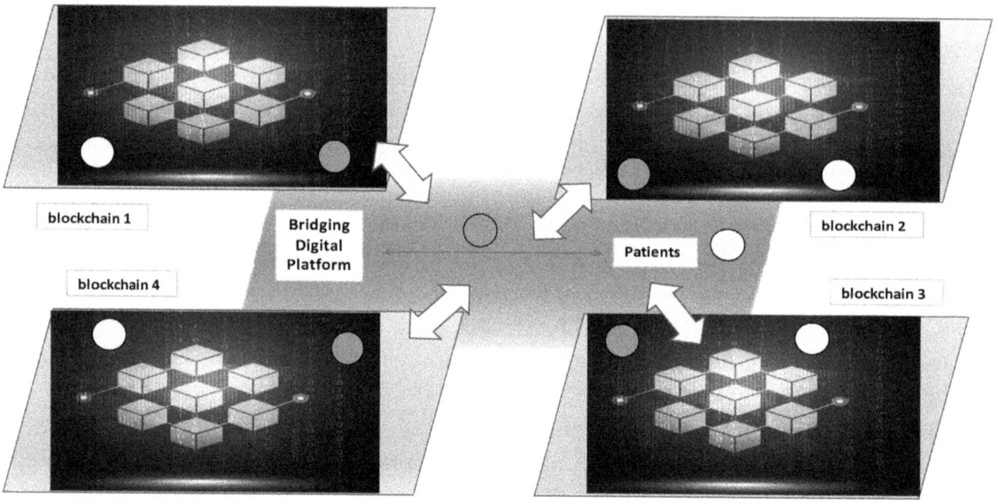

FIGURE 8.9
Multilayer networks: Digital platforms connecting different blockchains.

8.8 Concluding Remarks

A blockchain is a growing list of records, called blocks, that are linked using cryptography. By design, a blockchain is resistant to any modification of the data, therefore being suitable for sensitive healthcare applications. It has been recalled that blockchains can extensively be applied well beyond their initial background, represented by cryptocurrencies. A huge amount of data is being generated every day from patients' medical checkups, treatments, symptoms, etc., which are to be handled with care as they are very crucial and can be tampered with by hackers which can lead to serious problems. Therefore, such critical data must need to be secured with blockchain as it makes it difficult to tamper with the data (Gupta et al., 2020).

Today's healthcare data management systems are facing key challenges in terms of data transparency, traceability, immutability, audit, data provenance, flexible access, trust, privacy and security. Blockchain is an emerging and disruptive decentralized technology that has the potential to significantly revolutionize, reshape and transform the way data are being handled in the healthcare industry (Yaqoob et al., 2021).

Whereas the utilization of blockchains in healthcare has been subject to increasing scrutiny—as witnessed by the many surveys that show the evolution and stratification of research—little if any attention has been paid to some frontier topics. Among those issues, this chapter analyzes the reinterpretation of the healthcare blockchain in network terms, using digital platforms as a catalyzer of the stakeholders' interaction.

Within the healthcare ecosystem, patients unsurprisingly represent the prioritizing stakeholder. Blockchain applications should accordingly be patient-friendly, encouraging a patient-centric vision.

The main conclusion of this chapter is that if input information (amassed in "big" data) is already expressed in a digital form, it is (obviously) fitter for blockchain digital applications. Digitalization of the healthcare ecosystem (Moro-Visconti & Morea, 2020) surrounding the blockchains should so be encouraged.

A further consideration concerns the potential synergies that many patient-centric healthcare applications may show (e.g., electronic health recording linked to IoT sensors applied to diagnostic equipment). These apps may conveniently be interpreted in network terms, bringing sophisticated multilayer network analysis. These frontier topics deserve further investigation and may shed additional light on the extensions of a technology whose potential is still largely unexplored, especially in sensitive industries—such as healthcare—where data validation is a priority.

Bibliography

Agbo, CC and Mahmoud, QH. (2019). Comparison of Blockchain Frameworks For Healthcare Applications, *Internet Technology Letters*, July.

Agbo, CC, Mahmoud, QH and Eklund, JM. (2019). Blockchain Technology in Healthcare: A Systematic Review, *Healthcare*, April.

Agrawal, R, Chatterjee, JM, Kumar, A and Rathore, PS. eds. (2020). *Blockchain Technology in Business and Healthcare Opportunities and Innovation*, September, Boca Raton, FL: CRC Press.

Angraal, S, Krumholz, HM and Schulz, WL. (2017). Blockchain Technology: Applications in Health Care, *Circulation: Cardiovascular Quality and Outcomes*, 10, September.

Aumasson, J. (2017). *Serious Cryptography: A Practical Introduction to Modern Encryption*, San Francisco: No Starch Press.

Bapat, RB. (2011). *Graphs and Matrices*, Berlin: Springer.

Barabási, A. (2016). *Network Science*, Cambridge: Cambridge University Press.

Bianconi, G. (2018). *Multilayer Networks*, Oxford: Oxford University Press.

Bittins, S, Kober, G, Margheri, A, Masi, M, Miladi, A and Sassone, V. (2021). Healthcare Data Management by Using Blockchain Technology. In Namasudra, S and Deka, GC. (eds) *Applications of Blockchain in Healthcare. Studies in Big Data*, 83, Singapore: Springer.

Blossey, G, Eisenhardt, J and Hahn, G. (2019). Blockchain Technology in Supply Chain Management: An Application Perspective, Proceedings of the 52nd Hawaii International Conference on System Sciences. http://hdl.handle.net/10125/60124

Bogoeva, A. (2018). *Blockchain Technology in Healthcare: Opportunities and Challenges*, Master Thesis, University of Mannheim.

Caldarelli, G and Catanzaro, M. (2011). *Networks. A Very Short Introduction*, Oxford: Oxford University Press.

Chen, HS, Jarrell, JT, Carpenter, KA, Cohen, DS and Huang, X. (2019). Blockchain in Healthcare: A Patient-Centered Model, *Biomed Journal of Scientific & Technological Resources*, 20(3), 15017–15022.

Ciampi, M, Esposito, A, Marangio, F, Sicuranza, M and Schmid, G. (2021). Modernizing Healthcare by Using Blockchain. In: Namasudra, Sand Deka, GC (eds). *Applications of Blockchain in Healthcare. Studies in Big Data*, 83, Singapore: Springer.

Cong, LW and He, Z., (2018). Blockchain Disruption and Smart Contracts, NBER Working Paper No. 24399, April.

Constantinides, P, Henfridsson, O and Parker, GG. (2018). Platforms and Infrastructures in the Digital Age, *Information Systems Research*, 29(2), 381–400.

De Aguiar, EJ, Faiçal, BS, Krishnamakari, B and Ueyama, J. (2020). A Survey of Blockchain-Based Strategies for Healthcare, *ACM Computing Surveys*, 53(2), June, 1–27.

Deloitte. (2018). Breaking Blockchain Open- Deloitte's 2018 Global Blockchain Survey. *Deloitte Insights*, 48. https://doi.org/10.1002/ejoc.201200111

de Reuven, M, Sørensen, C and Basole, RC. (2018). The Digital Platform: A Research Agenda, *Journal of Information Technology*, 33, 124–135.

Dhillon, V, Metcalf, D and Hooper, M. (2021). Blockchain in Healthcare. In: *Blockchain Enabled Applications*, Berkeley, CA: Apress.

Dimitrov, DV. (2019). Blockchain Applications for Healthcare Data Management, *Healthcare Informatics Research*, January, 25(1), 51–56.
Dujak, D and Sajter, D. (2019). *Blockchain Applications in Supply Chain*, Berlin: Springer Verlag.
The Economist (2015). Blockchains. The Great Chain of Being Sure About Things, October 31. https://www.economist.com/briefing/2015/10/31/the-great-chain-of-being-sure-about-things.
Engelhardt, M. (2017), Hitching Healthcare to the Chain: An Introduction to Blockchain Technology in the Healthcare Sector, *Technology Innovation Management Review*, 7, 22–34.
Erdős, P and Rényi, A. (1959). On Random Graphs, *Publicationes Mathematicae*, 6, 290–297.
Esposito, C, De Santis, A, Tortora, G, Chang, H and Choo, KKR. (2018). Blockchain: A Panacea for Healthcare Cloud-Based Data Security and Privacy? *IEEE Cloud Computing*, 5(1), 31–37. https://doi.org/10.1109/MCC.2018.011791712
Estrada, E and Knight, PA. (2015). *A First Course in Network Theory*, Oxford: Oxford University press.
Fan, T, He, Q, Nie, E and Chen, S. (2017). A Study of Pricing and Trading Model of Blockchain & Big Data-based Energy-Internet Electricity, IOP Conference Series, Earth and Environmental Science.
Ferretti, S and D'Angelo, G. (2019). On the Ethereum Blockchain Structure: A Complex Networks Theory Perspective. To appear in *Concurrency and Computation: Practice and Experience*, NJ: Hoboken. Wiley.
Gawer, A. (2014). Bridging Differing Perspectives on Technological Platforms: Toward an Integrative Framework, *Research Policy*, 43(7), 1239–1249.
Gawer, A and Cusumano, MA. (2014). Industry Platforms and Ecosystem Innovation, *The Journal of Product Innovation Management*, 31, 3.
Gordon, WJ and Catalini, C. (2018). Blockchain Technology for Healthcare: Facilitating the Transition to Patient-driven Interoperability, *Computational and Structural Biotechnology Journal*, 16, 224–230.
Griggs, KN, Ossipova, O, Kohlios, CP, Baccarini, AN, Howson, EA and Hayajneh, T. (2018). Healthcare Blockchain System Using Smart Contracts for Secure Automated Remote Patient Monitoring, *Journal of Medical Systems*, 42(7), 1–7.
Gupta, S, Malhotra, V and Singh, SN. (2020). Securing IoT-Driven Remote Healthcare Data Through Blockchain. In: Kolhe, M, Tiwari, S, Trivedi, M and Mishra, K. (eds) *Advances in Data and Information Sciences*. Lecture Notes in Networks and Systems, 94, Singapore: Springer.
Gupta, M, Jain, R, Kumari, M and Narula, G. (2021). Securing Healthcare Data by Using Blockchain. In: Namasudra, S Deka, GC. (eds) *Applications of Blockchain in Healthcare. Studies in Big Data*, 83, Singapore: Springer.
Hagiu, A and Wright, J. (2015). Multi-sided Platforms, *International Journal of Industrial Organization*, 43(C), 162–174.
Hasselgren, A et al. (2020). Blockchain in Healthcare and Health Sciences-A Scoping Review, *International Journal of Medical Informatics*, 134, February, 1–10.
Hölbl, M, Kompara, M, Kamišalíc, A and NemecZlatos, L. (2018). A Systematic Review of the Use of Blockchain in Healthcare, *Symmetry*, 10, 470.
Hussien, HM, Yasin, SM Udzir, SNI, Zaidan, AA and Zaidan, BB. (2019). A Systematic Review for Enabling of Develop a Blockchain Technology in Healthcare Application: Taxonomy, Substantially Analysis, Motivations, Challenges, Recommendations and Future Direction, *Journal of Medical Systems*, 43, 320.
Jackson, MO. (2008). *Social and Economic Networks*, Princeton: Princeton University Press.
Jacobides, MG, Cernamo, C and Gawer, A. (2018). Towards a Theory of Ecosystems, *Strategic Management Journal*, 39, 8.
Jin Z., Lichtenstein, Y. and Gander, J. (2015) Designing Scalable Digital Business Models. In: Baden-Fuller, C. and Mangematin, V., (eds.) Business Models and Modelling. Bingley, U.K. : Emerald Group Publishing Limited. 241–277. (Advances in Strategic Management, (33)).
Junaid Gul, M, Subramanian, B, Paul, A and Kim, J. (2021). Blockchain for Public Health Care in Smart Society, *Microprocessors and Microsystems*, 80, February, 103524.
Kennet, DY, Perc, M and Boccaletti, S. (2015). Networks of Networks – An Introduction, *Chaos, Solitons & Fractals*, 80, 1–6.

Kenney, M and Zysman, J. (2016). The Rise of the Platform Economy, *Issues in Science and Technology*, 32, 3.
Khatoon, A. (2020). A Blockchain-Based Smart Contract System for Healthcare Management, *Electronics*, 9, 94.
Khezr, S, Moniruzzaman, M., Yassine, A and Benlamri, R. (2019). Blockchain Technology in Healthcare: A Comprehensive Review and Directions for Future Research, *Applied Sciences*, April, 9(9), 1736.
Kim, S and Deka, GC. (2019). *Advanced Applications of Blockchain Technology*, Springer Nature, Singapore.
Korpela, K, Hallikas, J and Dahlberg, T. (2017). Digital Supply Chain Transformation toward Blockchain Integration, Proceedings of the 50th Hawaii International Conference on System Sciences. https://scholarspace.manoa.hawaii.edu/handle/10125/41666.
Kumar, V. (2019). Blockchain in Healthcare Market Research Report 2023, *Healthcare*, September
Kuo, TT, Kim, HE and Ohno-Machado, L. (2017). Blockchain Distributed Ledger Technologies for Biomedical and Health Care Applications, *Journal of the American Medical Informatics Association*, 24, 1211–1220.
Kuo, T, Zavaleta Rojas, H and Ohno-Machado, L. (2019). Comparison of Blockchain Platforms: A Systematic Review and Healthcare Examples, *Journal of the American Medical Informatics Association*, 26(5), 462–478.
Ismail, L, Materwala, H and Zeadally, S. (2019). Lightweight Blockchain for Healthcare, *IEEE Access*, October
Lee, KM, Min, B and Goh, K-I. (2015). Towards Real-World Complexity: An Introduction to Multiplex Networks. *European Physical Journal B*, 88, 2.
Lotti, L. (2016). Contemporary Art, Capitalization and the Blockchain: On the Autonomy and Automation of Art's Value. *Finance and Society*, 2(2), 96.
Lui, PT. (2016). Medical Record System Using Blockchain, Big Data and Tokenization. Paper Presented at the Information and Communications Security, 18th International Conference, 254–261.
Malagihal, SS. (2019). Decoding Blockchain for Healthcare Sector, *BIMS International Research Journal of Management and Commerce*, 3(2), June 23663–23673.
Mao, D, Wang, F, Hao, Z and Li, H. (2018). Credit Evaluation System Based on Blockchain for Multiple Stakeholders in the Food Supply Chain, *International Journal of Environmental Research and Public Health*, 15, 8.
Mazlan, AA, Mohd Daud, S, Mohd Sam, S, Abas, H, Abdul Rasid, SZ and Yusof, MF. (2020). Scalability Challenges in Healthcare Blockchain System - A Systematic Review, *IEEE Access*, 8, 23663–23673.
Meinert, E et al. (2019). Blockchain Implementation in Health Care: Protocol for a Systematic Review, *JMIR Research Protocols*, 8(2), February 1–8.
Miah, SJ. (2019). Blockchain in Healthcare, *Australasian Journal of Information Systems*, July.
Mišic, VB., Mišic, J and Chang, X. (2019). Towards a Blockchain-Based Healthcare Information System, Conference Paper, July.
Moro-Visconti, R and Martiniello, L. (2019). Smart Hospitals and Patient-Centered Governance, *Corporate Ownership & Control*, 16, 2.
Moro-Visconti, R. (2019). Combining Network Theory with Corporate Governance: Converging Models for Connected Stakeholders, *Corporate Ownership & Control*, 17, 1.
Moro-Visconti, R. (2020). *The Valuation of Digital Intangibles*, Cham: Palgrave-Macmillan.
Moro-Visconti, R, Larocca, A and Marconi, M. (2017). Big data-driven Value Chains and Digital Platforms: From Value Co-creation to Monetization. In: Somani, AK and Deka, G (eds), *Big Data Analytics: Tools, Technology for Effective Planning*, Boca Raton: CRC press.
Moro-Visconti, R and Morea, D. (2019). Big Data for the Sustainability of Healthcare Project Financing, *Sustainability*, 11(3748), July, 1–17.
Moro-Visconti, R and Morea, D. (2020). Healthcare Digitalization and Pay-For-Performance Incentives in Smart Hospital Project Financing, *International Journal of Environmental Research and Public Health*, 17(2318), 1–25.

Muneeswaran, V, Nagaraj, P, Dhannushree, U, Ishwarya Lakshmi, S, Aishwarya, R and Sunethra, B. (2021). A Framework for Data Analytics-Based Healthcare Systems. In Raj, JS, Iliyasu, AM, Bestak, R and Baig, ZA (eds). *Innovative Data Communication Technologies and Application. Lecture Notes on Data Engineering and Communications Technologies*, 59, Singapore: Springer.

Norman, MD, Karavas, YG and Reed, H. (2018). The Emergence of Trust and Value in Public blockchain networks. https://www.researchgate.net/publication/325552991_The_Emergence_of_Trust_and_Value_in_Public_Blockchain_Networks

Onik, MH, Aich, S, Yang, J, Kim, C and Kim, H. (2019). Privacy Protection and Management of Medical Records Using Blockchain Technology. In Dey N. et al. eds. *Big Data Analytics for Intelligent Healthcare Management*, Chapter 8, Academic Press, San Diego, USA.

Prokofieva, M and Miah, SJ. (2019). Blockchain in Healthcare, *Australasian Journal of Information Systems*, 23, Research Note, 1–22.

Raj, P and Deka, GC. (2018). *Blockchain Technology: Platforms, Tools and Use Cases*, Vol. 111, Academic Press, Elsevier. https://www.elsevier.com/about/locations.

Roehrs, A, da Costa, CA, da Rosa Righi, R, Alex, R, Costa, CA and Righi, RR. (2017). OmniPHR: A Distributed Architecture Model to Integrate Personal Health Records, *Journal of Biomedical Informatics*, 71, 70–81.

Ribitzsky, R et al. (2018). Pragmatic, Interdisciplinary Perspectives on Blockchain and Distributed Ledger Technology: Paving the Future for Healthcare, *Blockchain in Healthcare Today*, March.

Saberi, S, Kouhizadeh, M, Sarkis, J and Shen, L. (2018). Blockchain Technology and Its Relationships to Sustainable Supply Chain Management, *International Journal of production research*, 57(7), 1–19.

Saharan, Rand Prasad, R. (2021). Blockchain Technology for Healthcare Data. In: Rathore, VS, Dey, N, Piuri, V, Babo, R, Polkowski, Z and Tavares, JMRS (eds). *Rising Threats in Expert Applications and Solutions. Advances in Intelligent Systems and Computing*, 1187, Singapore: Springer.

Sater, S. (2018). Blockchain Transforming Healthcare Data Flows. https://ssrn.com/abstract=3171005

Schallmo, DRA and Williams, CA. (2018).*Digital Transformation of Business Models, Digital Transformation Now!*, Springer Briefs in Business, Cham: Springer.

Schumacher, A. (2017). Blockchain & Healthcare – 2017 Strategy Guide for the Pharmaceutical Industry, Insurers & Healthcare Providers. https://www.researchgate.net/publication/317936859

Schreieck, M, Hein, A, Wiesche, M and Krcmar, H. (2018). The Challenge of Governing Digital Platform Ecosystems. In Linnhoff-Popien, C, Schneider, R and Zaddach, M (eds). *Digital Marketplaces Unleashed*, Berlin: Springer.

Sharma, L, Olson, J, Guha, A and McDougal, L. (2021). How Blockchain Will Transform the Healthcare Ecosystem, *Business Horizons*, February.

Shifrin, M, Khavtorin, A, Stepurin, V and Zingerman, B. (2019). Blockchain as a Process Control Tool for Healthcare, July. https://www.researchgate.net/publication/334731683

Shing Liu, PT. (2016). Medical Record System Using Blockchain, Big Data and Tokenization. In: Proceedings of the Information and Communications Security: 18th International Conference, 254–261.

Sleiman, MD, Lauf, AP and Yampolskiy, R. (2015).Bitcoin Message: Data Insertion on a Proof-of-Work Cryptocurrency System. In Proceedings of the 2015 International Conference on Cyberworlds (CW), Visby, Sweden, 7–9 October, 332–336.

Spagnoletti, P, Resca, A and Lee, G. (2015). A Design Theory for Digital Platforms Supporting Online Communities: A Multiple Case Study, *Journal of Information Technology*, 30(4), 364–380.

Sutherland, Wand Jarrahi, MH. (2018). The Sharing Economy and Digital Platforms: A Review and Research Agenda, *International Journal of Information Management*, 43, 328–341.

Tanwar, S, Parekh, K and Evans, R. (2020). Blockchain-based Electronic Healthcare Record System for Healthcare 4.0 Applications, *Journal of Information Security and Applications*, 50, February, 102407.

Tiwana, A. (2014). *Platform Ecosystems: Aligning Architecture, Governance, and Strategy*, Morgan Kaufmann, Amsterdam. https://www.scirp.org/(S(i43dyn45teexjx455qlt3d2q))/aboutus/index.aspx.

Tiwana, A, Konsynsky, B and Bush, AA. (2010). Platform Evolution: Coevolution of Platform Architecture, Governance, and Environmental Dynamics, *Information Systems Research*, 21(4), 675–687.

Tomasini, M. (2015). An Introduction to Multilayer Networks, BioComplex Laboratory, Florida Institute of Technology. https://www.researchgate.net/profile/Marcello_Tomasini/publication/321546271_An_Introduction_to_Multilayer_Networks/links/5a26fe48aca2727dd8839dee/An-Introduction-to-Multilayer-Networks.pdf

Van Steen, M. (2010). Graph Theory and Complex Networks. An Introduction, Maarten Van Steen.

Veuger, J. (2018). Trust in a Viable Real Estate Economy with Disruption and Blockchain, *Facilities*, 36(1/2), 103–12.

Xu, M, Chen, X and Kou, G. (2019). A Systematic Review of Blockchain, *Financial Innovation*, 5, 27.

Yaqoob, I, Salah, K, Jayaraman, Rand Al-Hammadi, Y. (2021). Blockchain for Healthcare Data Management: Opportunities, Challenges, and Future Recommendations, *Neural Computing & Applications*, January.

Yermack, D. (2017). Corporate Governance and Blockchains, *Review of Finance*, 21(1), 7–31.

Yoon, H. (2019). Blockchain Technology and Healthcare, *Healthcare Informatics Research*, April, 25(2), 59–60.

Zhang, Y and Wen, J. (2016). The IoT Electric Business Model: Using Blockchain Technology for the Internet of Things, *Peer-to-Peer Network Applications*, April.

Zhang et al. (2017). Metrics for Assessing Blockchain-based Healthcare Decentralized Apps, Computer Science, IEEE 19th International Conference on e-Health Networking, Applications and Services (Healthcom).

Zhang, P, Schmidt, DC, White, J and Lenz, G. (2018). Blockchain Technology Use Cases in Healthcare. In Deka G (eds). *Blockchain Technology: Platforms, Tools, and Use Cases*, Cambridge, MA: Academic Press.

Zheng, Z, Xie, S, Dai, H, Chen, X and Wang, H. (2017). An Overview of Blockchain Technology: Architecture, Consensus, and Future Trends. In Proceedings of the 2017 IEEE International Congress on Big Data (Big Data Congress), Boston, MA, USA, 11–14 December; 557–564.

Zheng, Z, Xie, S, Dai, H, Chen, X Wang, H. (2018). Blockchain Challenges and Opportunities: A Survey, *International Journal of Web and Grid Services*, 14(4).

9

Security of Healthcare Data Using Blockchains

Mayank Pandey, Rachit Agarwal, Sandeep K Shukla and Nishchal K Verma

CONTENTS

9.1 Introduction

With the advancements in technology, various tools and methodologies exist that facilitate the efficient and effective functioning of the healthcare sector. The influx of large volumes of data coming from healthcare-related Internet of Things (IoT)-based devices further catalyzes its functioning. For example, IoT devices provide a way to transform hand-written diagnostic and other related reports into digital reports. They also provide a way to make the storage and sharing of such reports convenient with different stakeholders (such as patients, doctors, pharmaceutical suppliers, health insurance people and healthcare administrators). On top of this, analytics on healthcare-related data pave the way for many related services to coexist. For example, in the case of a pandemic like Covid-19, vaccine development is based on the available genetic data (Le et al., 2020), while the use of Remdesivir for treatment is based on clinical trial data (Beigel et al., 2020). Further, as another example, in Brown et al. (2020), the authors propose using smartphones to capture and analyze cough sounds for identifying potential infection with Covid-19. Apart from this, analysis of the day-to-day healthcare data provides policymakers with the necessary inputs to make policies.

A significant healthcare data component comprises Electronic Healthcare Records (EHRs) (Stafford & Treiblmaier, 2020). EHRs contain private medical diagnosis information of a patient. Apart from EHRs, there are various other types of healthcare data. These include (a) personal health record (PHR) (Bietz et al., 2016) that contains data such as the physiological

DOI: 10.1201/9781003133179-9

health parameters and allergy information of the patient, (b) pharmaceutical/medicine data that includes information on the manufactured medications and its clinical trial data (Burbidge et al., 2001), (c) health insurance data that comprises information related to the insurance policy of the patient, payment information and data on the availed insurance-related services (Moulis et al., 2015) and (d) data generated and used for research in healthcare such as those of cough sounds for Covid-19 detection (Brown et al., 2020) and X-ray images for pneumonia classification (Stephen et al., 2019). Such immense data help doctors gain more understanding of their patients and provide better healthcare services to them. Nonetheless, different stakeholders exploit different healthcare data for (a) enhancing their services, such as pharmaceutical representatives influencing doctors (Fugh-Berman & Ahari, 2007) or (b) engaging in illegal activities such as drug abuse (Berenson & Rahman, 2011).

A major challenge with such healthcare data is to ensure its security from various cyber-attacks such as unauthorized access and tampering. In Kumar and Walker (2017), the authors provide in-depth analysis of: (a) what threats exist (such as EHRs in hospitals not being well protected) for the healthcare data, (b) how many people and organizations providing healthcare services are affected by the breach (such as the Athena Group hack) and (c) the behavior responsible for the success of such attacks (such as the habit of personal internet surfing and social media access on workplace computers along with low cybersecurity awareness). Security of healthcare data has recently been the focus of many policy-makers due to various cyberattack incidents, such as the one on the University of Vermont (UVM) Medical Centre and the Ryuk ransomware attack in October 2020. In Dyrda (2020), the author provides an analysis of the significant cyberattacks that happened in 2020 on healthcare data and reiterates the necessity of data security education and awareness among the people working in the healthcare sector.

As the threats to such data increase, preventive measures and research to improve healthcare data security are highly critical. One viable solution for improving healthcare data security is to use blockchain technology, which ensures the integrity, immutability and traceability of the data. Blockchain technology was first introduced in 2008 (Nakamato, 2008) with the introduction of bitcoin as an alternative to the existing centralized banking and payment structures. Here, the author presented blockchain as a decentralized ledger with the capability of storing the transaction records in blocks that are serially and sequentially connected. Blockchain operates as a decentralized peer-to-peer network, where the participants (or the nodes in the network) carry out transactions, transaction verification and mining and willing participants have a copy of the blockchain stored with them, providing redundancy.

In healthcare, applications of blockchain technology are in the field of data management and sharing (Hölbl et al., 2018), pharmaceutical supply chain management (Khezr et al., 2019) and secure medical data storage and log management (De Aguiar et al., 2020). In Shi et al. (2020), the authors survey and discover the research opportunities regarding the collaboration of blockchain technology with other emerging technologies such as big data, machine learning, and the IoT. In Tariq et al. (2020), the authors examine blockchain technology's role in the data security of resource-constrained medical IoT devices. The authors identify that such devices are vulnerable to attacks such as forgery and data tampering. They also survey blockchain-based solutions that address the security issues faced by the healthcare systems. In Hardin and Kotz (2019), the authors provide an analysis of the challenges faced during the implementation of blockchain technology in healthcare systems in terms of security parameters such as integrity, confidentiality, access control and interoperability. The authors identify that such technology benefits for healthcare security come with their own sets of challenges, such as deciding on data requirements and individual privacy. In Radanović and Likić (2018), the authors explore the opportunities for blockchain technology in medicine and argue that such technology can mitigate the shortcomings related to different types of data, such as EHRs. They also provide a discussion on the benefits of blockchain technology, not only with respect to data security but also with respect to other factors such as processing time reduction, cost reduction and transparency. Note that, henceforth, in this chapter, we refer to blockchain technology as blockchain.

In terms of healthcare data security, all the aforementioned work focuses on the solutions for securing EHR data. Pharmaceuticals, administration and health insurance are also useful as the organizations relevant to these components are part of the healthcare domain and are actively involved in sharing, accessing and using the generated data. Healthcare data security also encompasses protecting information such as medical diagnosis data, health insurance data, pharma supply chain data and biomedical research data.

In this chapter, we assess the role of the blockchain in strengthening healthcare data security through the fundamental questions, why, what, who, when and how, i.e., 4W and 1H. More specifically, we answer why we need a blockchain for the security of healthcare data? What (which type) are the healthcare data areas we need a blockchain for implementing? Who (which organizations and individuals) need a blockchain for protecting their healthcare data? When do we need a blockchain for the security of healthcare data, and how do we implement a blockchain for this?

Based on the above questions, our key contributions through this chapter are:

- **Survey**: Using the 4W1H methodology, we present an understanding on what data, when we need, why we need, who needs and how state-of-the-art techniques use blockchains to secure healthcare data. We also identify the gaps present in the state-of-the-art methods related to the implementation of blockchain in healthcare data from the security perspective and survey them. We also provide a survey of technical and regulatory challenges faced in the process of the implementation of blockchain-based healthcare data security systems. We identify that a proper user interface for the blockchain-based systems is warranted. Also, the immutability of data on the blockchain is in direct contention with the right to be forgotten, which comes under the right to privacy.
- **Application-specific**: We explore blockchain's role in healthcare data security in pandemic situations like Covid-19.
- **Research perspectives**: Based on the survey, we provide prospective future research and development directions that can benefit authorities and researchers in the field.

The remainder of the chapter is organized as follows. First, in Section 9.2, we provide an understanding of the healthcare data types and their managing institutions. Then, in Section 9.3, we provide services that are rendered using such healthcare data. In Section 99.4, we discuss and explain the different security issues present when using conventional healthcare data storage and management systems. In Sections 9.5 and 9.6, we provide the security parameters required for healthcare data protection and an overview of healthcare-relevant blockchain functionalities and advantages, respectively. In Section 9.7, we discuss the functionality of different state-of-the-art blockchain-based solutions that enable data security. In Sections 9.8 and 9.9, we present various technical limitations and regulatory challenges that exist while implementing a blockchain-based solution for healthcare data security, respectively. In Section 9.10, as a case study, we study how blockchains can help in achieving data security in the case of a pandemic such as Covid-19. Finally, in Section 9.11, we present the conclusion and perspective to future research directions.

9.2 Types of Healthcare Data Systems and Managing Institutions

Healthcare data is a pool of all the information relevant to the organizations and people associated with the healthcare sector. Before we discuss blockchain implementation for healthcare data security, we provide details of the healthcare sector data. This section provides a brief discussion on the different categories of data associated with the healthcare sector and their managing institutions. In the healthcare sector, data systems operate through the functionalities comprising the generation, access control and individual health data storage.

We broadly categorize the healthcare data into three categories: Personal data, pharmaceutical data and insurance-based data. We further classify personal data into patient data and healthcare professional data. Among the patient data, the most common and frequently generated patient records are the **Electronic Health Records** (EHRs) (Hayrinen et al., 2008). An EHR contains personal details, physiological health parameters, medical history, laboratory-generated medical test results and pharmaceutical prescription data of a patient. Healthcare institutions such as hospitals and clinics generate EHR data based on the healthcare professionals' and laboratories' diagnoses. Specialist third-party companies and vendors generally do the storage and management of the EHRs, while the healthcare institutions and professionals are their clients (Mandl & Kohane, 2012).

Other than EHRs, **Personal Health Records** (PHRs) are the records generated and owned by the patients (Win et al., 2006) where each patient provides access to their PHR information based on need. A PHR is usually generated using smartphones and various other IoT-based wearable medical devices. It contains information on the general wellbeing of a patient, including data about blood pressure, heart rate, body temperature, allergies, vaccination history and previous surgeries. PHRs pave the way for remote assistance and decrease the response time in case of an emergency. The healthcare professionals render their advice to the patients based on the data available in both EHRs and PHRs. PHR data is managed by the individuals themselves with the help of specialized third-party tools. For example, the use of smartphone-based applications, web-based storage services (such as HealthVault (Sunyaev et al., 2010)) and specialized software for data storage (Carrion et al., 2011).

In the personal data category, another type of data is the information about the **healthcare professionals, administrative staff and researchers** (Fugh-Berman & Ahari, 2007). This data contains personal details, professional qualifications, work timings and the details of their professional tasks. The data containing these details is vital for the smooth day-to-day operations of healthcare organizations. The respective institutions to which the person is affiliated manage the storage and management of such personal information.

Besides the personal data, the **data on pharmaceuticals** is also vital. The pharmaceutical data have different attributes, such as those related to clinical trial data, medication manufacturing information and pharma supply chain data containing the distribution information. The clinical trial data is essential for the invention of new treatment methods in the form of medications and vaccines. Medication manufacturing information includes the medication's composition, information related to side effects and allergies and clinical trial data for research and development activities. In addition, data on manufacturing date, expiry date and dosage information for manufactured medications is also critical. The information on medications for various ailments is essential for doctors to proceed with treatment. On the other hand, the supply chain is also a crucial part of the pharmaceutical industry. The supply chain data is essential in the distribution of raw material and the final product. It constitutes information such as the list of distributors, quantity, distribution, product storage and transportation-related condition information. Such pharmaceutical data is stored and managed by the pharmaceutical companies either by themselves or through specialist third-party organizations.

For the smooth processing of patient treatment, **health insurance information and the related data** are also essential (Pitacco, 2014). Such data is usually shared between insurance companies and hospitals. This data contains both the health and financial information of a patient along with the information on availed insurance facilities. More specifically, it includes details such as personal details, medical history and insurance plan preference. Such data is stored and managed by insurance companies.

In summary, in this section, we discussed different healthcare data types (summarized in Figure 9.1) and the institutions that store and manage them. Here, we see that the scope of healthcare data goes beyond just the medical diagnosis reports and personal health information and involves data belonging to pharma, health insurance and details of healthcare professionals.

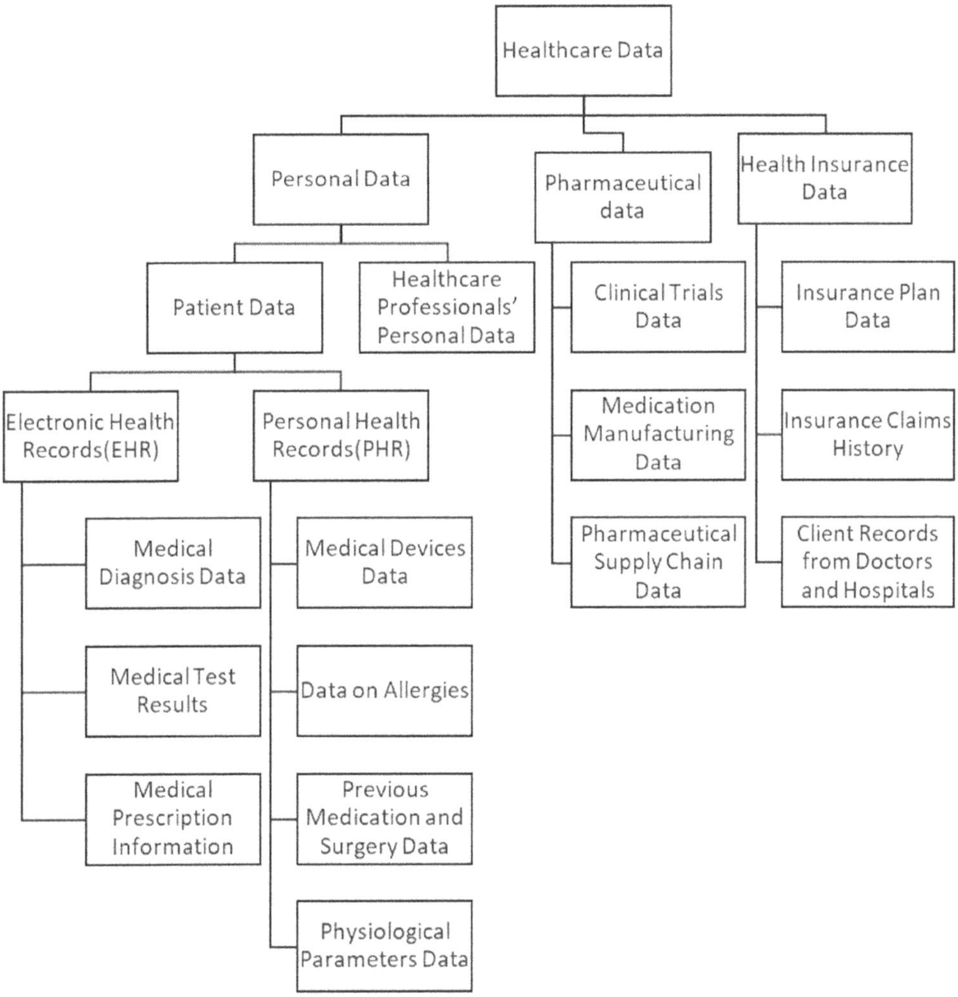

FIGURE 9.1
Healthcare data types.

9.3 Healthcare Data-Related Services

In Section 9.2, we detailed different healthcare data categories. Since the healthcare data goes beyond just the medical reports and the personal health information, the related services also go beyond diagnosis by doctors and medical tests. The scope of these services is diverse. They range from individual patients via diagnosis to organizational and national level via healthcare resource deployment. Apart from this, the functioning of the services related to healthcare research programs, pharmaceutical distribution and health insurance procedures require diverse healthcare data as a vital input. Healthcare data-related services are broadly classified as medical-related services, distribution services and commercial activity-related services. In this section, we discuss such healthcare data-related services in detail.

The most significant healthcare service (medical-related service) based on the healthcare data is the **patient diagnosis** and treatment plan. The doctors affiliated to a hospital or operating in an individual capacity assisted by nurses primarily provide such services (Hayrinen et al., 2008). The doctors thus require data from the sources such as EHRs and PHRs to prescribe treatment through methods such as medication and surgery.

Healthcare Research and Development (R&D) plays a vital role in developing healthcare-related services (medical-related services) based on healthcare data. Apart from the primary task of diagnosis, doctors and other researchers contribute to the healthcare research activities based on their domain expertise and daily experience (such as mobile health applications, as in Brown et al., (2020). For pharmaceutical companies, research for new medications is an essential component of their operations, along with clinical trials for new medications. These trials generate large quantities of data vital to the discovery of new forms of medication and treatment. Data such as EHRs and pharmaceutical research data in the healthcare domain are essential for improving the medication for various ailments, healthcare monitoring devices and even the guidelines related to daily lifestyle (Koh & Tan, 2005). Also, healthcare data is an essential input for artificial intelligence (AI)-based research in the healthcare domain. For example, the use of surgical robots, which find their utility through minimally invasive and precise incisions during the surgery process (Bergeles & Yang, 2014). Another example is the application of IBM Watson, a supercomputer for clinical decision support systems (Ahmed et al., 2017). In addition to new treatments, healthcare data aid the research on discovering new diseases, bacteria and viruses.

In addition to the data described in Section 9.2, the aforementioned services also contribute a significant amount of healthcare data (Dash et al., 2019). In Dash et al. (2019) the authors discuss the commercial **big data analytics services** platforms operating in the healthcare sector, such as Ayasdi,* IBM Watson Health† and Enlitic,‡ that use and generate a significant amount of healthcare data for both medical-related and commercial services. These platforms provide services in a number of applications such as **healthcare monitoring, prediction, knowledge and recommendation systems** (Bahri et al., 2019).

Apart from such services, there are services related to the **supply chain in the healthcare sector and resource deployment**. The EHR and PHR data of different patients from

* Ayasdi Care is a software package for healthcare solutions, providing efficient data-based patient care strategies for doctors and hospitals.

† IBM Watson Health combines human experts and AI to help healthcare researchers provide patient care decisions based on big data analytics.

‡ Enlitic uses deep learning algorithms on clinical data to help radiologists with illness diagnosis.

a specific geographical region consolidate to provide an overview of the health conditions prevailing in that region. Healthcare institutes and professionals deploy their resources to perform medical-related services based on the requirement deduced from the local EHR and PHR data (Landry et al., 2016). For example, the overwhelming number of patients due to community transfer of Covid-19 prompted an increase in intensive care unit (ICU) capacity. The doctors and nursing staff were redeployed to provide medical services such as critical care units with immediate training (Lee et al., 2020). In another similar approach, in Ethiopia, the government deployed medical staff based on healthcare data such as child immunization, child mortality rate, maternal mortality rate and presence of skilled manpower in different areas of the country (Teklehaimanot & Teklehaimanot, 2013). The resource deployment's objective was to achieve the results according to the World Health Organization's (WHO) Millennium Development Goals. The consolidated EHR and PHR data, along with pharmaceutical manufacturing data, is an essential input for the pharmaceutical companies for distribution services, marketing, manufacturing and sales for healthcare-related products (Jaberidoost et al., 2013).

Another commercial activity service related to the healthcare sector is the **Health Insurance Service** (Pitacco, 2014). Different health insurance-related decisions such as premium amount, healthcare insurance plan and whether to offer insurance or not for a patient is based on his/her healthcare data components such as medical history, ailments, allergies and previous claim history.

In summary, in this section, we classified various healthcare data-related services into three classes (also summarized in Figure 9.2 using different color codes). We further identify that doctors play an essential role in diagnosis services. Non-medical professionals also form a significant part of the healthcare workforce and are involved in various other related services. All the aforementioned services require storage of different types of healthcare data as well as sharing amongst themselves. As such services are essential and critical, it is important that healthcare-related organizations, which are both public and private, receive accurate data and take proper measures to secure the data they generate.

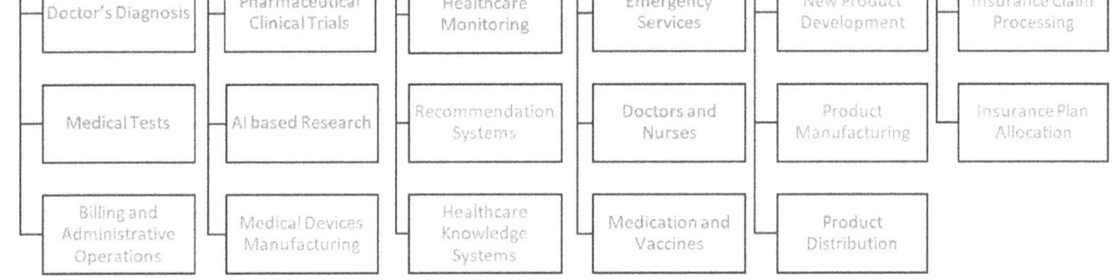

FIGURE 9.2
Healthcare data related services. Here, encoding represents the three classes: Medical-related services, distribution services and commercial activity.

9.4 Security Issues in Conventional Healthcare Data Storage Systems

In Sections 9.2 and 9.3, we discussed different healthcare data types and the services built using them. Due to the sensitive nature of the data involved, security is of utmost importance. As there is a significant increase in healthcare data generation, the data storage systems have transformed from paper-based record keeping to cloud-based storage. However, there are still security issues that are storage-centric, device-centric and services-centric. In Filkins (2014), the author analyzed the cyberthreat to healthcare organizations in terms of the level of compromise and malicious traffic. Most malicious activities mainly affect healthcare providers such as hospitals (72%), health insurance providers (6.9%) and pharmaceutical companies (2.9%). The total cost of compromised healthcare data, including factors such as recovery, legal actions and new security investments, was more than US$142 million in 2013 for the US healthcare sector. The compromise in PHR and health insurance data resulted in the loss of US$12 billion for two million US citizens in 2013. The main factors behind the compromise of healthcare data were identified as unsecured medical device networks, storage and lack of data security awareness among citizens. We discuss the security issues and challenges faced by healthcare data storage and management as we proceed.

The storage-centric security issues arise primarily due to centralized storage and management by healthcare-related organizations and are further classified into vulnerabilities and threats. A significant security limitation with respect to centralized healthcare data storage systems is the **vulnerability due to a single point of control.** Since the healthcare data also consists of personal and critical information of a patient and healthcare professionals, such control points are always targeted by cybercriminals. Stealing such healthcare data and selling it illegitimately for financial gain is the prime motivation for cybercriminals (Fugh-Berman & Ahari, 2007), (Hathaliya & Tanwar, 2020). A successful cyberattack on the control point can compromise the data integrity and confidentiality of all the associated systems.

Ambiguity in patient data ownership causes privacy-related issues and the problem of unauthorized access to stored data. For example, an EHR, although generated by the hospitals and the doctors, concerns a patient. Currently, such data is also managed by specialist third-party companies (Mandl & Kohane, 2012). Thereby it raises an issue of who owns the data (doctors, hospitals or patients). Similarly, the patients' health insurance data is managed either by the insurance companies themselves or through specialist cloud-based storage companies. This brings up the privacy issue related to who owns the data (insurance companies or patients) and in what sense the data can be used. The ownership decisions related to healthcare data, such as access control, access rights and modification privileges, are a significant issue affecting the security and privacy of healthcare data storage systems (Huda et al., 2009).

Due to such vulnerabilities, cloud-based healthcare data storage systems are under constant threat of various **cyberattacks.** The attempt to gain unauthorized access is through different methods such as Denial-of-Service (DoS) attacks, password attacks, malware attacks and social engineering attacks (Dogaru & Dumitrache, 2017). Attackers perform the DoS attacks (Hussain et al., 2003) to shut down a hospital's network by flooding it with false requests. Similarly, attackers conduct a social engineering attack (Krombholz et al., 2015) to carry out insurance fraud and steal patient records through a careless insider. Further, attackers steal the passwords (Raza et al., 2012) through techniques such as brute force and phishing to gain unauthorized access to patients' healthcare records. Moreover, in a malware attack (Spence et al., 2018), the attackers plant malicious code in either the healthcare data storage systems or medical devices to disrupt the functioning. A significant malware attack was the WannaCry ransomware attack (Hsiao & Kao, 2018) which took place worldwide. It locked the files in systems which were using the older Windows operating system and demanded payment of bitcoin cryptocurrency to unlock them. Since the beginning of the Covid-19 outbreak, attackers have performed several similar attacks on hospitals (Muthuppalaniappan & Stevenson, 2021). In Seh et al. (2020), the authors analyze financial losses suffered by the US healthcare sector due to data breaches owing to these attacks. They report that, in the last 15 years, around 249 million people were affected due to different data breach incidents. In 2019, 2,013 incidents were reported in 86 countries. The average cost of a healthcare data breach is US$6.45 million worldwide, with cost in the US being highest at around US$15 million, according to an IBM report (Alder, 2019). Such a large-scale financial loss prompts proper measures to secure the healthcare system.

Apart from the attacks on the healthcare system from the outside, **malicious insiders** are also a significant issue threatening healthcare data security (Hathaliya & Tanwar, 2020). An attempt at unauthorized access to medical information is either carried out by someone inside the system or from outside the system taking advantage of a careless insider. An insider with the required credentials but not the authorization to see the healthcare data can misuse his/her privilege.

Apart from the storage-related issues, there are threats to healthcare data due to **vulnerabilities present in specialized or related healthcare devices** (such as CT scanners, X-ray machines and MRI machines (Dogaru & Dumitrache, 2017) and those involved in mobile health, more commonly known as mHealth). A major device-centric security issue related to healthcare data protection is the vulnerability of such devices and the data generated using them. For example, the procedure to send the data involves connecting these devices to the cloud, where the aggregated information is stored and managed (Plachkinova et al., 2015). These devices are also vulnerable to potential network-based attacks, such as false data injection attacks (Ahmed & Ullah, 2018), DoS attacks, and medjacking attacks (Djenna & Eddine Saidouni, 2018). The individuals using these devices to record and send their physiological and healthcare data generally lack awareness about cybersecurity, making their devices and data vulnerable. In Kawamoto (2017), the author analyses the incidents of data breaches in IoT devices through a survey in which about 47.2% of the respondents from the healthcare sector accepted data breaches from their medical IoT devices.

In addition to the storage and device-related data security challenges, service-centric issues also cause healthcare data threats. Several issues arise in the big data analytics-based services in the healthcare domain (Abouelmehdi et al., 2018). These issues are due to parallel data storage and analysis across multiple servers. The computations on this also run parallel at multiple clusters. The compromise of even one such cluster can lead to wrong analysis (Gahi et al., 2016). Therefore, in addition to storage, the **vulnerability of computational analysis algorithms** is also a significant security issue.

In addition to medical data security issues, the protection of pharmaceutical supply chain data is also challenging. Pharmaceutical products are distributed to hospitals, clinics and medical stores through a wide network of supply chains. For pharmaceutical companies, the protection of their supply chain information to prevent **pharmaceutical counterfeiting** is a significant challenge (Coustasse et al., 2010). The data on manufactured medications, including composition, manufacturing date, expiry date and supply information, is vulnerable due to a single point of its storage and access. Pharmaceutical companies must mitigate the **risks of data breach attempts** from outside as well as inside the system to ensure the smooth operation of their services (Jaberidoost et al., 2013). Any breach of the product distribution information enables activities such as **stealing for misuse** and counterfeiting of the drugs (Urciuoli et al., 2013). Therefore, the protection of pharmaceutical supply chain information is essential for the healthcare sector's proper functioning. The same applies to the companies producing biomedical devices for hospitals and doctors.

This section discussed healthcare data-related security issues around various healthcare affiliated organizations and their tasks (also summarized in Figure 9.3). We identify that the healthcare sector's vulnerabilities related to data security can either be storage-based, device-based or services-based. The storage-based vulnerabilities arise primarily due to centralized control, while the device-based vulnerabilities owe their presence to the security resource-constrained specialized medical devices. The services-related vulnerabilities occur due to reasons such as parallel data storage and computation requirements. To mitigate the security threats caused by vulnerabilities, in the next section, we describe security parameters that are essential.

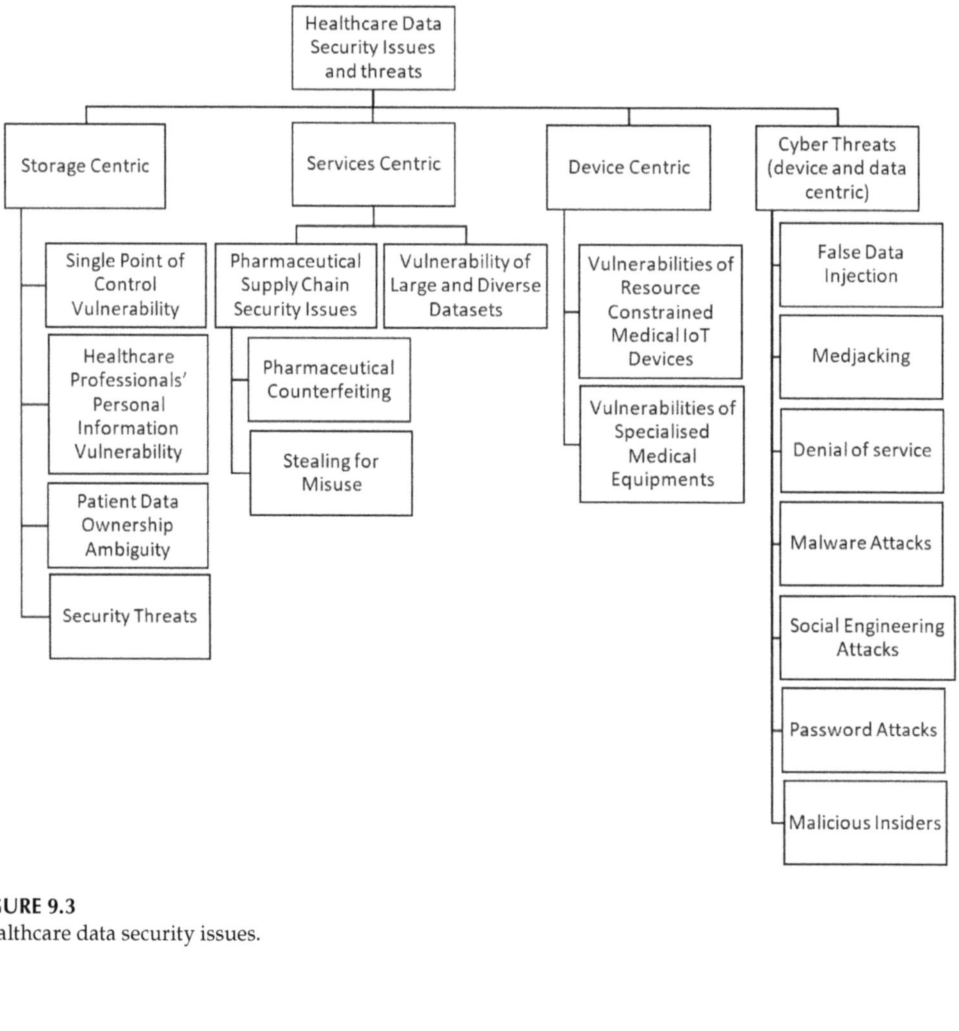

FIGURE 9.3
Healthcare data security issues.

9.5 Types of Security Parameters vis-à-vis Healthcare Sector

The security of healthcare data is essential for the stakeholders in the healthcare sector. Overall healthcare data protection encompasses a range of security parameters such as access control, data integrity and traceability (Hardin & Kotz, 2019). In this section, we describe these parameters in detail.

An essential security parameter in the healthcare sector is **access control** to preserve healthcare data privacy (Abouelmehdi et al., 2017). The medical records of a particular patient should be accessed only by doctors who are involved in the treatment of the individual in question. Apart from the doctors, healthcare organizations' administrative staff access patient data from time to time for billing and insurance-related processing. Different countries have different data privacy laws, such as the Health Insurance Portability and Accountability Act (HIPAA) in the US specifically for healthcare data, general data protection laws like the Personal Information Protection and Electronic Documents act in Canada and the General Data Protection Regulation (GDPR) in European Union. These laws mandate the organizations storing healthcare data to obtain the concerned person's consent through a disclosure form before using his/her data and enforcing data privacy. They make access control of the healthcare data essential so that any unauthorized access can be prevented (Dagher et al., 2018). Therefore, the healthcare data storage and management systems should have proper access control measures to comply with the privacy laws enforced in the country in which they operate. The same applies to healthcare insurance companies, medical research organizations and pharmaceutical companies trying to access the medical data for their functioning and research activities. The consent of a patient for healthcare data access is also essential in such cases to prevent its misuse.

Currently, many patients consult different doctors across multiple hospitals either for different ailments or for acquiring a second opinion for the same condition. Further, various healthcare-related organizations collaborate for different data-related services. For example, the collaboration between the University of Oxford and the AstraZeneca pharmaceutical company for developing a vaccine for protection against Covid-19 (Mullard, 2020). Such aspects need a common platform where **data are secure, interoperable** and have proper access control (Iroju et al., 2013).

In addition to access control, **preserving data integrity** is an essential parameter for healthcare data security (Pandey et al., 2020). Data integrity refers to the process of maintaining the accuracy and reliability of data over their entire utility cycle. In the healthcare domain, this includes maintaining the accuracy and integrity of the healthcare data, which, if lost, is catastrophic. Thus, the authorities should regulate any unauthorized modification in healthcare data.

To identify the source of data in healthcare data storage and management systems, **traceability and auditability** (Hardin & Kotz, 2019) of the stored information are essential security parameters. Every day, a considerable amount of healthcare data either get created or updated. Even after the proper measures, some of this data might be unauthorized and malicious. For instance, someone with credentials to access the healthcare data storage systems inserts incorrect information in the records file. Therefore, a secure healthcare data storage system must have the provisions for identifying the source of each new entry and modification in it.

Finally, **protection against cyberattacks** is the most significant security parameter for healthcare data storage and management systems. There are several security threats to the healthcare sector in the form of cyberattacks discussed in Section 9.4. The objectives of such attacks are diverse, including stealing data through unauthorized access, corrupting the data, making the network inaccessible or causing the system to malfunction. Any successful attack causes a significant amount of damage due to the sensitive nature of the data. Therefore, the healthcare data management systems must be robust enough to thwart such attacks successfully.

In this section, we summarized the various security parameters that are essential while creating healthcare data storage and management systems. The access control for healthcare data management systems should be strictly requirements-based, such as doctors for diagnosis and administrative staff for billing to preserve healthcare data privacy. A proper design for inter-organizational operability should be there for the smooth operating of healthcare-related services without compromising on data security. Besides, healthcare organizations must have adequate auditing mechanisms for their stored data. Finally, the system must be robust enough to resist outsider as well as malicious insider attacks successfully. As we proceed, we discuss blockchain's utility in implementing these parameters for data security in the healthcare sector.

9.6 Blockchain Components and Properties for Improvement in Data Security

Blockchain technology is based on decentralized networks introduced initially as a channel for cryptocurrency generation and payments (Nakamato, 2008). A blockchain is a distributed ledger consisting of data stored in the form of blocks sequentially linked to each other through hash values of block data. Once the data gets recorded on the ledger, it is hard to modify it due to its **immutability property**. It **prevents unauthorized modification** as well as **providing for traceability** of healthcare data. There is no centralized storage of the blockchain data. Instead, each participating node in the decentralized network maintains a copy of the blockchain stored with it. At present, many applications use blockchain technology, including healthcare (Engelhardt, 2017). The use of blockchain in the healthcare sector has the potential to improve the transparency and security of healthcare data (Agbo et al., 2019).

The security of a blockchain network is linked to the permission level for new participants. Based on the permission rules for new participants joining, there are two categories of a blockchain-enabled platform: **Permissionless** and **permissioned blockchain** (Wust & Gervais, 2018). In a **permissionless blockchain**, any person is allowed to join and transact with other users without any pre-authentication and central authority. For **permissionless** blockchains, there is **no single point of control,** and hence the scenario of a system malfunction due to the failure of a centralized administrator is not present. The blockchain for bitcoin cryptocurrency was the first instance of a permissionless blockchain (Nakamato, 2008). A permissionless blockchain is always public. On the other hand, a **permissioned blockchain** is for a single group or organization only. Here a **central authority is present** for tasks such as providing permission to join, assigning roles, and granting privileges to the network's nodes. However, the other operations are carried out internally without interference from the authority. For example, Walmart Canada uses a permissioned blockchain for food supply chain management (Smith et al., 2020) using the Hyperledger Fabric framework (Androulaki et al., 2018). Since the number of nodes able to participate is limited in number, the time required to verify data and create a block is less than in a permissionless blockchain. A permissioned blockchain is either a private permissioned blockchain or a public permissioned blockchain. A **private permissioned blockchain** has the criteria for entry as well as roles and specified tasks for each user. On the other hand, a **public permissioned blockchain** (Ruiz, 2020) has entry criteria but no discrimination over access. An example of a public-permissioned blockchain is Alastria (Ibáñez & Moccia, 2020), a non-profit multi-sector blockchain-based organization. A permissioned blockchain between multiple organizations is a **consortium blockchain** (Zhang & Lin, 2018).

The blockchain participants carry out the addition of new data in the form of blocks to the agreed-upon blockchain through the **consensus protocol**. The objective is to **get rid of a single controlling authority** with respect to decisions related to healthcare data storage and management. A proper consensus protocol should be resilient enough to function correctly against the issues such as failure of nodes, malicious nodes, delay in communication and data corruption. In a consensus mechanism, a participant is selected either through a competition like solving a puzzle or through a randomized selection process. In Xiao et al. (2020), the authors provide a detailed survey on consensus protocols in the blockchain. Among these protocols, **Proof of Work (PoW)** is the first significant consensus procedure (Nakamato, 2008). In this case, the participant nodes compete amongst themselves to find the solution to a cryptographic puzzle through a brute-force-based process. In another consensus protocol, **Proof of Stake (PoS)**, a node is selected from a group of validators for the block formation with selection probability depending on cryptocurrency units staked into the network (Saleh, 2021). Both PoW and PoS work in both permissionless and permissioned blockchains. **Practical Byzantine Fault Tolerance (PBFT)** (Hao et al., 2018) and the **Raft Consensus Protocol** (Ongaro & Ousterhout, 2014) are the consensus mechanisms designed only for those permissioned and consortium blockchain platforms with the property of byzantine fault tolerance (Castro & Liskov, 2002). Their functioning involves one node selected as the leader to initiate the block formation based on the feedback from the rest of the follower nodes regarding the validity of transactions. The objective is to reach a consensus with the correct information despite the presence of malicious and faulty nodes sending false information. The blockchain-based networks use several other methods such as Proof of Authority (PoA), Proof of Capacity (PoC), and Tendermint.

Another critical function of the blockchain is **hashing of the data through hash algorithms**. A hash algorithm converts a data string of any length into a fixed output of binary data. For blockchain, the hash algorithms used are SHA-256 (Gueron et al., 2011) and ethash (Han et al., 2019). It is nearly impossible to predict the input data from the hashed output. In a blockchain, each block has the previous block hash value stored as part of its data. The property of **hash-based linking of blocks** makes it difficult to alter the block data by predicting the ever-increasing chain of hash values. Apart from this, blockchain also uses public-key cryptography to create node addresses and digitally signing transactions. Some of the encryption techniques used for transactions in blockchain networks are elliptic curve cryptography (Hankerson et al., 2006), zero-knowledge proof (Partala et al., 2020) and ring signatures.

Blockchain technology has been constantly evolving since its introduction. A significant stage in evolution is the conception of blockchain 2.0 through the Ethereum blockchain platform. Blockchain 2.0 identifies and implements blockchain as a programmable decentralized trust platform (Kehrli, 2016) by introducing smart contracts (Ulieru, 2016). **Smart contracts** are self-enforceable autonomous programs containing predefined conditions for executing a transaction on an Ethereum Virtual Machine. Smart contracts provide an agreement between the nodes participating in blockchain transactions. Once they get added to the blockchain, no-one is able to modify them. When a smart contract is called for carrying out a transaction, each validating node executes it to verify the transaction's correctness and to reach a consensus. Due to verification by each node, a smart contract should be deterministic and verifiable. The conditions executed through smart contracts get recorded as transactions during addition into the blockchain.

As discussed in Section 9.4, there are different types of services such as medical diagnosis, conducting medical tests and administrative tasks in healthcare. The assigning of different roles and privileges to the participating nodes based on which service they carry out is essential in this case. Therefore, permissioned blockchains are deemed more suited for healthcare data security. While implementing blockchain in the healthcare sector for data security, one requires several initialization operations. One such operation is assigning predefined roles and privileges to the entities such as doctors, staff and patients. In addition to initialization, there are tasks related to the functioning after implementation, such as adding, modifying and accessing healthcare data.

By defining healthcare data access control through smart contracts, blockchain **enables patient ownership and control** over his/her data. A patient is able to see the history of their data concerning the activities such as addition to and access of the records. In addition to patients, if the different hospitals use blockchain for inter-organizational interaction and sharing of healthcare data, it **enables a secure standard format** for efficient processing of healthcare-related services. The integration of hospitals with pharmaceutical and health insurance companies through blockchain provides a secure platform for efficiently carrying out services such as the medication distribution chain and insurance claim processing.

Estonia is one of the first countries that is officially incorporating blockchain in its healthcare sector functioning (Heston, 2017) to ensure data security and its ease of availability for patients. To do so, Estonia collaborates with Guardtime (a private data security company) to secure its citizens' health records through blockchain. Government-authorized entities provide the decentralized storage. Auditing is error-free due to the blockchain's immutability property. Within the blockchain, the medical researchers get anonymized data rewards in exchange for mining services.

Next, we answer the fundamental questions related to the what, who, when and why (4W) of blockchain technology. We first answer the "**what**" and "**why**" questions. For securing the healthcare data such as EHRs, PHRs, pharmaceutical data, health insurance data and data generated by the services (discussed in Section 9.3), blockchain technology is one solution. Blockchains provide access control, integrity, traceability and immutability to the healthcare data, which is currently missing from the traditional healthcare system that usually stores the data in a centralized manner. Healthcare institutions such as hospitals, clinics, pharmaceutical companies and health insurance companies that manage data should implement blockchain-based solutions and are thus the ones **who** need blockchain to secure the healthcare data they are storing and the data their services are generating. Finally, we answer the "**when**" question. To carry out healthcare-related services, the people involved, such as doctors, staff members and patients, perform different tasks such as uploading, modifying and accessing healthcare data components. When used in the healthcare sector, blockchain securely performs these tasks, leading to improved healthcare data security.

In a blockchain, copies of data get distributed across the nodes of the network. This distribution, along with immutability, creates the problem of maintaining the privacy of data. The blockchain-embedded encryption technique enables user privacy, but it does not guarantee the data's privacy. In the healthcare segment, as the data contains medical history, diagnostic information and medical test reports in the form of text and images, it has a large volume and is sensitive. For this reason, as a solution, only lightweight values such as hashes, pointers and metadata are stored on the ledger.

Additionally, **to enable privacy protection in a blockchain-based healthcare data storage system, different encryption and authentication techniques are used on top of blockchain-provided encryption.**

This section discussed the advantages of blockchain and its properties vital in establishing healthcare data security. The immutability of blockchain prevents any unauthorized modification of healthcare data. The ability to operate without a centralized authority by establishing a general majority-based consensus procedure provides for a transparent functioning of the healthcare sector. Proper use of smart contract functionality enforces the security parameters, such as access control for healthcare-related services, inter-organizational operability of healthcare organizations and traceability of healthcare data. In the next section, we answer **how** different state-of-the-art approaches implement blockchain to improve healthcare data security.

9.7 Blockchain for Improvement in Healthcare Data Security

In this section, we survey different proposed systems that implement blockchain to improve healthcare data security through its inherent properties and functionalities.

In Zhuang et al. (2020), the authors propose a permissioned blockchain framework for creating a patient-centric health information exchange system with an objective to provide patients with **control** of their data. In the proposed system, the EHR reports are encrypted and stored on the respective hospital's servers, while their hash values are stored on the ledger to prevent tampering. The hospital administrators also create the pointers to each patient's EHR data, referred to as touchpoints, and store them on the ledger. The patient provides data access to a doctor by adding him/her to the "allowed list" through the smart contract. Any mismatch between the stored records and their hash values on the blockchain gets marked. Like Zhuang et al. (2020), in Shahnaz et al. (2019), the authors use the permissioned blockchain and smart contracts to **secure healthcare records by defining access rules.** The EHR data is stored using the interplanetary file system (IPFS) protocol (Benet, 2014), while the ledger stores the hash values of the EHRs. In the proposed system, smart contracts define patient, doctor and administrator roles in the healthcare network and implement the health records' storage and management functions. A blockchain transaction in the proposed system defines the roles, adding, viewing, updating and deleting health records. The administrator provides entry to the doctors in the system through a transaction. Once assigned as a doctor, a node performs the transactions related to adding, viewing and updating the EHR data. The access control for the transaction activities is directly related to the defined roles. Any form of unauthorized tampering traces back to the user who performed the transaction.

Similarly, in Shen et al. (2020), the authors propose a system for the secure sharing of collaborative healthcare data. The system consists of three stakeholders, third parties, data owners and miners operating on a consortium blockchain. Here, the third parties are referred to as the entities that perform data analysis-related tasks based on the requests and charge for them. The requested data are stored on the blockchain by the owners and accessed by the authorized third party. The data owners and miners receive their share of the services' generated revenue through smart contracts and a revenue model based on the Shapley value method (An et al., 2019). It provides for a secure and predefined incentive mechanism for healthcare data analysis services. In another similar work, in Qiao et al. (2020), the authors propose a solution for the secure sharing of medical data between organizations from different regions using cross-chain communication between multiple consortium medical blockchains.

In addition to organization-centric data security, blockchain technology is also used for **secure storage and management solutions for home-based healthcare monitoring devices**. In Li et al. (2020), the authors propose chain software-defined infrastructure (ChainSDI), combining permissioned blockchain with SDI for healthcare to ensure regulation compliance by medical institutions. The compliance system is used for patient-generated sensor data from wearable devices in addition to EHR data. The authors claim that their system is compliant with the US Government's HIPAA. In the proposed system, the stakeholders are the administrators that manage the data storage, data user (e.g., researcher) and patients. Their system invokes direct communication between a patient and the data user for access rights. The admin nodes verify whether the data user and patient are on the list registered on the blockchain. The admin node grants a data user's request to access data after receiving approval from the concerned patient. All these activities are enabled through smart contracts and get recorded on the ledger as transactions.

Third-party independence is another parameter in which healthcare data security is improved. In Wang et al. (2019), the authors combine blockchain with attribute-based encryption and cloud storage to **enable PHR sharing without relying on a third-party**. The hash values of encrypted PHR data get stored on the blockchain, along with an index linking to the patient's ID and data stored in the smart contract. The stakeholders of the system are patients, users and cloud server organizations. The PHR data stored is encrypted using attribute-based encryption (Bethencourt et al., 2007). When a user requests a patient for data access, the patient generates attribute-based keys according to user requirements. These keys enable the user to access the required data stored on the server. Therefore, it allows the patients to have requirement-based access control on their data without relying on a third party.

Similarly, in Madine et al. (2020), the authors propose a system for **patient-controlled secure PHR management** without dependence on the third party. Their solution works on both permissioned and permissionless blockchains and uses an IPFS system for data storage. The patients, doctors, hospitals and other healthcare-related organizations are registered on the blockchain as nodes through a controller smart contract. The request and permission for accessing records are enabled through smart contracts and get stored as transactions on the ledger. The system enables the patient to generate a symmetric key used to encrypt his/her PHR data. Then the blockchain-provided public key is used to encrypt the symmetric key. While granting access, the patient's private key is combined with the doctor's public key to generate a re-encryption key. This re-encryption key is used to encrypt the symmetric key. The symmetric key is then obtained using the doctor's blockchain-provided private key followed by the doctor accessing the requested data. Therefore, the proposed system provides an extra layer of data privacy and enhances security. The hash values of PHRs are stored on the blockchain, and any unauthorized change is detected. Similarly, in Meena et al. (2019), the authors propose a Hyperledger Fabric-based healthcare ecosystem consisting of hospitals, insurance companies, pharmacies and patients. The objective is to establish the patient's control over his/her data. A vital component of the proposed system is maintaining user and data privacy while forwarding the shared data in a computationally efficient manner through a proxy re-encryption algorithm.

Besides the techniques mentioned above, there are often emergencies when a patient is not able to provide consent for access to PHR data. In such a case, access is critical for emergency response staff and doctors involved in treatment, thereby needing **secure temporary access for emergency cases**. In Rajput et al. (2019), the authors propose a Hyperledger Fabric-based emergency access control management system (EACMS) for such situations. In EACMS, the patients grant emergency rights for access of their data to emergency doctors through smart contracts at the time of registration in the system. In EACMS, there are three registered stakeholders: A patient, a doctor and an emergency doctor (ED), apart from the system administrator. Here a doctor is referred to as the regular doctor. During an emergency, the administrator assigns a registered ED to the concerned patient. After verifying the authenticity, the tasks performed by ED, such as accessing patient records and doing modifications, are recorded as transactions on the blockchain and are immutable. There is no dependence on a third party for emergency access procedures in the proposed system as the registered patients have already defined the access policy through the smart contract.

In Wang et al. (2019), the authors propose a consortium-based blockchain along with cloud-assisted storage of EHRs to prevent unauthorized access. Their proposed system has four stakeholders, the data owners (DO), which are patients; data providers (DP), which are doctors; cloud servers (CS) and data requesters (DR). The health records are encrypted and uploaded on the cloud by DP after getting authorization from the concerned DO. The DP creates the keywords and index of data and stores them on the blockchain. The DR requests data through the keywords provided by the DP to locate the relevant EHR index on the blockchain. Then DO authorize the access request.

Besides access control and data management, blockchain also finds its usage for **securing mutual communication** between patients and data-sharing between doctors from different hospitals (Liu et al., 2019). Here, a typical transaction stored on the blockchain consists of the medical data shared along with the granter and requester node's ID. In the approach, there are three stakeholders: The system manager, hospitals and the users such as doctors and patients. This solution uses an improved version of delegated proof of stake (DPoS) consensus. In the consensus mechanism, the doctors act as delegates in DPoS while the hospital server acts as a verifier supernode. For each doctor, a score based on shared records' authenticity is also calculated and stored on the ledger.

Apart from the access control, **secure inter-organization authentication** is an essential parameter for secure sharing of healthcare data because patients often visit multiple doctors and hospitals for either different ailments or to get a second opinion. In Yazdinejad et al. (2020), the authors propose a public blockchain-based authentication system for distributed hospital networks. The hospital nodes act as validators and perform the task of adding members such as staff and patients to the blockchain and generating encryption keys for them. The creating and sharing of the keys are done based on the authentication of the concerned patient's device MAC address. The same encryption keys get used for migration across the hospitals. The transaction data recorded on the blockchain includes the patient health data linked with the registration information. Such a mechanism removes the dependency on the third-parties as well as decreasing the time required for authentication.

Note that the solutions mentioned above do not consider the **direct participation of medical devices** in sharing the data. In Zghaibeh et al. (2020), the authors propose SHealth, which overcomes this limitation and allows direct participation of medical devices. SHealth is a private multi-layered Hyperledger-based blockchain system. Here, the nodes are classified into five groups based on the privileges. Group 1 includes partners such as the government, while Group 2 consists of providers such as hospitals and pharmacies.

Group 3 comprises all individual users such as doctors, nurses and patients. While nodes that belong to Groups 4 and 5 are the addresses of stored records and IoT terminals, respectively. User privilege assignment and full data storage are done by nodes in Group 1, while Group 2 nodes maintain the blockchain and participate in the consensus process. The Group 3 nodes are the service consumer nodes and use smart contracts related to health records access. All the stakeholders access the relevant data without compromising authenticity. Patients also use smart contracts for requests and queries related to appointments, prescriptions and medical history. The proposed system enables the confidentiality of the activities such as doctor visits and enables secure and smooth data portability among healthcare organizations.

In Nguyen et al. (2019), the authors discuss the security of medical data exchanged through mobile devices by enabling blockchain-based transactions. In the proposed system, the mobile data (i.e., EHR, PHR, wearable devices data) gets stored in a distributed IPFS file system. The patient nodes are provided with an area ID based on their location, while each area has an EHR manager node. The blockchain stores the tuple (containing patient ID, patient area ID, transaction type and mobile data hash). The transaction types involve uploading, modification and access of EHR data. Smart contracts define and enable the functioning of these transactions. In the proposed system, admin nodes provide access to the EHR manager nodes and define their access roles. EHR managers upload encrypted EHR data of their patients in the IPFS file system after receiving data. The data storing process gets recorded as the transactions.

Other than the access control, **the interaction between wearable devices and associated smartphone applications also needs to be secured**. In Tomaz et al. (2020), the authors provide a lightweight non-interactive zero-knowledge proof authentication mechanism for resource-constrained mobile healthcare devices. The proposed blockchain-based system shares medical data for remote health monitoring along with the provision of attribute-based encryption for patient-controlled data privacy. The metadata of health records is stored on the blockchain, while the authenticity of accessing nodes is established through smart contracts.

In Xu et al. (2019), the authors propose a blockchain-based solution called Healthchain for **protecting the privacy of large-scale health data** uploaded through medical IoT devices. It consists of two sub-blockchains, Userchain, which is public, and Docchain, which is a consortium blockchain. The Docchain records doctors' diagnoses and contains the associated transactions. The Userchain records the transactions related to uploading medical IoT devices' data and accessing their own diagnosis records. The transactions on these chains include data from IoT devices, keys for access control and doctors' diagnoses. It protects the interest of patients by keeping the information confidential and ensuring accountability through record keeping.

The healthcare sector is regarded as an essential service. The healthcare data is sensitive and crucial for the smooth functioning of medical facilities. Such aspects cause the healthcare data storage and management systems to be constantly under attack from outside as well as inside the system. The objective of such attacks varies from data theft to DoS. The threat is much more severe in the case of medical IoT device networks. In Meng et al. (2020), the authors propose a blockchain-based solution for **protection against malicious attacks**. Here, they focus on collaborative intrusion detection systems (IDS)-based trust management for preventing insider attacks. Each user has the IDS system installed on their device, having traffic monitor components, communication components and a blacklist of malicious nodes. In the proposed system, there are two layers: The medical smartphone network (MSN) layer and the chain layer. The MSN layer deals with the interaction of smartphone devices with centralized storage. The chain layer consists of a consortium blockchain that helps users upload the unwanted and malicious feature/data packets information. Based on the provided information, the central server calculates dynamic trust values through Bayesian inference (Sun et al., 2006). Based on the trust values, each user can record its own blacklist of malicious nodes. The data recorded on the blockchain is immutable, and hence the list of malicious nodes cannot be manipulated by anyone.

In Zhu et al. (2020), the authors propose a solution to **prevent counterfeiting** medication information in the supply chain. Here, blockchain technology is used to track the medication distribution within the nodes comprising manufacturers, distributors, pharmacies, hospitals, doctors and regulators. If an issue gets detected at any stage of the supply chain, it is traced to the source of origin using the blockchain's stored information.

In another solution targeting malicious activities (Saldamli et al., 2020), the authors use blockchain for **insurance fraud detection**. The authors point out the lack of coordination between health insurance companies with respect to data-sharing and show that most of the financial loss is due to instances of fraudulent claims through fake healthcare information. In Saldamli et al. (2020), the authors propose linking insurance claims data using BigchainDB to create a distributed database on blockchain concepts. For the patients, they propose two different identifications, patient ID and billing ID. The billing ID is linked to a patient ID and is unique for each healthcare service the patient has availed. Whenever a health insurance company processes a claim with respect to a billing ID, it is recorded on the ledger. Then the amount in the claims file and billing file is compared to check for authenticity of the insurance claim. Due to blockchain data's immutability, it is impossible to avail insurance for the same billing ID twice. However, the proposed work assumes that the billing information generated from the healthcare service provider is authentic. Therefore, the development of methodology of verifying medical bills' authenticity is a potential future research problem.

We provide a summary of the blockchain-based solutions for healthcare data security in Table 9.1. in which we summarize and discuss the specific issues present in the state-of-the-art solutions. Besides the specific issues, there are general blockchain-based limitations that are common across all the proposed solutions. We discuss those limitations in the next section. In summary, in this section, we discuss how blockchain technology is applied to achieve healthcare data security. The use of blockchain enables security-based functionalities such as access control, inter-organizational operability and preventing counterfeiting. Regarding user and data privacy, proposed blockchain-based systems use additional data encryption techniques for enabling privacy preservation.

9.8 Technical Limitations in the Implementation of Blockchain in Healthcare

For healthcare data security, blockchain use provides a significant edge over cloud-based data storage and management systems. However, its implementation in the healthcare sector has several challenges and limitations. Some of these challenges are generic, i.e., applicable to blockchain regardless of the application, while some are healthcare-sector specific.

TABLE 9.1

List of Proposed State-of-the-Art Blockchain-Based Solutions for Healthcare Data Security. Here, P_r: Private blockchain, P_u: Public blockchain, C.: Consortium-based blockchain, C.C.: Cross Consortium-based blockchain, -: "No mention of," ⸸: Only hashes and transactions stored on-chain, †: Only shared data and transactions stored on-chain and "‡": All data and transactions stored on-chain.

	Blockchain		Functionality								
Approaches	Types	Storage	Storage	Exchange	Independence	Incentives	Emergency	Privacy	IoT Device-Based	Malicious Detection	Issues
(Zhuang et al., 2020)	P_r	⸸	✓	✓	✓						Setup is required to be installed at each healthcare facility.
(Shahnaz et al., 2019)	-	⸸	✓	✓	✓						No defined specification of organizational involvement.
(Nguyen et al., 2019)	P_r	⸸	✓	✓	✓				✓		Solution for low-network latency in wearable devices networks not provided.
(Shen et al., 2020)	C	†	✓	✓	✓	✓					Multiple transactions are required for each sharing request due to the massive volume of data.

(Continued)

TABLE 9.1 (CONTINUED)

List of Proposed State-of-the-Art Blockchain-Based Solutions for Healthcare Data Security. Here, P_r: Private blockchain, P_u: Public blockchain, C.: Consortium-based blockchain, C.C.: Cross Consortium-based blockchain, -: "No mention of," ⸸: Only hashes and transactions stored on-chain, †: Only shared data and transactions stored on-chain and "‡": All data and transactions stored on-chain.

	Blockchain		Functionality								
Approaches	Types	Storage	Storage	Exchange	Independence	Incentives	Emergency	Privacy	IoT Device-Based	Malicious Detection	Issues
(Qiao et al., 2020)	C.C	⸸	✓	✓	✓						The analysis provided is on a limited scale with few nodes. There is no clarity on real-time performance and the cost of building the system.
(Li et al., 2020)	C	⸸	✓	✓	✓				✓		Databases storing healthcare data are assumed to be compliant with privacy laws (HIPAA).
(S. Wang et al., 2019)	-	⸸	✓	✓	✓						There is no mechanism to verify cloud server response to the requirement related to PHR data management.

(Continued)

TABLE 9.1 (CONTINUED)

List of Proposed State-of-the-Art Blockchain-Based Solutions for Healthcare Data Security. Here, P_r: Private blockchain, P_u: Public blockchain, C.: Consortium-based blockchain, C.C.: Cross Consortium-based blockchain, -: "No mention of," ⸸: Only hashes and transactions stored on-chain, †: Only shared data and transactions stored on-chain and "‡": All data and transactions stored on-chain.

	Blockchain		Functionality								
Approaches	Types	Storage	Storage	Exchange	Independence	Incentives	Emergency	Privacy	IoT Device-Based	Malicious Detection	Issues
(Madine et al., 2020)	P_u+P_r	⸸	✓	✓	✓						Multiple deployments of the same smart contract are required for it to work across different countries. No integration of a patient's PHR in case of consultations in other countries.
(Rajput et al., 2019)	P_r	⸸	✓	✓	✓		✓				The system assumes that the person given access to PHR data in case of emergency is not malicious.

(Continued)

TABLE 9.1 (CONTINUED)

List of Proposed State-of-the-Art Blockchain-Based Solutions for Healthcare Data Security. Here, P_r: Private blockchain, P_u: Public blockchain, C.: Consortium-based blockchain, C.C.: Cross Consortium-based blockchain, -: "No mention of," ⸸: Only hashes and transactions stored on-chain, †: Only shared data and transactions stored on-chain and "‡": All data and transactions stored on-chain.

	Blockchain		Functionality								
Approaches	Types	Storage	Storage	Exchange	Independence	Incentives	Emergency	Privacy	IoT Device-Based	Malicious Detection	Issues
(Wang et al., 2019)	C	⸸	✓	✓	✓						The computational performance of smart contract algorithms depends on the length of EHR data keywords (pointers) stored on the blockchain.
(Zghaibeh et al., 2020)	P_r	⸸	✓	✓	✓				✓		A new node joins through a bureaucratic procedure that involves government nodes physically verifying the candidate against a government database. A

(Continued)

TABLE 9.1 (CONTINUED)

List of Proposed State-of-the-Art Blockchain-Based Solutions for Healthcare Data Security. Here, P_r: Private blockchain, P_u: Public blockchain, C.: Consortium-based blockchain, C.C.: Cross Consortium-based blockchain, -: "No mention of," ⸸: Only hashes and transactions stored on-chain, †: Only shared data and transactions stored on-chain and "‡": All data and transactions stored on-chain.

	Blockchain		Functionality								
Approaches	Types	Storage	Storage	Exchange	Independence	Incentives	Emergency	Privacy	IoT Device-Based	Malicious Detection	Issues
											patient can get his/her health record updated through a partner, which refers to a health insurance organization.
(Liu et al., 2019)	P_r	‡	✓	✓	✓			✓			Medical data to be shared must be lightweight due to on-chain sharing.
(Tomaz et al., 2020)	-	⸸	✓	✓	✓			✓	✓		The proposed system works on the assumption that the initial device registration is done in a secure environment.

(Continued)

TABLE 9.1 (CONTINUED)

List of Proposed State-of-the-Art Blockchain-Based Solutions for Healthcare Data Security. Here, P_r: Private blockchain, P_u: Public blockchain, C.: Consortium-based blockchain, C.C.: Cross Consortium-based blockchain, -: "No mention of," ⸸: Only hashes and transactions stored on-chain, †: Only shared data and transactions stored on-chain and "‡": All data and transactions stored on-chain.

	Blockchain		Functionality								
Approaches	Types	Storage	Storage	Exchange	Independence	Incentives	Emergency	Privacy	IoT Device-Based	Malicious Detection	Issues
(Xu et al., 2019)	P_u+C	⸸	✓	✓	✓			✓	✓		The system assumes that any adversary working to crack the encryption key has limited computing power. Also, the off-chain channel between patients and medical IoT devices is assumed to be secure.
(Meena et al., 2019)	P_r	‡	✓	✓	✓			✓			Money transfer is done outside the network, while the insurance and pharmacy-related bills are stored on the ledger.

(Continued)

TABLE 9.1 (CONTINUED)

List of Proposed State-of-the-Art Blockchain-Based Solutions for Healthcare Data Security. Here, P_r: Private blockchain, P_u: Public blockchain, C.: Consortium-based blockchain, C.C.: Cross Consortium-based blockchain, -: "No mention of," ⸸: Only hashes and transactions stored on-chain, †: Only shared data and transactions stored on-chain and "‡": All data and transactions stored on-chain.

	Blockchain		Functionality								
Approaches	Types	Storage	Storage	Exchange	Independence	Incentives	Emergency	Privacy	IoT Device-Based	Malicious Detection	Issues
(Yazdinejad et al., 2020)	P_u	‡	✓	✓	✓						Patient control over his/her healthcare data is not present.
(Meng et al., 2020)	C	⸸	✓	✓	✓					✓	The impact of external attacks such as DoS on the system is not considered. Also, the experiment and analysis are done with a very limited number of nodes.
(Zhu et al., 2020)	P_u+P_r	‡	✓	✓	✓					✓	The proposed system assumes that the medication information uploaded on the blockchain is authentic, and each node is honest.

(Continued)

TABLE 9.1 (CONTINUED)

List of Proposed State-of-the-Art Blockchain-Based Solutions for Healthcare Data Security. Here, P_r: Private blockchain, P_u: Public blockchain, C.: Consortium-based blockchain, C.C.: Cross Consortium-based blockchain, -: "No mention of," ⸸: Only hashes and transactions stored on-chain, †: Only shared data and transactions stored on-chain and "‡": All data and transactions stored on-chain.

	Blockchain		Functionality								
Approaches	Types	Storage	Storage	Exchange	Independence	Incentives	Emergency	Privacy	IoT Device-Based	Malicious Detection	Issues
(Saldamli et al., 2020)	P_u	⸸	✓	✓	✓					✓	The blockchain technology used (BigchainDB) does not have a stable version and community support.

This section discusses the technological limitations in the current blockchain-based systems concerning the healthcare sector.

The **scalability issues for the large networks** are one of the blockchain technology's functional limitations (Yli-Huumo et al., 2016). This issue is much more severe in the case of healthcare data storage. In the healthcare sector, the data generated is of greater volume than financial transaction data due to the presence of images such as X-ray and CT scans (Esposito et al., 2018). Storage of such a large amount of data at every node is cumbersome. To resolve this issue, in Xia et al. (2017), the authors propose to store only partial data such as metadata, hash values and pointers on the blockchain while other data is on the servers.

Apart from scalability, another issue is healthcare **data privacy** (Nawari & Ravindran, 2019). As a blockchain operates in a distributed network, each node stores a copy of the ledger. However, it is not in the interest of a patient to have copies of his/her medical diagnosis reports shared across the network. Therefore, the issue of data privacy is also one of the reasons for a blockchain-based hybrid data storage system in the healthcare sector. However, even if the whole data is not shared across the network, the transaction information linked to the nodes' IDs is available for everybody on the blockchain. Therefore, the blockchain by itself cannot protect the privacy of activities carried out by nodes. As we discussed in the previous section, several encryption techniques are applied in addition to blockchain-based encryption to achieve user privacy. Various policies related to access control are defined in state-of-the-art blockchain-based systems to address data privacy limitations. Although these policies get embedded into the system through storage on the blocks, there is **no way to enforce them within the network** without functionalities outside the blockchain properties (Hardin & Kotz, 2019). To handle such limitations, some nodes are given more privileges than the rest by giving them administrative powers. Such a requirement, of providing some nodes more privilege than the others, is one reason why most of the proposed frameworks for healthcare data security are based on permissioned blockchains. This leads to **centralization** within the blockchain-based networks (Nawari & Ravindran, 2019).

Apart from the overall functionality limitations, there are also specific **limitations associated with various consensus algorithms** used in blockchain (Zhang & Lee, 2020), which are generic and equally applicable to blockchain in healthcare applications. The proof of work needs computational resources, which in most cases are outside the scope of individual patients as well as some small hospitals. The requirement of computational resources works against the principle of participants' equality, even for the permissioned blockchains. For the PBFT consensus used in Hyperledger blockchain, the large number of messages required to be sent between the nodes causes network congestion. Nowadays, patients send their personal healthcare data recorded through various medical IoT devices and smartphones. The requirements for full participation force these resource-constrained devices to be mere spectators in the blockchain networks. Similarly, proof-of-stake consensus favors financially strong healthcare institutions. The disadvantage of such favors gives disproportionate power to big institutions with respect to discretion regarding inclusion or exclusion of certain transactions.

The functions like access control, privacy, recording, modification and seeing the healthcare data get executed through smart contracts. Smart contracts play an essential role in the automation of tasks. However, there are several **smart contract limitations** (Zou et al., 2019) that directly affect the functioning of healthcare data security. Once a smart contract gets recorded on the blockchain, no one can change its code. Due to this, the developers need to check for vulnerabilities before deploying. Anytime these contracts are called to execute a task, every validating node runs it to verify the transactions. It again creates a privacy issue as every node has access to all the data used by the code. Therefore, extra care must be taken while developing a smart contract in deciding how much data and the encryption keys to provide.

Due to the above limitations, there are several **security risks** associated with blockchains, such as double spending (a participant creates a parallel transfer of the same data to two different participants leading to an invalid transaction), 51% attacks (occur when a participant or a group controls most computational resources and tries to tamper with the blockchain data) and risks associated with encryption techniques used in blockchain (Nawari & Ravindran, 2019). The risks related to the encryption techniques are due to the progress of computational technology. For instance, quantum computing's fast progress has the potential to make current blockchain encryption techniques obsolete against quantum attacks (Fernandez-Carames & Fraga-Lamas, 2020).

In this section, we discussed the technology-related limitations of blockchain implementation for healthcare data security. These include the blockchain's limitations in general and the constraints due to the healthcare data structure and functioning. The two main issues are scalability and data privacy, for which additional measures such as the hybrid storage model and re-encryption of data are additionally applied, as discussed in the previous section.

9.9 Regulatory Challenges for Blockchain in Healthcare Data Security

Apart from the technology-based limitations, there are several legal and regulatory challenges while applying blockchain to improve healthcare data security. From the perspective of governments and their relevant departments, there are many issues to be resolved.

A significant one amongst these is related to the issue of privacy. If an individual patient or an organization decides to leave the blockchain-based network, their previous data cannot get erased due to its immutability property. It goes against the structure of the "**right to be forgotten**" granted under privacy rights in most countries (Gabison, 2016). This right explicitly enables an individual to get his/her data removed in the event of opting out of the organization. It creates a regulatory challenge for the stakeholders involved.

Blockchain-based healthcare data storage systems are **not yet officially standardized** (Yeoh, 2017). The different state-of-the-art systems get adopted by the organizations according to their requirements. The healthcare organizations using blockchain have their specific data storage format, encryption techniques and consensus algorithms. It leads to **interoperability issues** across the blockchains, causing it to become difficult for hospitals and other healthcare organizations to collaborate. It becomes an issue for the patients due to the need to migrate their data across the chains. Therefore, standard guidelines for blockchain operations are warranted.

There is also the **issue of jurisdiction for permissionless blockchains** that go beyond national boundaries (Yeoh, 2017). It is a general issue of blockchain but equally affects healthcare, as in any other sector. In the systems operating through permissionless blockchains, a patient can get a diagnosis from a doctor in different countries, and the information gets stored on the ledger. The jurisdiction regarding ownership of healthcare data, payment information and taxation is not defined for such cases. Although only the metadata or hash values get stored on the blockchain in most cases, the issue of ownership is still present. To avoid this issue, most of the proposed systems run on permissioned blockchains. However, even for permissioned blockchains, a clear regulatory code specifying the **laws of functioning, data ownership, compliance, etc., is warranted** for most nations. It reduces blockchain to an experimental and assisting technology for existing healthcare data management systems.

A significant issue in the way of widespread adaptation of blockchain for healthcare data security is the **lack of training and awareness** (Kramer, 2019). From the perspective of healthcare organizations such as hospitals, they have their share of concerns regarding the adoption of blockchain for data security. For migrating to the blockchain, the patients, doctors and administrative staff need to undergo training to learn the secure usage for data storage and access. With the technology still evolving, the proper user interfaces for blockchain-based systems are still not in place, making it challenging for non-technical personnel to adjust to its functioning. The stakeholders must learn about the security aspects like the use of encryption keys, calling proper smart contract functions and protection of their information to ensure data security. Hence, adequate training is essential for the widespread adoption of blockchain.

Overall, the healthcare organizations, government departments and blockchain-developing organizations need to coordinate amongst themselves to make blockchain a mainstream technology in healthcare.

9.10 Blockchain's Role in Pandemics like Covid-19 for Largescale Data Security and Management

At the time of writing, all nations are struggling to cope with the pandemic caused by coronavirus disease (Covid-19), known as severe acute respiratory syndrome coronavirus-2 (SARS-CoV-2). It was first detected in the Wuhan region of China in December 2019. Since then, it has found its way into almost all nations worldwide due to its infectious nature of spreading through close contact and respiration. It was declared a worldwide pandemic by the WHO in March 2020 (Kalla et al., 2020). At the time of writing, the total detected infections had passed 100 million worldwide, causing more than two million deaths. It has caused an unprecedented strain on economies worldwide, with the healthcare sector being most affected. To counter and wipe out the virus, efforts are being made on all fronts in healthcare, including emergency services, treatment facilities, medication and research on dealing with such pandemics through vaccination. All the mentioned fields require the processing of data for their functioning. The data includes the components, such as patient's health records, data on hospital resources, information on persons infected with coronavirus, research data for developing medication and vaccines. The security of this data generated on such a large scale is a challenge for governments, healthcare organizations and research laboratories. In this regard, blockchain performs a key role in managing Covid-19-related healthcare data.

A significant application where blockchain finds its use is contact tracing for Covid-19. A patient's anonymity is preserved using blockchain-generated IDs while alerting the persons who were in close contact through Bluetooth-based technology. For this purpose, the authors in Xu et al. (2021) propose a blockchain-based contact tracing solution named BeepTrace.

The traceability property also provides for tracking passenger movements. To facilitate this, a blockchain-based solution for issuing immunity certificates has been proposed

(Hasan et al., 2020). Using smart contracts, it issues medical passports for people with a negative in the Covid-19 medical test. Combined with an IPFS, it ensures the security of patient data. Since blockchain data is immutable, it cannot be manipulated by either of the stakeholders. Apart from this, by using smart contracts, the procedure for health insurance approval is made faster with lower processing costs.

A blockchain-based app Civitas (Wright, 2020), is used in Canada to control the impact of Covid-19. It maps people to blockchain to find out whether they are in quarantine or not. It also aids with the ideal time to go out of the house for essential tasks.

Besides, blockchain also aids in research for finding medication and vaccines to prevent and treat coronavirus disease. Currently, the medical records for Covid-19 are managed by each healthcare institution independently. In Yu et al. (2021), the authors provide a blockchain-based secure data sharing platform for carrying out collaborative medical research and clinical trials. The hospitals and medical research institutions are the nodes in the decentralized network. All data is attached to blockchain-based pseudonyms instead of real-world identities to protect the patient's privacy.

Overall, blockchain plays a vital role in ensuring the security of healthcare data-related operations for pandemic situations. It prevents information manipulation and provides the patients with the control of their data without relying on an independent third party.

9.11 Conclusion and Perspective on Future Research Directions

The decentralization of systemic functioning has become a major objective for healthcare systems to achieve complete security, privacy and accountability for the relevant data. The use of blockchain-based peer-to-peer networks plays a significant role in accomplishing this. The requirement of cryptographic verification and majority consensus before adding new blockchain blocks brings transparency and joint accountability to the healthcare system where sensitive patient data is involved. It has several benefits to the patients in terms of monitoring the access and use of their data. It also streamlines the operations of doctors, healthcare institutions and medical research centers in terms of acquiring the relevant information by removing the bottlenecks associated with the system's centralized operations. For the security of the data, blockchain puts the responsibility on all the stakeholders through individual encryption and removes the need for a trusted third party.

However, none of the proposed blockchain-based networks functioning in the healthcare sector are entirely decentralized. These systems have interference in the form of administrative nodes, which warrants the research required to achieve pure decentralization for full transparency. Blockchain-based systems in the healthcare sector also need a sustainable incentive generation scheme and sharing for the miners/validators to keep the network running. Specific to the healthcare sector, it is currently cumbersome to store all the data on the blockchain. Besides, data privacy is equally crucial. Therefore, instead of storing all healthcare data, only the metadata and hash values are stored on the blockchain. For data privacy in such conditions, additional data encryption is applied above the blockchain-provided encryption. With the requirement of continuous research on scalability and encryption techniques, blockchain-based networks can play a vital role in data security for next-generation healthcare systems. Apart from the technology-based challenges, there are regulatory questions such as the jurisdiction regarding ownership of healthcare data and a standard inter-organizational functioning format requirement.

Technologically, we need an overhaul in the blockchain structure and functioning, specific to the healthcare sector's data types, functioning hierarchy and security issues. Our recommendation for the researchers and developers working towards achieving healthcare data security through blockchain is to first collaborate with the policymakers, healthcare organizations and different stakeholders on a large scale (e.g., country scale) to understand the ever-changing global needs rather than providing healthcare data security solutions for a specific organization with a particular need. As we understand, data privacy is a significant issue to be addressed to achieve healthcare data security. It warrants the need to incorporate additional privacy measures within blockchain architecture. One research direction that researchers could focus on is to modify the blockchain architecture to include a privacy module. Besides, blockchain functioning is computationally expensive. Developing countries or third world countries lack the resources for such a large-scale implementation of blockchain. Another research direction is to develop a resource-efficient blockchain that could guarantee the privacy of healthcare data as well. Also, a properly defined incentive scheme is required for the miners/validators to motivate them towards active participation. These incentives could be altruistic or financial aid from the government. Researchers could look into different incentive schemes and revenue-sharing models. Finally, the acceptance of blockchain for healthcare data security depends on the people's willingness to adopt it as a solution. Therefore, proper training and awareness among stakeholders are required for it to become a success.

Acknowledgments

This work is partially funded by the National Blockchain Project at IIT Kanpur sponsored by the National Cyber Security Coordinator's office of the Government of India and partially by the C3i Center funding from the Science and Engineering Research Board of the Government of India.

References

Abouelmehdi, K, Beni-Hessane, A and Khaloufi, H. (2018). Big healthcare data: Preserving security and privacy. *Journal of Big Data*, *5*(1), 1–18. https://doi.org/10.1186/s40537-017-0110-7

Abouelmehdi, K, Beni-Hssane, A, Khaloufi, H and Saadi, M. (2017). Big data security and privacy in healthcare: A Review. *Procedia Computer Science*, *113*, 73–80. https://doi.org/10.1016/j.procs.2017.08.292

Agbo, C, Mahmoud, Q and Eklund, J. (2019). Blockchain technology in healthcare: A systematic review. *Healthcare*, *7*(2), 56 (1–30). https://doi.org/10.3390/healthcare7020056

Ahmed, MN, Toor, AS, O'Neil, K and Friedland, D. (2017). Cognitive computing and the future of health care cognitive computing and the future of healthcare: The cognitive power of IBM Watson has the potential to transform global personalized medicine. *IEEE Pulse*, *8*(3), 4–9. https://doi.org/10.1109/MPUL.2017.2678098

Ahmed, M and Ullah, ASSMB (2017). False data injection attacks in healthcare, In *Australasian Conference on Data Mining*, pp. 192–202. Springer, Singapore. https://doi.org/10.1007/978-981-13-0292-3_12

Alder, S. (2019). 2019 cost of a data breach study reveals increase in U.S. healthcare data breach costs. *HIPAA Journal*. https://www.hipaajournal.com/2019-cost-of-a-data-breach-study-healthcare-data-breach-costs/

An, Q, Wen, Y, Ding, T and Li, Y. (2019). Resource sharing and payoff allocation in a three-stage system: Integrating network DEA with the Shapley value method. *Omega*, *85*, 16–25. https://doi.org/10.1016/j.omega.2018.05.008

Androulaki, E, Barger, A, Bortnikov, V, Cachin, C, Christidis, K, De Caro, A, Enyeart, D, Ferris, C, Laventman, G, Manevich, Y, Muralidharan, S, Murthy, C, Nguyen, B, Sethi, M, Singh, G, Smith, K, Sorniotti, A, Stathakopoulou, C, Vukolić, M and Yellick, J. (2018). Hyperledger fabric: A distributed operating system for permissioned blockchains. *Proceedings of the Thirteenth EuroSys Conference*, 1–15. https://doi.org/10.1145/3190508.3190538

Bahri, S, Zoghlami, N, Abed, M and Tavares, JMRS. (2019). Big data for Healthcare: A survey. *IEEE Access*, *7*, 7397–7408. https://doi.org/10.1109/ACCESS.2018.2889180

Beigel, JH, Tomashek, KM, Dodd, LE, Mehta, AK, Zingman, BS, Kalil, AC, Hohmann, E, Chu, HY, Luetkemeyer, A, Kline, S, Lopez de Castilla, D, Finberg, RW, Dierberg, K, Tapson, V, Hsieh, L, Patterson, TF, Paredes, R, Sweeney, DA, Short, WR and Lane, HC. (2020). Remdesivir for the treatment of Covid-19 — Final report. *New England Journal of Medicine*, *383*(19), 1813–1826. https://doi.org/10.1056/NEJMoa2007764

Benet, J. (2014). *IPFS - Content Addressed, Versioned, P2P File System*, 1–11. http://arxiv.org/abs/1407.3561

Berenson, AB and Rahman, M. (2011). Prevalence and correlates of prescription drug misuse among young, low-income women receiving public healthcare. *Journal of Addictive Diseases*, *30*(3), 203–215. https://doi.org/10.1080/10550887.2011.581984

Bergeles, C and Yang, G-Z. (2014). From passive tool holders to microsurgeons: Safer, smaller, smarter surgical robots. *IEEE Transactions on Biomedical Engineering*, *61*(5), 1565–1576. https://doi.org/10.1109/TBME.2013.2293815

Bethencourt, J, Sahai, A and Waters, B. (2007). Ciphertext-Policy Attribute-Based Encryption. *2007 IEEE Symposium on Security and Privacy (SP '07)*, 321–334. https://doi.org/10.1109/SP.2007.11

Bietz, MJ, Bloss, CS, Calvert, S, Godino, JG, Gregory, J, Claffey, MP, Sheehan, J and Patrick, K. (2016). Opportunities and challenges in the use of personal health data for health research. *Journal of the American Medical Informatics Association*, *23*(e1), e42–e48. https://doi.org/10.1093/jamia/ocv118

Brown, C, Chauhan, J, Grammenos, A, Han, J, Hasthanasombat, A, Spathis, D, Xia, T, Cicuta, P and Mascolo, C. (2020). Exploring automatic diagnosis of COVID-19 from crowdsourced respiratory sound data. *Proceedings of the 26th ACM SIGKDD International Conference on Knowledge Discovery & Data Mining*, 3474–3484. https://doi.org/10.1145/3394486.3412865

Burbidge, R, Trotter, M, Buxton, B and Holden, S. (2001). Drug design by machine learning: support vector machines for pharmaceutical data analysis. *Computers & Chemistry*, *26*(1), 5–14. https://doi.org/10.1016/S0097-8485(01)00094-8

Carrion, I., Aleman, JLF and Toval, A. (2011). Assessing the HIPAA standard in practice: PHR privacy policies. *2011 Annual International Conference of the IEEE Engineering in Medicine and Biology Society*, 2380–2383. https://doi.org/10.1109/IEMBS.2011.6090664

Castro, M and Liskov, B. (2002). Practical byzantine fault tolerance and proactive recovery. *ACM Transactions on Computer Systems*, *20*(4), 398–461. https://doi.org/10.1145/571637.571640

Coustasse, A, Arvidson, C and Rutsohn, P. (2010). Pharmaceutical counterfeiting and the RFID technology intervention. *Journal of Hospital Marketing & Public Relations*, *20*(2), 100–115. https://doi.org/10.1080/15390942.2010.493369

Dagher, GG, Mohler, J, Milojkovic, M and Marella, PB. (2018). Ancile: Privacy-preserving framework for access control and interoperability of electronic health records using blockchain technology. *Sustainable Cities and Society*, *39*, 283–297. https://doi.org/10.1016/j.scs.2018.02.014

Dash, S, Shakyawar, SK, Sharma, M and Kaushik, S. (2019). Big data in healthcare: Management, analysis, and future prospects. *Journal of Big Data*, *6*(1), 1–25. https://doi.org/10.1186/s40537-019-0217-0

De Aguiar, EJ, Faiçal, BS, Krishnamachari, B and Ueyama, J. (2020). A survey of blockchain-based strategies for healthcare. *ACM Computing Surveys*, *53*(2), 1–27. https://doi.org/10.1145/3376915
Djenna, A and Eddine Saidouni, D. (2018). Cyber attacks classification in IoT-based-healthcare Infrastructure. *2018 2nd Cyber Security in Networking Conference (CSNet)*, 1–4. https://doi.org/10.1109/CSNET.2018.8602974
Dogaru, DI and Dumitrache, I. (2017). Cyber security in healthcare networks. *2017 E-Health and Bioengineering Conference (EHB)*, 414–417. https://doi.org/10.1109/EHB.2017.7995449
Dyrda, L. (2020). The 5 most significant cyberattacks in healthcare for 2020. *Becker's Hospital Review*. https://www.beckershospitalreview.com/cybersecurity/the-5-most-significant-cyberattacks-in-healthcare-for-2020.html
Engelhardt, MA. (2017). Hitching healthcare to the chain: An introduction to blockchain technology in the healthcare sector. *Technology Innovation Management Review*, *7*(10), 22–34. https://doi.org/10.22215/timreview/1111
Esposito, C, De Santis, A, Tortora, G, Chang, H and Choo, KKR. (2018). Blockchain: A Panacea for healthcare cloud-based data security and privacy? *IEEE Cloud Computing*, *5*(1), 31–37. https://doi.org/10.1109/MCC.2018.011791712
Fernandez-Carames, TM and Fraga-Lamas, P. (2020). Towards post-quantum blockchain: A review on blockchain cryptography resistant to quantum computing attacks. *IEEE Access*, *8*, 21091–21116. https://doi.org/10.1109/ACCESS.2020.2968985
Filkins, B. (2014). *Health Care Cyberthreat Report: Widespread Compromises Detected, Compliance Nightmare on Horizon*. https://www.redwoodmednet.org/projects/events/20150731/docs/Norse-SANS-Healthcare-Cyberthreat-Report2014.pdf
Fugh-Berman, A and Ahari, S. (2007). Following the script: How drug reps make friends and influence doctors. *PLoS Medicine*, *4*(4), e150. https://doi.org/10.1371/journal.pmed.0040150
Gabison, G. (2016). Policy considerations for the blockchaintechnology public and private applications. *Science and Technology Law Review*, *19*(3), 327–350. https://scholar.smu.edu/cgi/viewcontent.cgi?article=1043&context=scitech
Gahi, Y, Guennoun, M and Mouftah, HT. (2016). Big data analytics: Security and privacy challenges. *2016 IEEE Symposium on Computers and Communication (ISCC)*, 952–957. https://doi.org/10.1109/ISCC.2016.7543859
Gueron, S, Johnson, S and Walker, J. (2011). SHA-512/256. *2011 Eighth International Conference on Information Technology: New Generations*, 354–358. https://doi.org/10.1109/ITNG.2011.69
Han, R, Foutris, N and Kotselidis, C. (2019). Demystifying crypto-mining: Analysis and optimizations of memory-hard PoW algorithms. *2019 IEEE International Symposium on Performance Analysis of Systems and Software (ISPASS)*, 22–33. https://doi.org/10.1109/ISPASS.2019.00011
Hankerson, D, Menezes, AJ and Vanstone, S. (2006). *Guide to Elliptic Curve Cryptography*. Springer-Verlag. https://doi.org/10.1007/b97644
Hao, X, Yu, L, Zhiqiang, L, Zhen, L and Dawu, G. (2018). Dynamic practical byzantine fault tolerance. *2018 IEEE Conference on Communications and Network Security (CNS)*, 1–8. https://doi.org/10.1109/CNS.2018.8433150
Hardin, T and Kotz, D. (2019). Blockchain in health data systems: A survey. *2019 Sixth International Conference on Internet of Things: Systems, Management, and Security (IOTSMS)*, 490–497. https://doi.org/10.1109/IOTSMS48152.2019.8939174
Hasan, HR, Salah, K, Jayaraman, R, Arshad, J, Yaqoob, I, Omar, M and Ellahham, S. (2020). Blockchain-based solution for COVID-19 digital medical passports and immunity certificates. *IEEE Access*, *8*, 222093–222108. https://doi.org/10.1109/ACCESS.2020.3043350
Hathaliya, JJ and Tanwar, S. (2020). An exhaustive survey on security and privacy issues in healthcare 4.0. *Computer Communications*, *153*, 311–335. https://doi.org/10.1016/j.comcom.2020.02.018
Hayrinen, K, Saranto, K and Nykanen, P. (2008). Definition, structure, content, use, and impacts of electronic health records: A review of the research literature. *International Journal of Medical Informatics*, *77*(5), 291–304. https://doi.org/10.1016/j.ijmedinf.2007.09.001
Heston, T. (2017). *A Case Study in Blockchain Healthcare Innovation* (AUTHOREA_213011_3643634).

Hölbl, M, Kompara, M, Kamišalić, A and Nemec Zlatolas, L. (2018). A systematic review of the use of blockchain in healthcare. *Symmetry*, *10*(10), 470. https://doi.org/10.3390/sym10100470

Hsiao, S-C and Kao, D-Y. (2018). The static analysis of WannaCry ransomware. *2018 20th International Conference on Advanced Communication Technology (ICACT)*, 153–158. https://doi.org/10.23919/ICACT.2018.8323680

Huda, MN, Sonehara, N and Yamada, S. (2009). A privacy management architecture for patient-controlled personal health record system. *Journal of Engineering Science and Technology (JESTEC)*, *4*(2), 154–170.

Hussain, A, Heidemann, J and Papadopoulos, C. (2003). A framework for classifying denial of service attacks. *Proceedings of the 2003 Conference on Applications, Technologies, Architectures, and Protocols for Computer Communications - SIGCOMM '03*, 99. https://doi.org/10.1145/863955.863968

Ibáñez, JW and Moccia, S. (2020). Designing the architecture of a blockchain platform: The case of Alastria, a national public permissioned blockchain. *International Journal of Enterprise Information Systems*, *16*(3), 34–48. https://doi.org/10.4018/IJEIS.2020070103

Iroju, O, Soriyan, A, Gambo, I and Olaleke, J (2013). Interoperability in healthcare: Benefits, challenges, and resolutions. *International Journal of Innovation and Applied Studies*, *3*(1), 262–270.

Jaberidoost, M, Nikfar, S, Abdollahiasl, A and Dinarvand, R. (2013). Pharmaceutical supply chain risks: A systematic review. *DARU Journal of Pharmaceutical Sciences*, *21*(1), 69. https://doi.org/10.1186/2008-2231-21-69

Kalla, A, Hewa, T, Mishra, RA, Ylianttila, M and Liyanage, M. (2020). The role of blockchain to fight against COVID-19. *IEEE Engineering Management Review*, *48*(3), 85–96. https://doi.org/10.1109/EMR.2020.3014052

Kawamoto, D. (2017). IoT security incidents rampant and costly. *Dark Reading*. https://www.darkreading.com/vulnerabilities---threats/iot-security-incidents-rampant-and-costly/d/d-id/1329367

Kehrli, J. (2016). Blockchain 2.0-from bitcoin transactions to smart contract applications. *NiceIdeas*. https://www.niceideas.ch/roller2/badtrash/entry/blockchain-2-0-from-bitcoin

Khezr, S, Moniruzzaman, M, Yassine, A and Benlamri, R. (2019). Blockchain technology in healthcare: A comprehensive review and directions for future research. *Applied Sciences*, *9*(9), 1736. https://doi.org/10.3390/app9091736

Koh, HC and Tan, G. (2005). Data mining applications in healthcare. *Journal of Healthcare Information Management: JHIM*, *19*(2), 64–72. http://www.ncbi.nlm.nih.gov/pubmed/15869215

Kramer, M. (2019). An overview of blockchain technology based on a study of public awareness. *Global Journal of Business Research*, *13*(1), 83–91.https://ssrn.com/abstract=3381119

Krombholz, K, Hobel, H, Huber, M and Weippl, E. (2015). Advanced social engineering attacks. *Journal of Information Security and Applications*, *22*, 113–122. https://doi.org/10.1016/j.jisa.2014.09.005

Kumar, V and Walker, C. (2017). Cyber-Attacks: Rising threat to healthcare. https://www.vasculardiseasemanagement.com/content/cyber-attacks-rising-threat-healthcare.

Landry, S, Beaulieu, M and Roy, J. (2016). Strategy deployment in healthcare services: A case study approach. *Technological Forecasting and Social Change*, *113*, 429–437. https://doi.org/10.1016/j.techfore.2016.09.006

Le, TT, Andreadakis, Z, Kumar, A, Gómez Román, R, Tollefsen, S, Saville, M and Mayhew, S. (2020). The COVID-19 vaccine development landscape. *Nature Reviews Drug Discovery*, *19*(5), 305–306. https://doi.org/10.1038/d41573-020-00073-5

Lee, CCM, Thampi, S, Lewin, B, Lim, TJD, Rippin, B, Wong, WH and Agrawal, RV. (2020). Battling COVID-19: Critical care and peri-operative healthcare resource management strategies in a tertiary academic medical centre in Singapore. *Anaesthesia*, *75*(7), 861–871. https://doi.org/10.1111/anae.15074

Li, P, Xu, C, Jin, H, Hu, C, Luo, Y, Cao, Y, Mathew, J and Ma, Y. (2020). ChainSDI: A software-defined infrastructure for regulation-compliant home-based healthcare services secured by blockchains. *IEEE Systems Journal*, *14*(2), 2042–2053. https://doi.org/10.1109/JSYST.2019.2937930

Liu, X, Wang, Z, Jin, C, Li, F and Li, G. (2019). A blockchain-based medical data sharing and protection scheme. *IEEE Access*, *7*, 118943–118953. https://doi.org/10.1109/ACCESS.2019.2937685
Madine, MM, Battah, AA, Yaqoob, I, Salah, K, Jayaraman, R, Al-Hammadi, Y, Pesic, S and Ellahham, S. (2020). Blockchain for giving patients control over their medical records. *IEEE Access*, *8*, 193102–193115. https://doi.org/10.1109/ACCESS.2020.3032553
Mandl, KD and Kohane, IS. (2012). Escaping the EHR trap — The future of health IT. *New England Journal of Medicine*, *366*(24), 2240–2242. https://doi.org/10.1056/NEJMp1203102
Meena, DK, Dwivedi, R and Shukla, S. (2019). Preserving patient's privacy using proxy re-encryption in permissioned blockchain. *2019 Sixth International Conference on Internet of Things: Systems, Management, and Security (IOTSMS)*, 450–457. https://doi.org/10.1109/IOTSMS48152.2019.8939226
Meng, W, Li, W and Zhu, L. (2020). Enhancing medical smartphone networks via blockchain-based trust management against insider attacks. *IEEE Transactions on Engineering Management*, *67*(4), 1377–1386. https://doi.org/10.1109/TEM.2019.2921736
Moulis, G, Lapeyre-Mestre, M, Palmaro, A, Pugnet, G, Montastruc, J-L and Sailler, L. (2015). French health insurance databases: What interest for medical research? *La Revue de Médecine Interne*, *36*(6), 411–417. https://doi.org/10.1016/j.revmed.2014.11.009
Mullard, A. (2020). COVID-19 vaccine development pipeline gears up. *The Lancet*, *395*(10239), 1751–1752. https://doi.org/10.1016/S0140-6736(20)31252-6
Muthuppalaniappan, M and Stevenson, K. (2021). Healthcare cyber-attacks and the COVID-19 pandemic: An urgent threat to global health. *International Journal for Quality in Health Care*, *33*(1), 1–4. https://doi.org/10.1093/intqhc/mzaa117
Nakamato, S. (2008). *Bitcoin: A Peer-to-Peer Electronic Cash System*. https://bitcoin.org/bitcoin.pdf
Nawari, NO and Ravindran, S. (2019). Blockchain and the built environment: Potentials and limitations. *Journal of Building Engineering*, *25*, 100832 (1–16). https://doi.org/10.1016/j.jobe.2019.100832
Nguyen, DC, Pathirana, PN, Ding, M and Seneviratne, A. (2019). Blockchain for secure EHRs sharing of mobile cloud based e-health systems. *IEEE Access*, *7*, 66792–66806. https://doi.org/10.1109/ACCESS.2019.2917555
Ongaro, D and Ousterhout, J. (2014). In search of an understandable consensus algorithm. *Proceedings of USENIX ATC '14: 2014 USENIX Annual Technical Conference.*, 305–319. https://www.usenix.org/system/files/conference/atc14/atc14-paper-ongaro.pdf
Pandey, AK, Khan, AI, Abushark, YB, Alam, MM, Agrawal, A, Kumar, R and Khan, RA. (2020). Key issues in healthcare data integrity: Analysis and recommendations. *IEEE Access*, *8*, 40612–40628. https://doi.org/10.1109/ACCESS.2020.2976687
Partala, J, Nguyen, TH and Pirttikangas, S. (2020). Non-interactive zero-knowledge for blockchain: A survey. *IEEE Access*, *8*, 227945–227961. https://doi.org/10.1109/ACCESS.2020.3046025
Pitacco, E. (2014). *Health Insurance*. Switzerland: Springer International Publishing. https://doi.org/10.1007/978-3-319-12235-9
Plachkinova, M, Andres, S and Chatterjee, S. (2015). A taxonomy of mHealth Apps -- Security and privacy concerns. *2015 48th Hawaii International Conference on System Sciences*, 3187–3196. https://doi.org/10.1109/HICSS.2015.385
Qiao, R, Luo, X-Y, Zhu, S-F, Liu, A-D, Yan, X-Q and Wang, Q-X. (2020). Dynamic autonomous cross consortium chain mechanism in e-Healthcare. *IEEE Journal of Biomedical and Health Informatics*, *24*(8), 2157–2168. https://doi.org/10.1109/JBHI.2019.2963437
Radanović, I and Likić, R. (2018). Opportunities for use of blockchain technology in medicine. *Applied Health Economics and Health Policy*, *16*(5), 583–590. https://doi.org/10.1007/s40258-018-0412-8
Rajput, AR, Li, Q, Taleby Ahvanooey, M and Masood, I. (2019). EACMS: Emergency Access Control Management System for personal health record based on blockchain. *IEEE Access*, *7*, 84304–84317. https://doi.org/10.1109/ACCESS.2019.2917976
Raza, M, Iqbal, M, Sharif, M and Haider, W. (2012). A survey of password attacks and comparative analysis on methods for secure authentication. *World Applied Sciences Journal*, *19*(4), 439–444. https://doi.org/10.5829/idosi.wasj.2012.19.04.1837

Ruiz, J. (2020). Public-permissioned blockchains as common-pool resources. *Linkedin*. https://www.linkedin.com/pulse/public-permissioned-blockchains-common-pool-resources-jesus-ruiz/

Saldamli, G, Reddy, V, Bojja, KS, Gururaja, MK, Doddaveerappa, Y and Tawalbeh, L. (2020). Health care insurance fraud detection using blockchain. *2020 Seventh International Conference on Software Defined Systems (SDS)*, 145–152. https://doi.org/10.1109/SDS49854.2020.9143900

Saleh, F. (2021). Blockchain without waste: Proof-of-Stake. *The Review of Financial Studies*, *34*(3), 1156–1190. https://doi.org/10.1093/rfs/hhaa075

Seh, AH, Zarour, M, Alenezi, M, Sarkar, AK, Agrawal, A, Kumar, R and Ahmad Khan, R. (2020). Healthcare data breaches: Insights and implications. *Healthcare*, *8*(2), 133. https://doi.org/10.3390/healthcare8020133

Shahnaz, A, Qamar, U and Khalid, A. (2019). Using blockchain for electronic health records. *IEEE Access*, *7*, 147782–147795. https://doi.org/10.1109/ACCESS.2019.2946373

Shen, M, Duan, J, Zhu, L, Zhang, J, Du, X and Guizani, M. (2020). Blockchain-based incentives for secure and collaborative data sharing in multiple clouds. *IEEE Journal on Selected Areas in Communications*, *38*(6), 1229–1241. https://doi.org/10.1109/JSAC.2020.2986619

Shi, S, He, D, Li, L, Kumar, N, Khan, MK and Choo, K-KR. (2020). Applications of blockchain in ensuring the security and privacy of electronic health record systems: A survey. *Computers & Security*, *97*, 101966. https://doi.org/10.1016/j.cose.2020.101966

Smith, B, Xiong, J and Medlin, D. (2020). Case study of blockchain applications in supply chain management- opportunities and challenges. *2020 Proceedings of the Conference on Information Systems Applied Research Virtual Conference*, 1501–1508.

Spence, N, Bhardwaj, N and Paul III, D. (2018). Ransomware in healthcare facilities: A harbinger of the future? *Perspectives in Health Information Management*, 1–22.

Stafford, TF and Treiblmaier, H. (2020). Characteristics of a blockchain ecosystem for secure and sharable electronic medical records. *IEEE Transactions on Engineering Management*, *67*(4), 1340–1362. https://doi.org/10.1109/TEM.2020.2973095

Stephen, O, Sain, M, Maduh, UJ and Jeong, D-U. (2019). An efficient deep learning approach to pneumonia classification in healthcare. *Journal of Healthcare Engineering*, *2019*, 1–7. https://doi.org/10.1155/2019/4180949

Sun, YL, Wei, Y, Zhu, H and Liu, KJR. (2006). Information theoretic framework of trust modeling and evaluation for ad hoc networks. *IEEE Journal on Selected Areas in Communications*, *24*(2), 305–317. https://doi.org/10.1109/JSAC.2005.861389

Sunyaev, A, Chornyi, D, Mauro, C and Krcmar, H. (2010). Evaluation framework for personal health records: Microsoft healthVault Vs. Google health. *2010 43rd Hawaii International Conference on System Sciences*, 1–10. https://doi.org/10.1109/HICSS.2010.192

Tariq, N, Qamar, A, Asim, M and Khan, FA. (2020). Blockchain and smart healthcare security: A survey. *Procedia Computer Science*, *175*, 615–620. https://doi.org/10.1016/j.procs.2020.07.089

Teklehaimanot, HD and Teklehaimanot, A. (2013). Human resource development for a community-based health extension program: A case study from Ethiopia. *Human Resources for Health*, *11*(1), 39. https://doi.org/10.1186/1478-4491-11-39

Tomaz, AEB, Nascimento, JC Do, Hafid, AS and De Souza, JN. (2020). Preserving privacy in mobile health systems using non-interactive zero-knowledge proof and blockchain. *IEEE Access*, *8*, 204441–204458. https://doi.org/10.1109/ACCESS.2020.3036811

Ulieru, M. (2016). Blockchain 2.0 and beyond: Adhocracies. In: Tasca, P, Aste, T, Pelizzon, L and Perony N (eds) *Banking Beyond Banks and Money* (pp. 297–303). Cham: Springer. https://doi.org/10.1007/978-3-319-42448-4_15

Urciuoli, L, Männistö, T, Hintsa, J and Khan, T. (2013). Supply chain cyber security – Potential threats. *Information & Security: An International Journal*, *29*, 51–68. https://doi.org/10.11610/isij.2904

Wang, S, Zhang, D and Zhang, Y. (2019). Blockchain-based personal health records sharing scheme with data integrity verifiable. *IEEE Access*, *7*, 102887–102901. https://doi.org/10.1109/ACCESS.2019.2931531

Wang, Y, Zhang, A, Zhang, P and Wang, H. (2019). Cloud-Assisted EHR sharing with security and privacy preservation via consortium blockchain. *IEEE Access*, *7*, 136704–136719. https://doi.org/10.1109/ACCESS.2019.2943153

Win, KT, Susilo, W and Mu, Y. (2006). Personal health record systems and their security protection. *Journal of Medical Systems*, *30*(4), 309–315. https://doi.org/10.1007/s10916-006-9019-y

Wright, T. (2020). Blockchain App used to track COVID-19 cases in Latin America. *Coin Telegraph: The Future of Money*. https://cointelegraph.com/news/blockchain-app-used-to-track-covid-19-cases-in-latin-america

Wust, K and Gervais, A. (2018). Do you need a Blockchain? *2018 Crypto Valley Conference on Blockchain Technology (CVCBT)*, 45–54. https://doi.org/10.1109/CVCBT.2018.00011

Xia, Q, Sifah, E, Smahi, A, Amofa, S and Zhang, X. (2017). BBDS: Blockchain-Based data sharing for electronic medical records in cloud environments. *Information*, *8*(2), 44. https://doi.org/10.3390/info8020044

Xiao, Y, Zhang, N, Lou, W and Hou, YT. (2020). A survey of distributed consensus protocols for blockchain networks. *IEEE Communications Surveys & Tutorials*, *22*(2), 1432–1465. https://doi.org/10.1109/COMST.2020.2969706

Xu, H, Zhang, L, Onireti, O, Fang, Y, Buchanan, WJ and Imran, MA. (2021). BeepTrace: Blockchain-enabled privacy-preserving contact tracing for COVID-19 pandemic and beyond. *IEEE Internet of Things Journal*, *8*(5), 3915–3929. https://doi.org/10.1109/JIOT.2020.3025953

Xu, J, Xue, K, Li, S, Tian, H, Hong, J, Hong, P and Yu, N. (2019). Healthchain: A Blockchain-based privacy preserving scheme for large-scale health data. *IEEE Internet of Things Journal*, *6*(5), 8770–8781. https://doi.org/10.1109/JIOT.2019.2923525

Yazdinejad, A, Srivastava, G, Parizi, RM, Dehghantanha, A, Choo, K-KR and Aledhari, M. (2020). Decentralized authentication of distributed patients in hospital networks using blockchain. *IEEE Journal of Biomedical and Health Informatics*, *24*(8), 2146–2156. https://doi.org/10.1109/JBHI.2020.2969648

Yeoh, P. (2017). Regulatory issues in blockchain technology. *Journal of Financial Regulation and Compliance*, *25*(2), 196–208. https://doi.org/10.1108/JFRC-08-2016-0068

Yli-Huumo, J, Ko, D, Choi, S, Park, S and Smolander, K. (2016). Where is current research on Blockchain technology? - A systematic review. *PLoS ONE*, *11*(10), 1–27. https://doi.org/10.1371/journal.pone.0163477

Yu, K, Tan, L, Shang, X, Huang, J, Srivastava, G and Chatterjee, P. (2021). Efficient and privacy-preserving medical research support platform against COVID-19: A blockchain-based approach. *IEEE Consumer Electronics Magazine*, *10*(2), 111–120. https://doi.org/10.1109/MCE.2020.3035520

Zghaibeh, M, Farooq, U, Hasan, NU and Baig, I. (2020). SHealth: A blockchain-based health system with smart contracts capabilities. *IEEE Access*, *8*, 70030–70043. https://doi.org/10.1109/ACCESS.2020.2986789

Zhang, A and Lin, X. (2018). Towards secure and privacy-preserving data sharing in e-health systems via consortium blockchain. *Journal of Medical Systems*, *42*(8), 1–18. https://doi.org/10.1007/s10916-018-0995-5

Zhang, S and Lee, J-H. (2020). Analysis of the main consensus protocols of blockchain. *ICT Express*, *6*(2), 93–97. https://doi.org/10.1016/j.icte.2019.08.001

Zhu, P, Hu, J, Zhang, Y and Li, X. (2020). A blockchain based solution for medication anti-counterfeiting and traceability. *IEEE Access*, *8*, 184256–184272. https://doi.org/10.1109/ACCESS.2020.3029196

Zhuang, Y, Sheets, LR, Chen, Y-W, Shae, Z-Y, Tsai, JJP and Shyu, C-R. (2020). A patient-centric health information exchange framework using blockchain technology. *IEEE Journal of Biomedical and Health Informatics*, *24*(8), 2169–2176. https://doi.org/10.1109/JBHI.2020.2993072

Zou, W, Lo, D, Kochhar, PS, Le, X-BD, Xia, X, Feng, Y, Chen, Z and Xu, B. (2019). Smart contract development: Challenges and opportunities. *IEEE Transactions on Software Engineering*, 1–1. https://doi.org/10.1109/TSE.2019.2942301

10

Electronic Medical Recordkeeping Application Using Blockchain Technology

Ujjawal Jain, Joythish Reddy, Yash Sarwaswa, Agya Pathak, Sameer Shrivastava and Malaya Dutta Borah

CONTENTS

DOI: 10.1201/9781003133179-10

10.1 Introduction

The concept of blockchain technology, introduced by Nakamoto, S. (2008) [1], initially became popular as a distributed ledger technology. Bitcoin, the first application of blockchain, facilitates the exchange of electronic coins/currency among the participants of a distributed and decentralized network, without the need of a centralized, trusted third party. One major advantage of this distributed network is a significantly reduced dependency on a trusted third party to facilitate the transactions. This in turn enables each of the clients of the network to take ownership of the data they push onto the network and, besides making the transactions public, it also makes them more secure as each of those clients have their own copies of the transactions.

Blockchain technology is fit for healthcare applications that deliver highly sensitive data requiring validation. Blockchain technology has a tremendous potential in healthcare, to meet the patient-centric approach. To connect disparate systems with the increasing accuracy of Electronic Healthcare Records (EHRs), blockchains are the best choice, since the blockchains are fully interoperable with e-health and m-health applications [2]. Some of the major aspects of the blockchain technology rendering it ideal for the healthcare sector include:

- Consistency of the shared data among the participant clients.
- Ownership of the data pushed into the blockchain by a client.
- Traceability of the historical evolution of a certain chain and protection against any unauthorized editing of the data/transactions.
- Decentralization, which prevents a central and/or hardly accessible entity to control and accumulate the data on the network.
- Transparency of the data, their author(s), editors and viewers are clearly reflected in the network.

10.1.1 Possible Research Questions (RQs) and Possible Mapping Decentralized Healthcare Applications

In order to research decentralized healthcare applications using blockchain technology, we enumerated the following RQs [3] and related findings. (Table 10.1, Table 10.2)

TABLE 10.1

Research Questions and Findings: Decentralized Healthcare Application Using Blockchain Technology

	Research Questions (RQs)	Descriptions
RQ1:	What are the current trends and use cases [3] of blockchain in healthcare?	This question is about applications and use cases of blockchain technology in the healthcare sector.
RQ2:	What are the challenges of utilizing blockchain in healthcare applications?	This can help to bridge the gaps between expectations from the application and its real time implementation.
RQ3:	How are the challenges being addressed currently?	This question is about current research scenario w.r.t. different approaches used the healthcare sector.

TABLE 10.2

Possible Mapping of RQ1

RQs	Possible Mapping
RQ1	Electronic Medical Record (EMR), Remote Patient Monitoring (RPM), Health Insurance Claims (HIC), Tracking Diseases and Others—Safeguarding Genomics.

10.1.2 Possible Mapping of RQs with Blockchain-Based Healthcare Applications

Mapping with RQ1:

- **Electronic medical record (EMR):** Healthcare data management is extremely important in the healthcare industry to provide holistic views of patients, personalize treatments, improve communication and enhance health outcomes. The fact that such a ledger will be immutable will protect medical records from being illegally accessed.
  - **EMR use cases:** Healthchain [5], Ancile [6] and MedRec [7], MedBlock [8], etc.,
- **Remote patient monitoring (RPM)**: EMRs can be retrieved in a secure and rapid fashion by medical personnel. Monitoring the status of patients outside of a traditional healthcare system like a hospital, for self-monitoring or home-based care can benefit from the same.
  - RPM use case: SMEAD [9].
- **Health insurance claims (HIC):** Matching a patient's EMR to the correct health insurance policy is still a challenge. Due to the unavailability of a unique identity, patient records can be easily tampered with by any of the parties. Also, there is no secure way for both hospitals and insurance providers to confirm whether the procedure is covered by insurance. Therefore, blockchain-based HIC is very important.
  - **HIC use case:** MIStore [10], which is developed using blockchain platform (Table 10.3).

Mapping with RQ2:

A couple of identified challenges are listed below:

- **Interoperability and scalability:** Interoperability is a primary concern stemming from the lack of a standard for blockchain implementation of healthcare platforms. This affects the exchange of information from one implemented platform to another. This directly impacts scalability.
- **Security and privacy:** Concerns regarding the fact that even after employment of encryption techniques possibilities exist of the identity of the patient being able to be pieced together by linking up certain data associated to the patient. The

TABLE 10.3

Possible Mapping of RQ2

RQs	Possible Mapping
RQ2	Interoperability and scalability, security and privacy, speed, scalability, patient engagement and immutability.

potential for malicious attacks by hackers or even government organizations that could compromise patient privacy and data integrity cannot be deterministically eliminated. In the past, attacks have taken place on cryptocurrency networks powered by blockchain. A leak of private key data can lead to unauthorized access and compromise health data.

- **Speed:** In the healthcare sector, the data load is bound to be significant. This will directly impact performance. Significant processing delays may be experienced. Such latency in this imperative application of blockchain is dangerous.
- **Scalability:** Scalability is directly impacted due to the large volume of data that is to be stored. This will lead to the degraded performance of such applications which can prove to be disastrous.
- **Patient engagement:** Generating social trust in this technology will not be an easy path. In particular, the elderly and the young will face issues and may not be able to manage their health-related data on such a platform. Also, they might simply not want to engage with such an application.
- **Immutability:** A concern arises from the property of immutability. A patient's health-related data may never be erased. This may prove to be counterproductive when it is desired to erase a patient's medical history (Table 10.4).

Mapping with RQ3:

A couple of propositions have aimed at working around some limitations and challenges [3]:

- **To counter the issue of scalability:** A proposition is in place to store health-related data off-chain. It implies that condensed information regarding accessing the data will be stored on the blockchain.
- **To counter the issue of security:** A private or consortium blockchain would be well suited to improve security. A huge number of threats can be combated by developing security measures.
- **To counter the issue of performance and enhance speed:** Permitting only selected nodes to participate in the consensus protocol can radically improve response times, unlike public blockchains where any node is allowed to participate in these protocols.

To address the above RQs this work proposed a system which highlights use of EMRs stored and accessed via a blockchain network, which makes it faster and more convenient for both the patients and doctors to be able to interact for all sorts of medical aids. For this particular purpose, the system employs storage of the digital records off-chain on a distributed platform called the InterPlanetary File System (IPFS) which is described later in the chapter. The system also facilitates the inclusion of pharmaceutical professionals which also helps monitor the drug-usage history of patients and keep a check on illegal or unprescribed incessant drug consumption.

TABLE 10.4

Possible Mapping of RQ3

RQs	Possible Mapping
RQ3	To counter the issue of scalability, to counter the issue of security, to counter the issue of performance and enhancing speed.

The system also employs cryptographic encryptions (which are discussed further), to secure the details of the clients using the blockchain network. Two particular algorithms that have been employed are Attribute-Based Encryption—to encrypt client details and Elliptic Curve Cryptography—which helps in generating a public key from a randomly generated private key. Cryptography ensures that the data being encrypted can be retrieved via invertible methods.

10.2 An Overview of the Technology Used in the Proposition

10.2.1 Ethereum [10]

An open and programmable blockchain platform "which allows developers to create arbitrary consensus-based applications that have the scalability, standardization, feature-completeness, ease of development and interoperability offered by these different paradigms all at the same time."

10.2.2 Smart Contracts [11]

A smart contract is a piece of code that includes a set of executable functions and states variables which reside on the blockchain and are identified by a unique address. It is like a cryptographic box that contains value and only unlocks if certain conditions are met.

10.2.3 InterPlanetary File System (IPFS) [12]

An implementation of a peer-to-peer distributed protocol, the IPFS is a versioned file storage system taking inspiration from platforms like Git. A distributed file system is one in which files may be stored and their versions successfully tracked. IPFS will potentially evolve the web as we know it uses its property of being a global, peer-to-peer file management system that is versioned. The web will be safer, faster and more open with the steady integration of IPFS. IPFS's integration into the web will augment the use of heavily used protocols such as HTTP.

10.2.4 Ciphertext-Policy Attribute-Based Encryption (CP-ABE) [13]

Attribute-Based Access Control (ABCL) is the central idea at work in CP-ABE which can revoke or provide access dynamically, based on the multiple attributes a user may have. The direct implication of this fact is that the decryption key of an attribute may be common amongst users. The encryptor may set the access in ways that define who may decrypt an encrypted message. Any encryptor can specify access control in terms of any access formula over the attributes in the system.

10.2.5 Truffle [14]

Truffle is a development environment that provides testing and asset pipelines for blockchains using Ethereum Virtual Machines (EVMs). It is used for compiling, linking and deploying the smart contracts. Truffle can also be used for testing the deployed contracts.

10.2.6 Metamask [15]

Metamask is a software cryptocurrency wallet developed to handle account management, store and manage keys, broadcast transactions, send and receive cryptocurrencies and tokens and securely connect to decentralized applications through a compatible web browser.

10.3 Proposed Application with Implementation Details

The blockchain system architecture proposes that the application can be easily accessed by users using any electronic device, such as computers and mobile devices such as phones and tablets. Portability has always been an important issue in electronic healthcare management. Applications that run on portable devices facilitate the transmission of information easily.

Our proposed implementation view shown in Figure 10.1 is designed as a multi-layered style. The user first uses a device such as computer, mobile, etc. to interact with the browser where the client application can be accessed. This client application connects to the web using Metamask which in turn connects the client to the Ethereum network. The Ethereum network contains the smart contracts, the storage space where the data is stored and also the events that trigger the contracts. The contracts are called using contract Application Programming Interface (API) calls which in turn modifies the initial Ethereum blockchain state or returns some data to the user.

10.3.1 EMR Management Using IPFS

Here, we are storing the data on the IPFS and the returned hashed address of the file location is encrypted and stored into the blockchain (Figure 10.2).

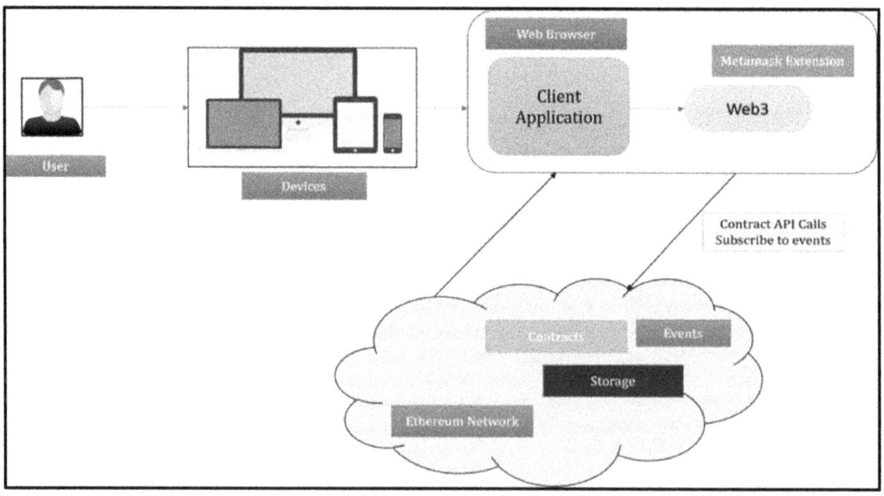

FIGURE 10.1
Proposed system.

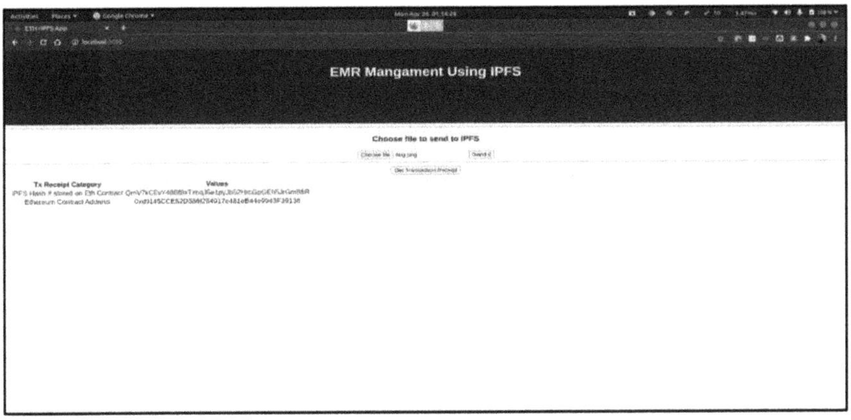

(a)

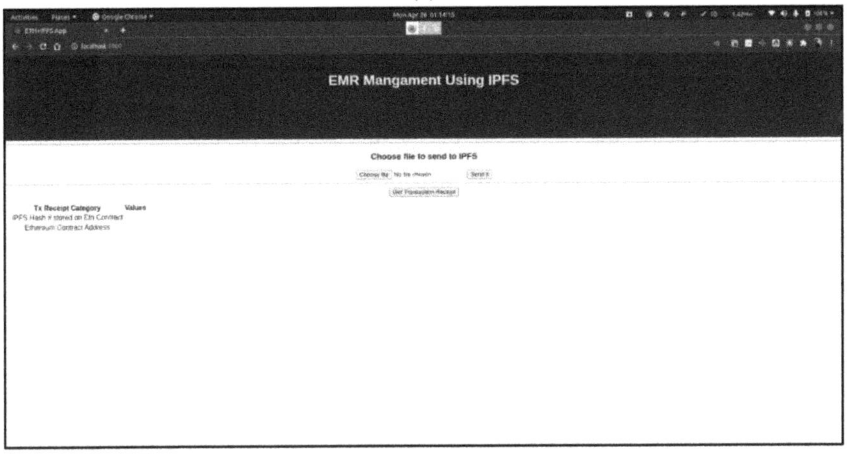

(b)

FIGURE 10.2
(a) Hash address return. (b) Data storing in IPFS.

10.3.2 The *addPatientInfo* Method

A patient registers onto the system using the *addPatientInfo* method. Forming the basis of the CP-ABE encryption algorithm, it triggers a smart contract to save the entered patient data on the blockchain Figure 10.3.

10.3.3 Generating *Public-Private Key* Pair

A set of attributes entered while registering onto the system is used as input to the ECDSA algorithm, that generates a *Public-Private Key* pair (Figure 10.4).

10.3.4 The *getPatientInfo* Method

The method allows a patient to access the information stored about a patient by querying using the *_adharCardNumber* in this implementation. It returns the data entered by a patient at the time of registration (Figure 10.5).

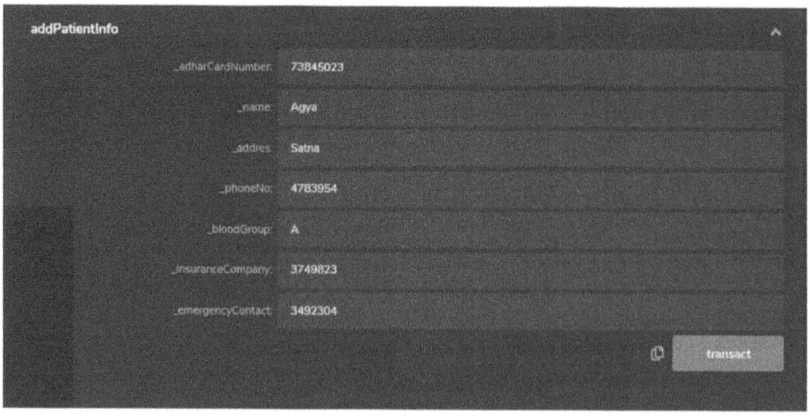

(a)

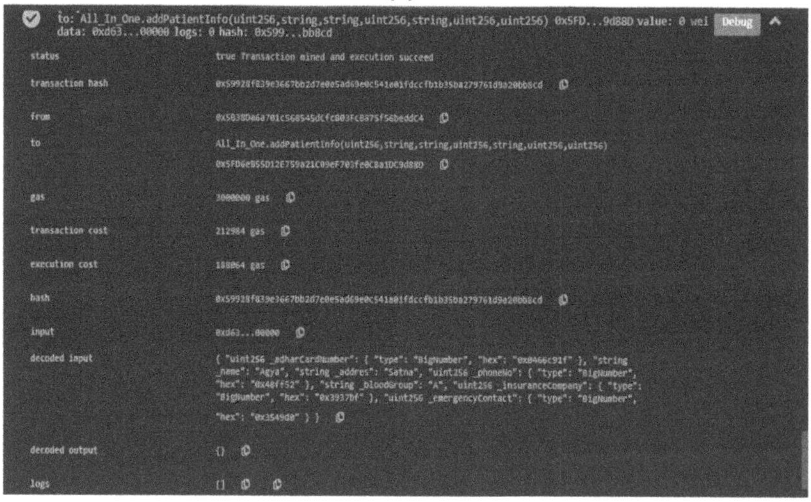

(b)

FIGURE 10.3
(a) Patient registration. (b) Output using CP-ABE encryption algorithm.

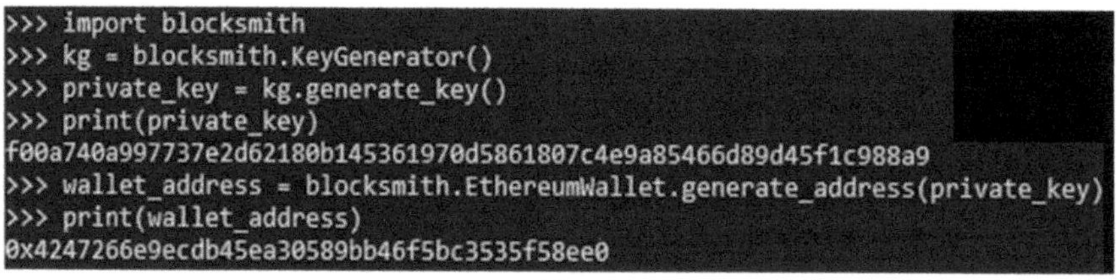
>>> import blocksmith
>>> kg = blocksmith.KeyGenerator()
>>> private_key = kg.generate_key()
>>> print(private_key)
f00a740a997737e2d62180b145361970d5861807c4e9a85466d89d45f1c988a9
>>> wallet_address = blocksmith.EthereumWallet.generate_address(private_key)
>>> print(wallet_address)
0x4247266e9ecdb45ea30589bb46f5bc3535f58ee0

(a)

Enter message: 73845023 Agya Satna 4783954 A
Encrypted: ((191583671121985594749303764087250856719201629171369335003480771344000749736 8, 1),
b'\xc9\x1bg\x9b\x9f\x13yr\xc9\x829\xf7\xb8\xb5ia\xae\xb0\x81\xd2\xf1\x95=\xab\xe5\xaepFq')
Decrypted: 73845023 Agya Satna 4783954 A

(b)

FIGURE 10.4
(a) Generation of private and public key. (b) Encrypted message.

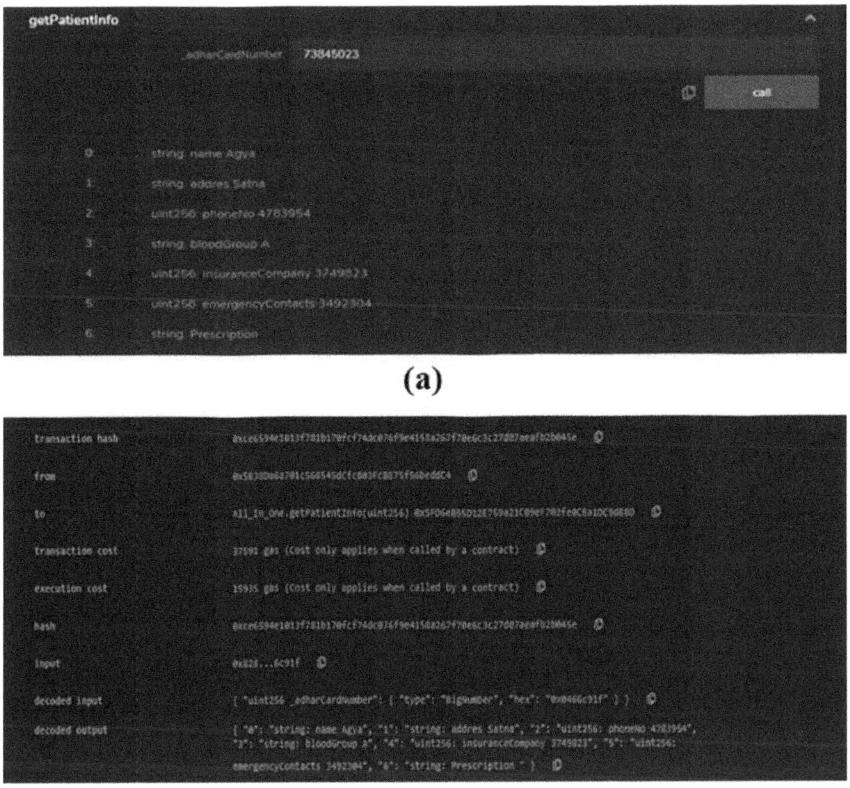

(a)

(b)

FIGURE 10.5
(a) Query using Adhar card no. (b) Decoded input and output.

10.3.5 The *addIPFSAddress* Method

This method is used to add the encrypted hashed IPFS addresses of medical records to the blockchain (Figure 10.6).

10.3.6 The *getIPFSAddress* Method

The *getIPFSAddress* method is utilized in accessing the encrypted hashed IPFS address of a medical record, in order to be able to view its content (Figure 10.7).

10.3.7 The *updatePrescription* Method

This method is used to update a patient's prescription after a chemist gives a patient the required medication (Figure 10.8).

10.3.8 The *addTreatmentDetails* Method

Creating and adding a new treatment to the blockchain with the address of the doctor and the patient (Figure 10.9).

(a)

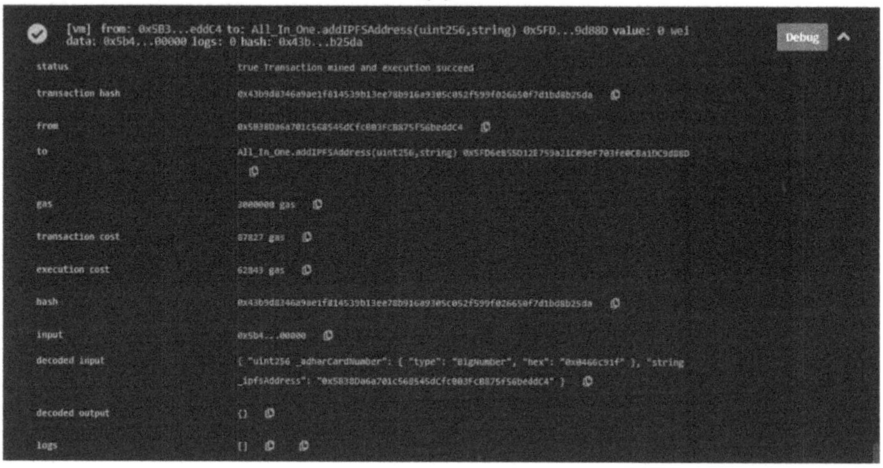

(b)

FIGURE 10.6
(a) Add the encrypted hashed IPFS. (b) Result after addition of data.

10.3.9 The *getTreatmentDetails* Method

This method is utilized to access the data regarding a patient's treatment, querying using the treatment ID defined when a doctor treats a patient (Figure 10.10).

10.3.10 The *addDoctor* Method

The *addDoctor* method is used to enter a doctor's details while registering them onto the system, before authentication by authorized personnel (Figure 10.11).

10.3.11 The *requestAccessToPatient* Method

A doctor, upon requiring access to the data of the patient they are treating, uses the *requestAccessToPatient* method to get that data. Only after the patient has verified the doctor's credentials do we use the CP-ABE scheme to add the doctor's attributes to the patient's data's encryption scheme. After this is done, the doctor may access a patient's data (Figure 10.12).

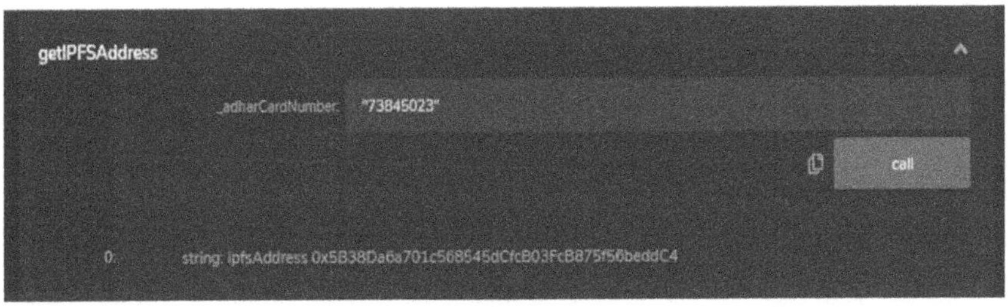

(a)

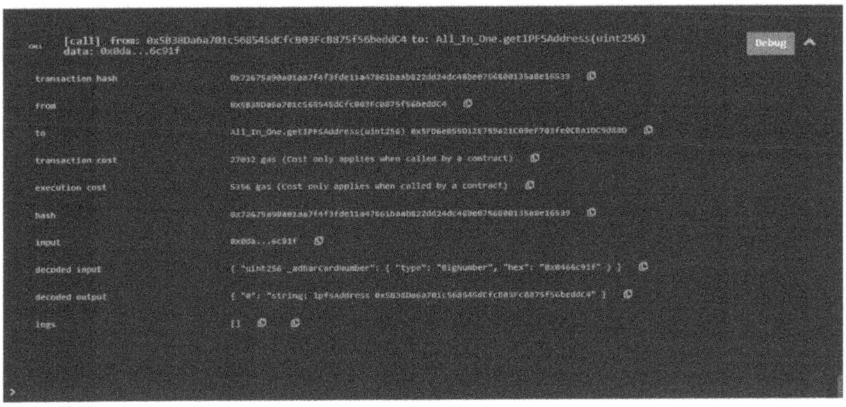

(b)

FIGURE 10.7
(a) *getIPFSAddress* method. (b) Encrypted hashed IPFS address of a medical record.

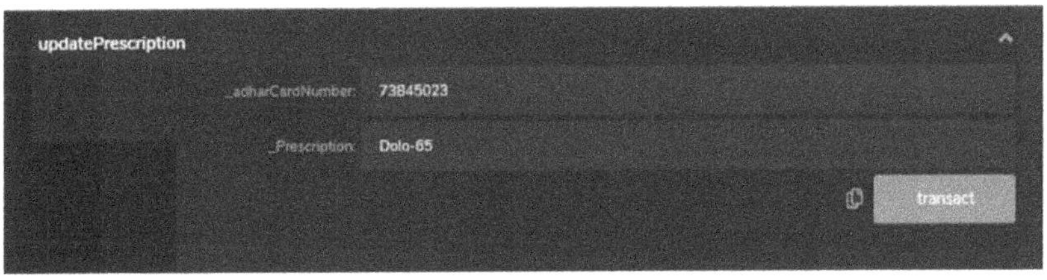

(a)

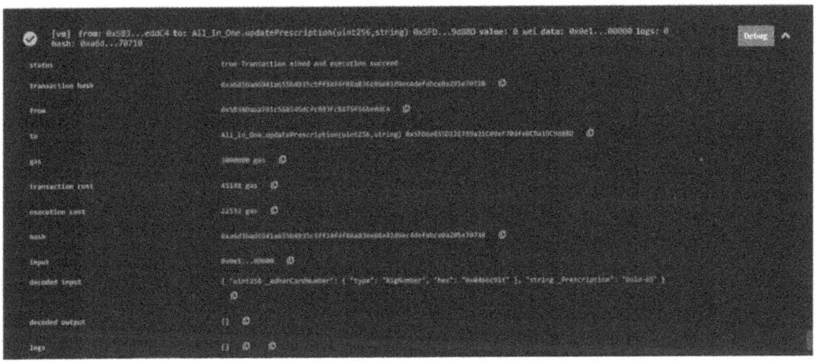

(b)

FIGURE 10.8
(a) Update a patient's prescription. (b) Records after update.

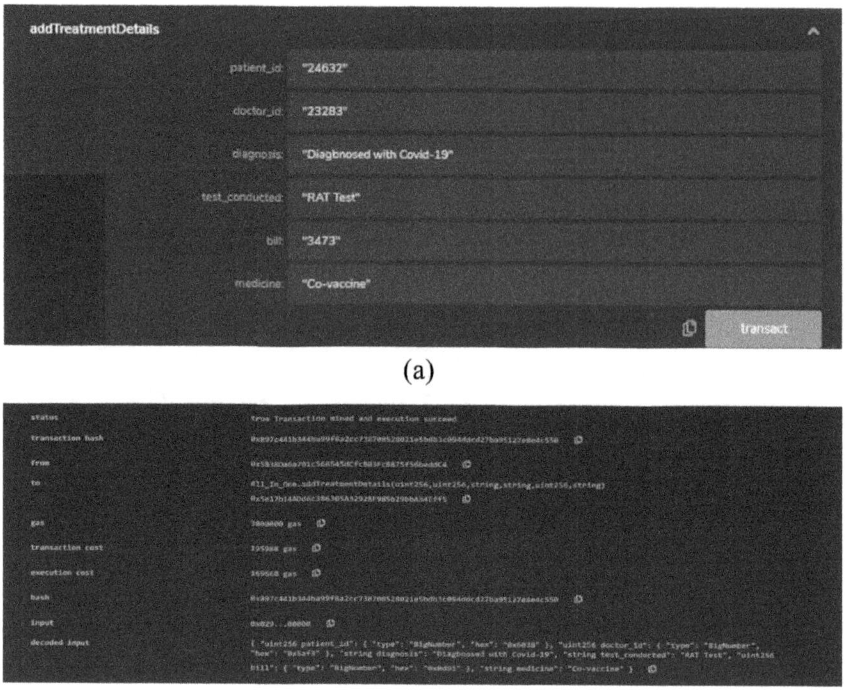

(a)

(b)

FIGURE 10.9
(a) Process of *addTreatmentDetails*. (b) Records after adding treatment details

10.3.12 The *addTreatmentDetails* Method

After having treated a patient, a doctor is to use the *addTreatmentDetails* method to add to the patient's database the details of the treatment they underwent. Once again, the data will only be added once the patient has verified it (Figure 10.13).

10.3.13 The *addChemistInfo* Method

A pharmacy will register onto our system using the *addChemistInfo* method. Their credentials will be verified by a board set up for the same purpose before adding them as suppliers onto our system (Figure 10.14).

10.3.14 System Testing

The decentralized blockchain application built has been tested on several use cases, covering all aspects of user interaction alongside several corner cases. All the functionalities and modules designed have been thoroughly tested and executed with a variety of different parameters and interactions and the system has been found to run successfully and seamlessly on all varied sets of input parameters.

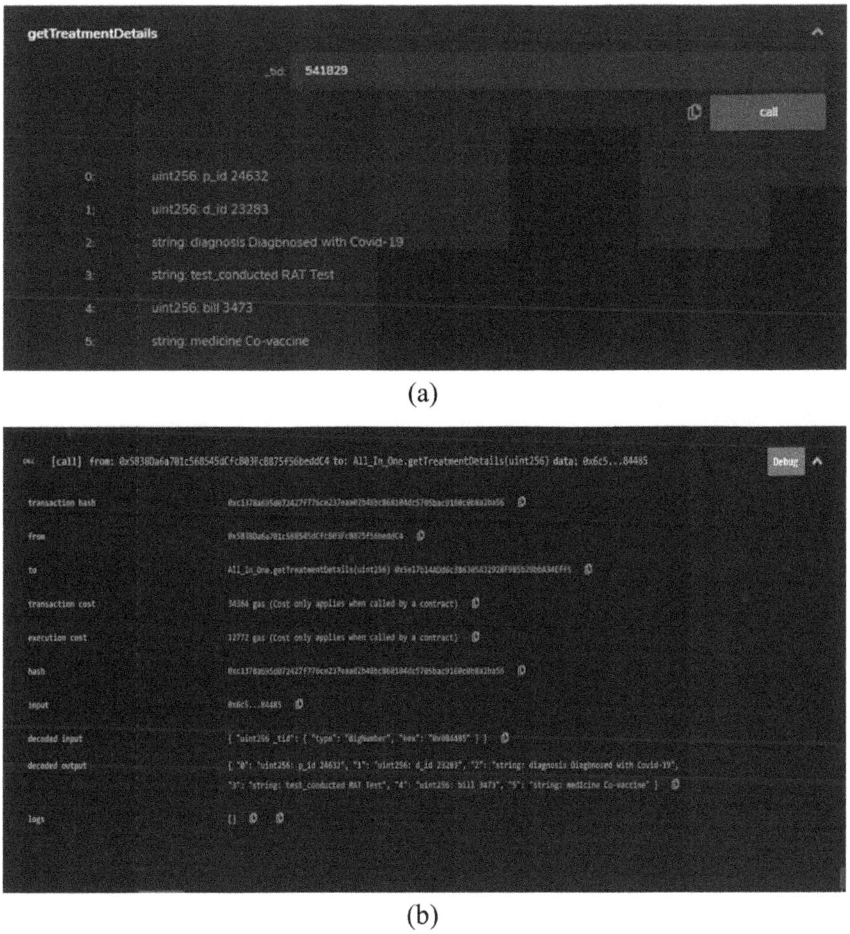

FIGURE 10.10
(a) Querying using the treatment ID. (b) *getTreatmentDetails.*

10.4 Discussions

This section describes the several limitations of the proposed system and also elaborates on areas of future research and similar open research topics that would prove significant in the actual up-scaled realization of the system.

The data encryption method used, the CP-ABE, is not a very popular data security algorithm and as such, there has not been a lot of research done that points out its flaws or measures its effectiveness. An incapacity of the system is that it includes no means to verify the credibility of a client registering as a doctor in the blockchain network. As such, any unverified node can end up being a part of the system.

One major limitation of the architecture is the heavy dependability on the IPFS system. Since a majority of the data are stored "off-chain" on the IPFS, the system crashes if there is a problem with the IPFS network/server.

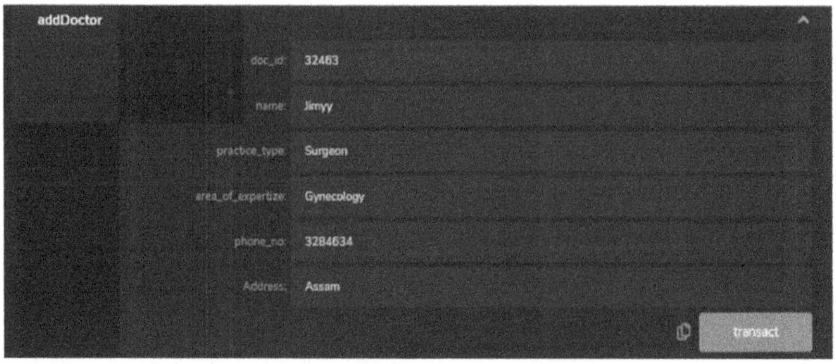

(a)

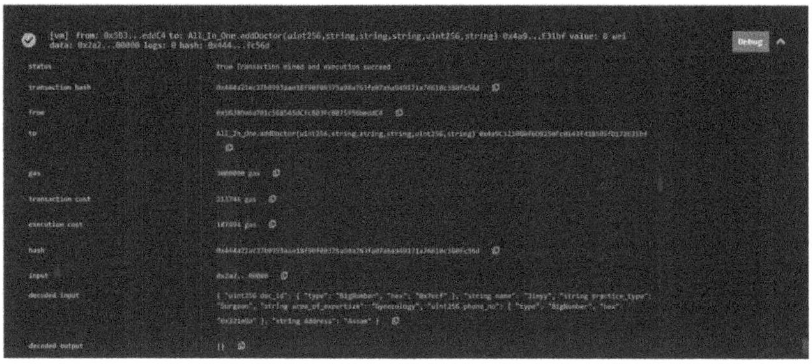

(b)

FIGURE 10.11
(a) *addDoctor*. (b) Decoded output.

(a)

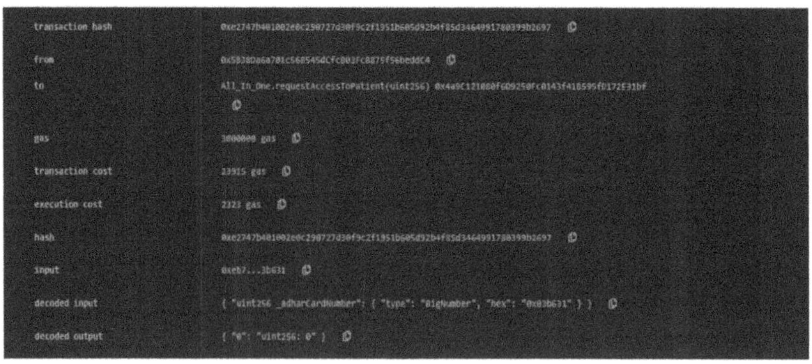

(b)

FIGURE 10.12
(a) *requestAccessToPatient*. (b) Accessing patient data.

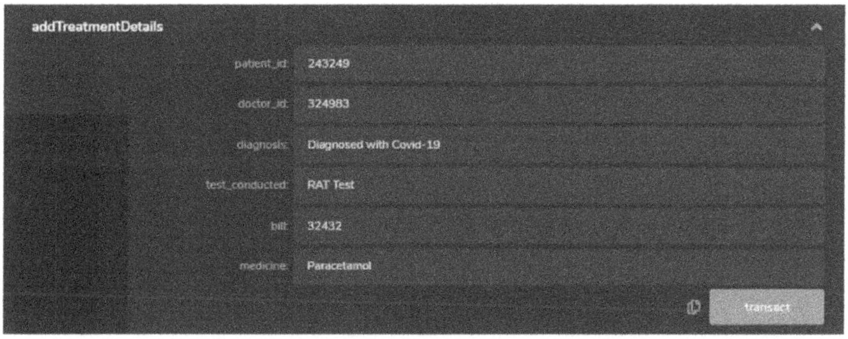

(a)

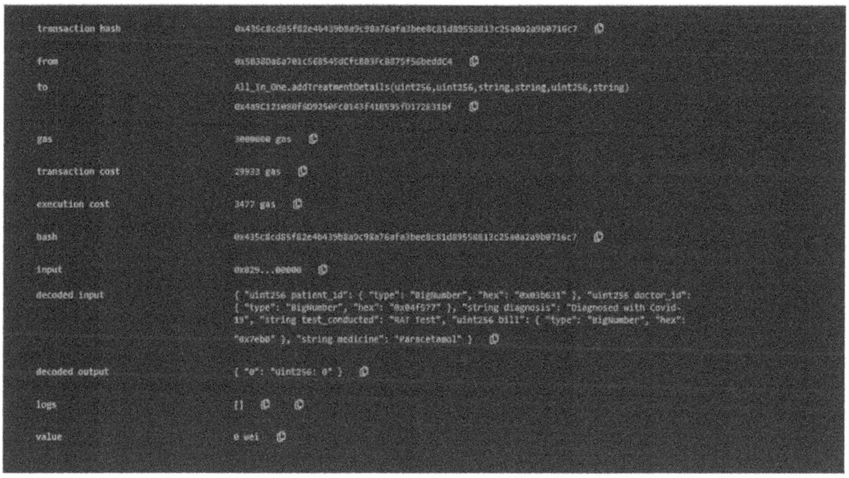

(b)

FIGURE 10.13
(a) Add to the patient database. (b) Decoded input and output of add record.

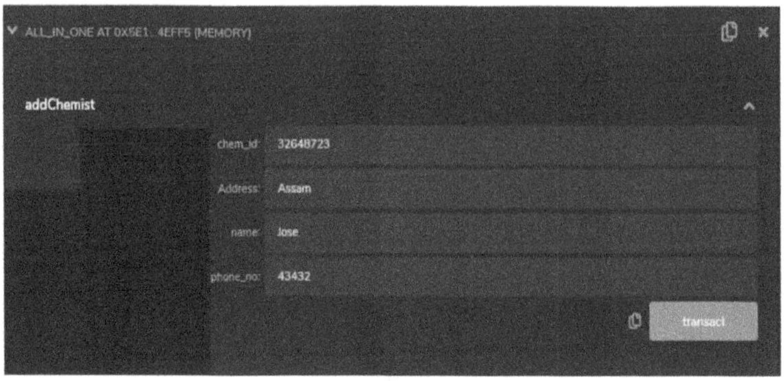

(a)

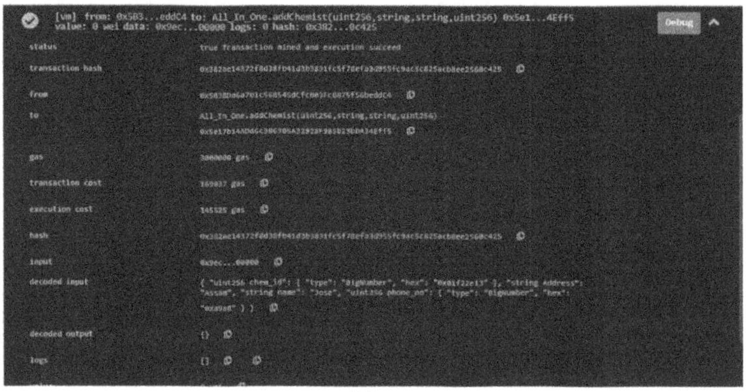

(b)

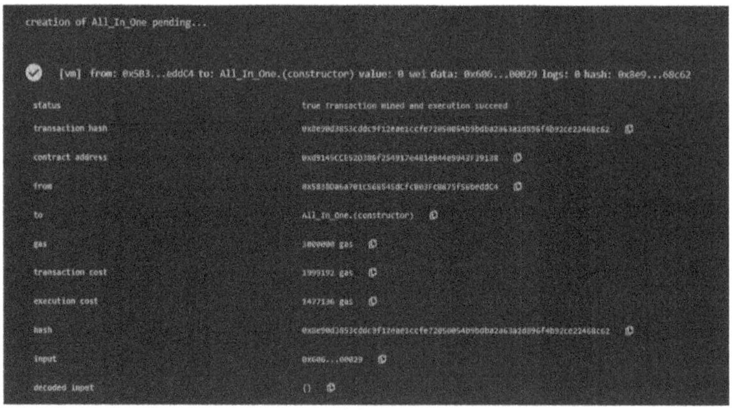

(c)

FIGURE 10.14
(a) Add chemist details. (b) Verification of credentials. (c) Data added to the system.

10.5 Conclusion

This work is based on blockchain-based EMRs which makes it faster and more convenient for both patients and doctors to be able to interact for all sorts of medical aids. The system uses blockchain-embedded technologies like Ethereum and IPFS and includes security-enforcing methods like data encryption and the use of public and private keys by the network clients.

References

1. Nakamoto, S. (2008). Bitcoin: A Peer-to-Peer Electronic Cash System. Retrieved from https://bitcoin.org/bitcoin.pdf.
2. Hussien, HM, Yasin, SM, Udzir, SNI, Zaidan, AA and Zaidan, BB. (2019). A Systematic Review for Enabling of Develop a Blockchain Technology in Healthcare Application: Taxonomy, Substantially Analysis, Motivations, Challenges, Recommendations and Future Direction. *J Med Syst*. 43(10), 320. doi:10.1007/s10916-019-1445-8. PMID:31522262.
3. Agbo, CC, Mahmoud, QH and Eklund, JM. (2019). Blockchain Technology in Healthcare: A Systematic Review. *Healthcare* 7(2), 56. doi:10.3390/healthcare7020056.
4. Zhou, L, Wang, L and Sun, Y. MIStore. (2018). A Blockchain-Based Medical Insurance Storage System. *J. Med. Syst.* 42, 149.
5. Ahram, T, Sargolzaei, A, Sargolzaei, S, Daniels, J and Amaba, B. (2017). Blockchain Technology Innovations. In Proceedings of the 2017 IEEE Technology & Engineering Management Conference (TEMSCON), Santa Clara, CA, USA, 8–10 June 2017; 137–141.
6. Dagher, GG, Mohler, J, Milojkovic, M, Marella, PB and Marella, B. (2018). Ancile: Privacy-Preserving Framework for Access Control and Interoperability of Electronic Health Records Using Blockchain Technology. *Sustain. Cities Soc.* 39, 283–297.
7. Azaria, A, Ekblaw, A, Vieira, T and Lippman, A. (2016). MedRec: Using Blockchain for Medical Data Access and Permission Management. In Proceedings of the 2016 2nd International Conference on Open and Big Data (OBD), Vienna, Austria, 22–24 August 2016; 25–30.
8. Fan, K, Wang, S, Ren, Y, Li, H and Yang, Y. (2018). MedBlock: Efficient and Secure Medical Data Sharing Via Blockchain. *J. Med Syst* 42, 136.
9. Saravanan, M, Shubha, R, Marks, AM and Iyer, V. (2017). SMEAD: A Secured Mobile Enabled Assisting Device for Diabetics Monitoring. In Proceedings of the 2017 IEEE International Conference on Advanced Networks and Telecommunications Systems (ANTS), Odisha, India, 17–20 December 2017; 1–6.
10. Buterin, V. Ethereum White Paper, A Next Generation Smart Contract & Decentralized Application Platform.
11. *Smart Contracts*. BlockchainHub. (2020), December 10. Retrieved from http://blockchainhub.net/smart-contracts/.
12. Benet, J., IPFS: Content Addressed, Versioned, P2P File System. Retrieved from https://ipfs.io/ipfs/ QmR7GSQM93Cx5eAg6a6yRzNde1FQv7uL6X1o4k7zrJa3LX/ ipfs.draft3.pdf.
13. Waters, B. (2011). Ciphertext-Policy Attribute-Based Encryption: An Expressive, Efficient, and Provably Secure Realization. In: D Catalano, N Fazio, R Gennaro and A Nicolosi (eds) *Public Key Cryptography – PKC 2011*. PKC 2011. Lecture Notes in Computer Science, vol. 6571. Springer, Berlin, Heidelberg. doi:10.1007/978-3-642-19379-8_4
14. Retrieved 31 May 2021, from http://truffle.readthecodes.io/
15. Metamask.io. (2021). *MetaMask*. [online] Retrieved from http://metamask.io/ [Accessed 31 May 2021].

11

Managing Health Insurance Using Blockchain Technology

Muralidhar Kurni and Mrunalini M

CONTENTS

DOI: 10.1201/9781003133179-11

11.1 Introduction

During the second decade of the 21st century, we saw rapid technological advancement take place at unmatched speed. In only ten years, a tremendous part of human life was digitized. This changed every industry on the planet. The insurance business was no different (ScaleFocus, 2108). The insurance business is moving to another plan of action by adjusting to trendsetting innovation (Hernandez, 2020). Advanced insurance technology is now an indispensable part of the Property and Casualty Insurance (P&C) industry, for both transporters and the insured. Getting a quote for insurance is as simple as clicking a button; managing coverage can regularly be accessed through a mobile app and paper insurance documents are almost gone. Insurance technology is ready to develop considerably more in the coming years. While a portion of these tools is now utilized by certain carriers, we see them turning out to be increasingly more common in the industry (Wargin, 2020).

Let's investigate the top trends that are molding the insurance industry and how blockchain is changing the business (WNS Global Services, 2018).

1. ***Trend 1.*** New models, personalized products—usage-based, on-request, "across the board," small scale and shared protection will turn out to be increasingly common.
2. ***Trend 2.*** AI and automation for faster claims—bots, fueled by artificial intelligence and robotic process automation, will mechanize strategy adjusting and guarantee executives quicker and customized client assistance.
3. ***Trend 3.*** Advanced analytics and proactiveness—insurers will use cutting edge information investigation to assemble granular individual hazard profiles, offer precise estimating and model practices and distinguish special cases.
4. ***Trend 4.*** InsurTech partnerships—mainstream safety net providers will purchase or tie up with InsurTech organizations to reconsider plans of action, help benefit and upgrade the client experience.
5. ***Trend 5.*** Mainstreaming blockchain—blockchain will encourage continuous client information, preparing for the vigorous approach of executives, spanning endorsing, approvals, claims handling and extortion location.

Indeed! The blockchain will be one of the most impressive innovation patterns to reform the insurance industry in the coming years (Mrunalini & D, 2020; Kumari et al., 2020). The requirement for colossal volumes of client information to be handled continuously by various insurance functions calls for a simple and secure exchange of information across associations and their different partners. Blockchain innovation gives the benefit of secure information across the board over different interfaces and partners without loss of quality. From identity management and endorsement to claims handling, misrepresentation of the executives and dependable information accessibility, the innovation offers decreased operational expenses. Decentralized Autonomous Organizations (DAOs) and smart agreements are extra advantages that blockchain can offer executives (WNS Global Services, 2018).

The blend of blockchain and insurance isn't just the subject of conversation but is also the high purpose of discussion among financial specialists, innovation suppliers and insurance providers. There are numerous reasons which make blockchain a subject of conversation. Each exchange in the blockchain is timestamped, making it simple for everyone in the framework to follow the root and goal. Every one of these highlights makes blockchain an appealing innovation. It additionally shapes the reason for different applications, which is another advantage (Sharma, 2018; Tropea, 2019).

11.1.1 Insurance Applications for Blockchain Technology

1. ***Property and loss protection***: Property and loss protection comprises principally of auto, business and home protection. Handling claims requires considerable manual intervention, which leaves space for human error. Blockchain innovation could make claims forms multiple times quicker and multiple times less expensive utilizing blockchain technology. By utilizing shared records and smart contracts (programming that checks for specific exchanges in the system and consequently executes activities dependent on predetermined conditions being met) to deliver insurance arrangements, the cases and installment procedures can be robotized to make them more proficient and accurate. Smart contracts can transform paper contracts into programmable code that mechanizes claims handling.
2. ***Medical coverage***: The healthcare coverage industry is full of inefficient aspects in its procedures, such as copied clinical records, a manual claims procedure and erroneous recordkeeping. There's a lot to be improved in terms of proficiency and accuracy. Along these lines, the interoperability of frameworks and gadgets is essential to guarantee that clinical experts give adequate consideration to patients, however, effectively accomplishing interoperability inside a clinical framework isn't simple. With blockchain, clinical records are cryptographically encoded and shared among wellbeing suppliers, advancing interoperability and expanded security inside the medical coverage biological system. Understanding clinical records can be stored securely and control of clinical information returned to patients, allows the business the chance to save cash and increase patient satisfaction.
3. ***Misrepresentation identification and risk mitigation***: An incomplete understanding of insurance business procedures leaves space for error and possible extortion. To combat this, insurance agencies could store claims data on a record that would assist them with conveying and recognizing dubious conduct.
4. ***Accident insurance***: There are two different ways through which blockchain can end up being valuable for the collision insurance industry. To begin with, it can interface all the clients and specialist organizations; with the assistance of a shared record, all the data will be readily accessible. It will help the auto safety providers in reducing risk and extortion. Second, with the assistance of smart contracts, the claim will fasten up.
5. ***Life coverage industry***: Life protection may sound like a simple procedure. Be that as it may, getting a policy from the insurance agency is an onerous task. It makes you face a succession of inquiries, a mass of paperwork and causes you to invest your time, cash and energy. Be that as it may, with the assistance of blockchain, we can expect some help here. By making a consortium of clinical offices, government organizations and so forth, one can get all the data without any problem. Also, insurance agencies can utilize smart contracts to give programmed pay-outs to clinical offices and different recipients.

The inbuilt highlights of blockchain offer a range of advantages such as restrictions to the insurance agencies, which incorporate the following (Tropea, 2019).

11.1.2 Advantages

- ***Enhances productivity***—because such a significant number of procedures are manual and tedious, blockchain can smooth out desk work for protection contracts.
- ***Increases trust***—cryptography in blockchain guarantees that exchanges are secure, validated and irrefutable, guaranteeing client protection.
- ***Claims preparation***—blockchain empowers ongoing information analysis and investigation, which could fundamentally accelerate claims handling and pay-outs.
- ***Smart contracts***—these agreements contain a method of reasoning that is consequently executed when conditions that were previously defined are met. "Since these contracts reduce administrative work, they will end up being what being could be compared to automated aircraft," said Jeff Stollman, Principal Consultant at Rocky Mountain Technical Marketing. "They will be easy to control and less expensive than increasingly substantial approaches, and installment can be quick."

11.1.3 Constraints

- ***Prone to digital assaults***—the worldwide blockchain network is expected to be worth US$20 billion in 2024. With such a significant number of new clients, blockchain is becoming progressively susceptible to digital assaults.
- ***Loss of respectability of information***—integrity of information must think about the legitimacy of each exchange, which brings fake exchanges into question. Blockchain must protect against false action to guarantee the trustworthiness of the information.
- ***Cost of tasks***—as blockchain becomes increasingly well known, it will turn out to be progressively costly for insurance agencies to receive this innovation by regular means.
- ***Blockchain protection***—in digital currency (like bitcoin), blockchain is freely accessible, which implies each exchange can be followed back to its unique source. That data can be accessed by criminals hoping to abuse that data.

11.2 Background of the Insurance Sector

11.2.1 Current Insurance Sector

11.2.1.1 What It Specifies

Insurance is an understanding that insures an individual, organization or other entity against loss of cash (Means et al., 2020). Insurance strategy specifies that the organization consents to remunerate the safeguarded individual (or other elements) for expected future misfortunes in such categories as wellbeing, home or vehicle, in return for the standard installment of expenses called premiums.

The purpose behind insurance is to secure the monetary prosperity of an individual, organization or other entity on account of an unexpected misfortune, for example, damage to a structure or the loss of wellbeing because of sickness or injury (Means et al., 2020). State and central governments can command that a few kinds of insurance, for example, accident coverage, be held; different kinds are discretionary.

Any risk that can be evaluated in some way no doubt has a sort of insurance to secure it. The most widely recognized categories of insurance are medical, vehicle, home and life security (Means et al., 2020). When the guaranteed policyholder pays the premium amount, medical protection will give the policyholder monetary help (for the most part the full or half the cost of specialist, emergency clinic and pharmaceutical charges identified with clinical consideration) if clinical treatment for a disease or injury is required. Collision protection offers monetary help in case of a car accident that harms the vehicle of the policyholder or of another person. Life coverage ensures payment to the recipients if the insured individual dies.

At the point when an insured individual or organization endures a misfortune, they record a claim to the insurer for measuring the loss (Means et al., 2020). At the point when the insurance agency repays the insured (or simply pays for the charges), the repayment comes out of a fund into which numerous policyholders have contributed premiums. That way, in the event of an individual's misfortune, the weight of paying the claim amount is distributed among numerous insurance agencies and doesn't impact on the individual or entity that has suffered a misfortune. The test for insurance agencies is to save enough cash for foreseen misfortunes with the goal that they provide benefits, because anything that remains over is called the edge.

Different insurance policies set up various terms of understanding (Means et al., 2020). Commonly, a policy will express the costs of the protected individual's premiums, how often they should be paid, who ought to benefit if the insured dies, what sorts of misfortune are secured and the timespan of the insurance cover and how much the organization will repay. Policies normally express that the policyholder is responsible for paying a portion of the claim, known as a deductible and that the insurance provider will pay what remains.

11.2.1.2 Types of Insurance Companies

Not all insurance agencies have the same plans for the same type of clients. Accident and health are among the largest categories for insurance agencies to work with; property and accident insurance providers; and monetary underwriters (Beers, 2019). The most well-known sorts of individual insurance arrangements are automobile, health, mortgage holders and life. Most people have one of these kinds of protection, and vehicle insurance is legally necessary.

Accident and health companies are likely the most notable, which are intended to help individuals who have been truly hurt. Life coverage organizations for the most part issue approaches that pay a death benefit as a singular amount upon the death of the guaranteed to their recipients. Life insurance policies might be sold as life terms, which is more affordable and terminates at the finish of the term or perpetual (entire life or general life), which is progressively costly yet endures forever and conveys a money accumulating element. Life insurance providers may likewise sell long-term disability insurance that guarantees the safeguarded salary in case they die or become disabled. Companies involved in property and loss safeguard the individual against misfortune of a non-physical nature. This can incorporate claim lawsuits, harm to individual resources, vehicle accidents and more.

Organizations are required to come up with exceptional insurance schemes that guarantee specific businesses against explicit kinds of danger. For example, a drive-through joint needs a scheme that takes care of it in case of an injury that might occur because of cooking with a fryer. An automobile seller doesn't require the above-mentioned policy yet will include it for the injury that could happen during test drives. There are, additionally, insurance schemes for specific necessities, for example, kidnap and ransom (K&R), clinical misbehavior and expert risk insurance and oversights insurance.

A few organizations take reinsurance to decrease hazards. Reinsurance protects the insurance agency against extreme misfortune because of the large number of claims at any one time. Reinsurance forms a fundamental part of insurance agencies' attempt to keep themselves afloat and to avoid losses due to pay-outs to companies and individuals.

11.2.1.3 Insurance Outlook for 2020 and Beyond

As guarantors adjust to new plans of action, client categories and innovation, the business's best days are ahead. Gone are the days when guarantors depended on just one channel to rovide cover. From insurance providers/agents to online media, these will be used to build up money-related education and security. All things considered, keep an eye out for insurance challenges. Shoppers are maturing and it's imperative to examine what their definite needs are to give tailored arrangements. This ought to likewise prepare for more client-driven encounters. Lastly, the cutting-edge innovation usually alluded to as the "disruptor," will be the empowering influence of development once it's embedded into better-than-ever insurance policy. Obviously, there will consistently be snags, yet we ought not expect to follow the business's old ways, the main way we're going is forward (Hernandez, 2020).

11.2.2 Rip-Offs in the Insurance Sector

Insurance should be a decent field, yet in all honesty, it once in a while takes after the much censured used vehicle business. In the two ventures, it's normal for forceful sales reps to pressure buyers into making inappropriate purchases. When taking out insurance, the conviction is that, as you are paying your monthly premium, you won't have to stress over any of the unanticipated circumstances in which you should utilize your policy. This is the thing that insurance is intended to do, all things considered. In reality, insurance agencies will do whatever they can to figure out how to avoid responsibility while overcharging their clients with high rates and some other strategy to take cash without accepting later liability.

Here are the most widely recognized ways you're getting overcharged by insurance companies (Brown, 2020):

1. ***Pointless travel insurance***: Every year, individuals burn through billions on travel insurance and once in a while it is even added to the final bill for their vacation. Trip specialists push to sell the travel insurance with accounts of lost luggage, canceled flights, etc., however, what they won't let you in on is that you may be secured by your mortgage holder's protection on charge cards, or the airline might be liable as a component of their legitimate commitments. The operator may likewise inform protection while at the same time having almost no genuine consideration about the way that your excursion will turn out.

2. ***Home insurance: Flood and wind***: After major climate events, property holders with policies try to claim for damage that was caused by the wind, yet the insurance agencies attempt to blame the damage on flooding—and flooding isn't secured by the policy holder's insurance. It has likewise been said that the representatives of the organizations are urged to think little of the cost of the claim with the goal that the organization won't need to pay what they ought to be on risk for.
3. ***Extra security settlements***: Extra security specialists have no motivation to get you the best arrangement when you choose to shop around for your disaster insurance to save some money and might be attempting to keep the purchaser of the approach upbeat. Although the agent will have their bonus in mind, they are ultimately not paying particular attention to you
4. ***Vehicle insurance and lowball offers***: If your vehicle is viewed as a write-off, your insurance policy may cover the value or even pay for a replacement. The insurance agency could attempt to offer a radically low sum while downplaying the vehicle's real condition. Furthermore, they may attempt to lower the estimation of the vehicle by utilizing one that is viewed as equivalent, but has an considerably higher mileage. Insurance agencies would appear to disregard your lower mileage to reduce the real estimation of the vehicle.
5. ***Whole life insurance as a "venture"***: Numerous specialists will push for whole life coverage as it tends to be viewed as a venture. The option in contrast to this is having term life coverage and taking care of your additional money as speculation. The merchants gain commission for selling these costly whole life policies. The more the client pays, the more profit the insurance specialist makes. This is their motivation to push for comprehensive protection and sell it as a picture of investment.
6. ***Medical coverage***: Sadly, lots of individuals feel that they have adequate medical coverage, however ordinarily the wellbeing specialist organization and the insurance agency will differ that the cases are legitimate. The client gets stuck between it and will end up covering a bill that is a lot larger than initially anticipated.

Here are the most well-known ways medical coverage organizations scam you (Hamer, 2018; Komarovsky, 2016).

i. *Denying claims*: Insurance agencies will pay for one test and overlook the other one, for which you will get a bill if you don't consider it an error and contest it with your doctor's finance office.
ii. *Changing coverage with little notice*: One of the most widely recognized grievances buyers have about medical coverage organizations ripping them off is an absence of notice for changes in coverage. In reality, organizations are required to inform you of changes, however, that doesn't mean the clarification is in every case clear. In a similar vein, insurance plans can likewise exclude certain medicines. Exclusions—like elective medication—are likely specified in your policy, yet the detail is in the fine print and loaded with language intended to confuse.
iii. *Employing out-of-network services*: The way that those secured by insurance must use out-of-organization services appears to be illogical. However, on the off-chance that you have a crisis during a vacation, or change occupations (and, in this way, insurance provider), you could be hit with out-of-arrangement costs you

never knew existed. Insurance agencies just settle on cost concurrences with specific doctors. Be cautious when seeing specialists in another state, or arranging meetings with nearby specialists not effectively "associated" with your insurer.

iv. *Sneaking in unnecessary hidden fees*: Your health insurance plan has been ripping off you and your boss with concealed expenses for a considerable length of time under categories such as, "supplier organization charges," "possibility expenses," "retiree overcharges," "out-of-policy appropriation expenses" and so forth.

v. *Over-inflating the costs of prescription drug service*: Many expect that paying a premium for a medicine-inclusive plan implies they'll naturally get the best costs. Lamentably, that doesn't generally occur as there are no set expenses for solutions. It is discovered that medications could cost up to many times more at one retailer than at another. Along these lines, it'd be shrewd to think about costs and arrange your prescriptions at numerous stores to stay away from such expensive tricks.

vi. *Committing billing "errors"*: Charging blunders are uncontrolled in the medical services industry—and they're not generally solved by the supplier. Upcoding, unbundling and double charging are for the most part basic ways medical coverage suppliers can control the coding framework to make you pay more for administration.

11.2.3 Types of Insurance Fraud

Insurance fraud is the most polished extortion on the planet. The insurance business, by its very nature, is vulnerable to misrepresentation. Insurance is a risk appropriation framework that requires the amassing of liquid resources as supports that are, thus, accessible to pay insurance claims. Insurance agencies amass a huge, consistent turnover of money through insurance premiums. Consistent income is a significant financial asset that is alluring and effectively maintained. Huge accumulation of liquid resources make insurance agencies attractive for fraudulent plans. Insurance agencies are under tremendous pressure to obtain the highest possible returns on the reserve fund investment, consequently making them defenseless against high yielding speculation plans (ACFE, 2018).

11.2.3.1 What Is Insurance Fraud?

Insurance extortion is an illicit follow-up on the part of either the purchaser or merchant of an insurance contract. Extortion from the guarantor (merchant) incorporates selling strategies from non-existent organizations, neglecting to submit premiums and menacing approaches to make more commissions. Purchaser extortion can comprise of overstated cases, adulterated clinical history, post-dated approaches, vertical misrepresentation, faked death or kidnap and murder (Chen, 2019).

11.2.3.2 How Does Insurance Fraud Work?

Insurance fraud is an attempt to misuse a contract (Chen, 2019). Insurance is intended to protect against loss, acting as a vehicle to benefit the insured. Although fraud happens, most cases have to do with the policyholder trying to get more cash by overstating a case. Extreme cases, for example, faking death or committing murder for the cash claim, are relatively uncommon.

11.2.3.3 Hard vs. Soft Fraud

Insurance fraud extortion can be called either hard or soft (ACFE, 2018). A hard fraud happens when a mishap, injury or robbery is thought up or planned to acquire cash from insurance agencies. At the point when a real misfortune happens, for example, the burglary of a mobile phone, and the insured adds something to the claim (e.g., a phone accessory) to cover the excess, it is viewed as a soft fraud. Soft fraud occurs when an authentic case is overstated.

11.2.3.4 Phases of Insurance Fraud

Fraud can happen at any phase of the insurance process by any of the following (ACFE, 2018):

- Application by individuals for insurance.
- Policyholders.
- Third-party claims.
- Middlemen.

11.2.3.5 Types of Insurance Frauds

Here are the five most common kinds of fraud in insurance.

1. ***Life insurance fraud***: Insurance fraud, when all is said in done, includes making bogus, misdirecting or deceptive explanations for the motivations behind inappropriately obtaining assets from an insurance agency (Sachon, 2018).

   The least difficult type of extra security extortion includes lying on an application for an insurance policy. On the off-chance that you cover genuine ailments for the purpose of meeting all requirements for a policy you wouldn't otherwise get, the insurance provider can deny the guaranteed death benefit when you die. If the misdirection is recognized before your death, the arrangement will be canceled. You could face indictment for extortion under these conditions; however, this sort of "delicate misrepresentation" probably isn't going to trigger similarly severe penalties from different kinds of life coverage extortion.

   While many insurance companies believe that stranger-directed life insurance is a scam, legislation is all over the place about whether it is illegal. Life insurance policies for the elderly focused on strangers are made available for purchase when sold to investors or hedge funds. People who are involved in the transaction are given a fee as a reward for it. A civil suit by the life insurance company is a possibility, as are criminal charges for all parties involved depending on the state's laws. People who fail to report the profit they made from selling something, unaware they are involved in a criminal act, could be charged with fraud.

   Some disaster protection misrepresentation tricks include extra security specialists who misuse customer premiums instead of buying life coverage or who advertise arrangements to individuals (typically seniors) that are inappropriate for their requirements.

   At last, faking death or disability, or causing the death of another person are significantly more serious offenses than other sorts of frauds. Both include complex plots, and both can trigger state or government charges that can prompt a lengthy jail sentence.

2. ***Healthcare fraud or health insurance fraud***: When a policyholder or a company tries to claim insurance by providing false information regarding health issues to the insurance company to gain a higher payout than what seems appropriate, this in turn will be a gain for the policy holder, third party or any other service provider. The offense can be committed at an individual or organizational level (PA Insurance Fraud Prevention Authority, 2020b).

   An individual supporter can submit medical coverage misrepresentation by:

   - Allowing another person to utilize their identity and insurance policy to acquire services.
   - Using advantages to pay for medicines that were not endorsed by their PCP.

   Social insurance suppliers can submit false acts by:

   - Monetary charges for services or supplies that were never given.
   - Charging more for administration facilities than were given.
   - Performing pointless administrations with the end goal of monetary benefit.
   - Misrepresenting non-secured medicines as a clinical need.
   - Falsifying a patient's results to legitimize tests, surgeries or different procedures.
   - Billing each stage of a treatment as though it were a different strategy.
   - Charging a patient more than the insurance terms.
   - Paying "payoffs" for referral of motor vehicle accident casualties for treatment.

3. ***Automobile insurance fraud***: This sort of misrepresentation involves somebody misleading an insurance agency about a case including their own or business vehicle. It can include giving out deceiving data or giving bogus documentation to help the case (PA Insurance Fraud Prevention Authority, 2020a).

   Accident protection misrepresentation can be divided into three significant classifications. In an extortion, an individual petitioner utilizes a real accident as a chance to create illegitimate benefits by purposely exaggerating the degree of harm caused by the accident. A fraudster submits a claim overcharging for the recovery transporte, increases the expenses of products and services required for vehicle repairs as well as for medical costs. In any case, the third kind of collision insurance misrepresentation, the planned claim, causes vehicle insurers the largest number of fraudulent claims, including, for instance, prearranged vehicle crashes and so forth.

4. ***Property insurance fraud***: Mortgage holders' protection misrepresentation or property protection extortion might be submitted against a property holder's insurance provider or a leaseholder's back-up plan (NY Criminal Defense, 2020). Property holders' and tenants' policies have subtle specific inclusion impediments. Mortgage holders and tenants likewise have a deductible that must be paid before a policy pays out on a claim.

   Whenever a property holder tries to avoid the necessary deductible, acquire inclusion that ought not to be secured or get a more higher valuation for remuneration than is covered by the policy, this is characterized as home insurance misrepresentation.

The misrepresentation ascends to the criminal level when an endeavor is made to misuse any assets from a guarantor. The insurance extortion shouldn't be beneficial at all for an individual who engineered the misrepresentation to face criminal indictment. Any individual engaged with any part of a property insurance extortion plan may likewise be accused of every criminal activity perpetrated by co-conspirators.

5. ***Workers' compensation fraud***: Workers' remuneration is insurance that pays for medical costs and compensation substitution if a representative is harmed or acquires an ailment at work. Be that as it may, the disease can't occur naturally or happen or a result of the worker breaching business procedures. Workers' compensation misrepresentation can come in a wide range of structures (NY Criminal Defense, 2020). Workers' compensation fraud is any falsehood or distortion made by a business, worker or supplier to profit monetarily. One to two percent of all specialists' remuneration installments are false. Workers' compensation insurance extortion can be the point at which a representative lies about their physical condition or sickness, when a business misclassifies workers to abstain from paying for workers' compensation insurance or when suppliers overstate a worker's symptoms to get more cash.

11.2.4 Fraud Detection and Risk Prevention

The discovery of insurance fraud generally occurs in two steps. The initial step is to distinguish dubious cases that have a higher chance of being false. This should be possible by automated measurable examination or by referrals from claims agents or insurance specialists. Moreover, people, in general, can give tips to insurance agencies, law enforcement agencies and different associations with regard to suspected, observed or conceded protection extortion executed by others. Despite the source, the following stage is to advise these cases to specialists for additional investigation.

Because of the sheer number of cases presented every day, it would be excessively costly for insurance agencies to have representatives check each claim for signs of extortion (Bolton & Hand, 2002). Rather, numerous organizations use PCs and factual examination to distinguish dubious cases for additional examination (Derrig, 2002). There are two fundamental sorts of measurable investigation devices utilized: Supervised and unsupervised (Bolton & Hand, 2002). In the two cases, dubious cases are distinguished by comparing information about the case with the expected qualities. The primary distinction between the two techniques how the normal qualities are determined (Bolton & Hand, 2002).

In a supervised method, the expected qualities are obtained by examining records of both deceitful and genuine cases (Bolton & Hand, 2002). Unsupervised methods for factual location include identifying claims that are unusual (Bolton & Hand, 2002). The two cases' agents and PCs can likewise be prepared to distinguish "warnings," or effects that in the past have frequently been related to false cases (Viaene et al., 2005). Factual location doesn't demonstrate that cases are false; it simply distinguishes dubious cases that must be explored further (Bolton & Hand, 2002). Fake cases can be one of two kinds (Lincoln, 2003), they can be in any case real cases that are misrepresented or "developed," or they can be bogus cases in which the harms asserted never really happened.

When a developed case is recognized, insurance agencies for the most part attempt to bring the case down to the proper sum (Derrig, 2002). Dubious cases can likewise be submitted to "extraordinary analytical units," or SIUs, for additional examination. These units by and large comprise experienced case agents with specialist training in analyzing fraudulent cases (Viaene et al., 2005). These agents search for specific features related to deceitful cases, or in any case search for proof of misrepresentation or something to that effect. This proof would then be able to be utilized to prevent claims or to indict fraudsters if the infringement is serious enough (Ghezzi, 1983).

At the point when an insurance agency's misrepresentation division examines an extortion attempt, it often continues in two phases: Pre-contact and post-contact (Morley et al., 2006). In the pre-contact stage, they dissect all accessible proof before they contact the suspect. They may audit submitted desk work, connect with outsiders and accumulate proof from accessible sources. At that point, in the "post-contact" stage, they meet the suspect to accumulate more data and, in a perfect world, get an implicating explanation. Insurance fraud examiners are prepared to scrutinize the suspect in a manner that blocks the suspect from raising a substantial resistance sometime in the future. For instance, inquiries regarding access to claim documentation block another individual from accessing the fake records. An example of a common defense that the suspect interview may preclude is that the suspect didn't know that their statement was false or that they lacked the intent to defraud (Podgor, 1999), or offered a vague expression that was later misconstrued (Parker et al., 2020). Complete honesty may add validity to a claimant's record of occasions, however, exclusions from exposure or bogus statements may reduce believability in later meetings or procedures (Parker et al., 2020). With regards to medical coverage, misrepresentation by medical coverage organizations is occasionally found by looking at incomes from premiums paid against the use by the healthcare coverage organizations on claims.

11.3 Revolution of Blockchain in the Insurance Sector

11.3.1 Need for Blockchain in the Insurance Sector

The insurance business, albeit settled and established, is presented with a few hazards that compromise its prosperity and efficiency. Information wastefulness, misrepresentation plans like misdirecting data, shared protection plans or concealing significant clinical findings, intermediate agents, human error because of manual input, etc. Issues are made two different ways—insurer controlling the information OR insured giving incorrect data to the organization.

Frauds can be caused in a number of ways. Phony and bogus processes to procure more benefits have been on the rise in the business. For instance, health insurance organizations face issues of fraudulent cases requesting payment for procedures not rendered by the clinic or specialist or overstating the number of procedures to guarantee higher benefits and so on. In other general insurance businesses, there have been examples of individuals concealing data of other insurance policies they hold to acquire double advantage or a separated couple applying for payment from a common advantage insurance policy. These are only a couple of cases, there are a lot of questionable policyholders with counterfeit records and numerous insurance plans for similar administrations and conditions. Will blockchain alleviate this hazard and eliminate extortion? Could blockchain innovation in insurance lead to a stage where information isn't presented to control? (Figure 11.1).

Then again, internal issues like manual handling of policies and claims, repetitive and complex techniques for information stockpiling and compromises that structure the center of insured activity, intermediaries blackmailing cash from organizations and clients the

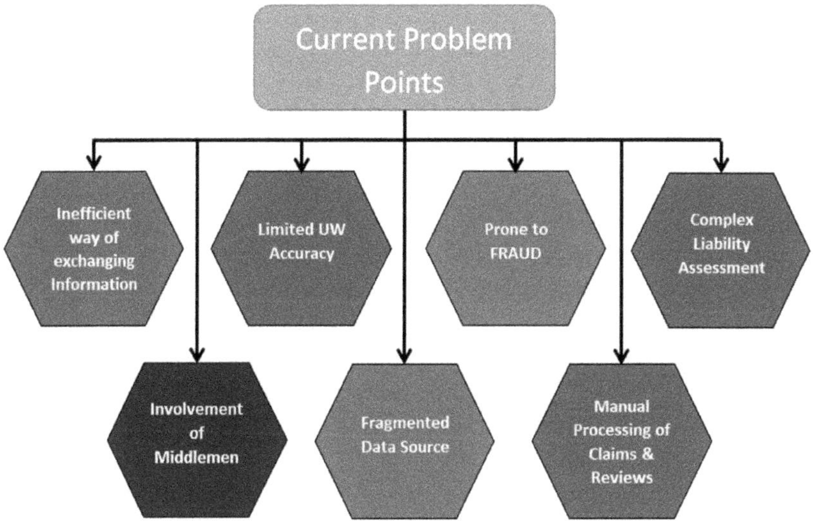

FIGURE 11.1
Current problem points in the insurance sector (image source: altoros.com).

same as commission, are numerous different elements influencing the insurance business from the inside. The privatization of insurance agencies and competition between them is a major concern. Information is dispersed; organizations would prefer not to divulge it to different parties because of the danger of losing a client. Without the sharing of information, it is difficult to distinguish counterfeit cases and policyholders. Could blockchain innovation in insurance with a decentralized system present an opportunity for the sharing of information between various insurance agencies?

This reluctance of insurance firms creates escape clauses in cybersecurity, presenting them to programmers and digital criminals which can lead to a data breach that reveals sensitive information. Additionally, delay in insurance applications and handling offer a great deal of time for programmers to complete their harmful exercises. Fraudsters have distinguished it as an appealing zone for information burglary and control, settling on digital security. Will blockchain innovation in insurance make a trusted and solid stage without digital assaults?

11.3.2 How Blockchain Benefits the Insurance Sector

Estimated to achieve a market share of US$2.3 billion in 2021 (Liu, 2019), much has been made about blockchain's utility across various businesses. Pundits assert that the innovation has insignificant publicity, that the distinction it makes is peripheral and not worth burning cash on. Supporters, then again, promptly concede that blockchain isn't the panacea being trumpeted in certain corners, yet also perceive that there are situations where it bodes well. It's the reason huge assets are being devoted to blockchain research by some of the world's biggest organizations.

Insurance is one such use case. Truth be told, blockchain is actually what is expected to infuse some development into an industry that has not changed much in decades. From global insurance plans down to new businesses, we are seeing a flood of new types of insurance, everything from flight delay insurance to improved risk warning.

The inbuilt highlights of blockchain offer a range of advantages to the insurance agencies. How about we investigate how blockchain is profiting the insurance sector (Lim, 2020)?

1. ***Data sharing***: Imagine a situation where insurance agencies can share know your client (KYC) data as opposed to researching each person that needs to purchase insurance. It could mean investment of thousands of dollars for every client. Blockchain makes this conceivable by permitting numerous insurance agencies to contribute data to the equivalent decentralized record. Furthermore, because the information is unchanging, the insurance agencies can believe that it is true. An example of such data is claims records. If insurance agencies contribute data to the equivalent blockchain, copy cases can without much of a stretch be distinguished.
2. ***Straightforwardness***: Generally, shopper information has been put away behind the dividers of insurance agencies. Buyers have no way to verify this information and rather are given just what the insurance agency chooses. What's more, if the data are imparted to outsiders, the shopper isn't advised about it. The open and decentralized nature of blockchain implies that purchasers will consistently have the option to see what information the insurance agency has and what that information is being used for.
3. ***Trust***: It isn't irregular for purchasers to doubt insurance agencies. Confusing policy terms, high premiums and long claim forms all add to this. The blockchain, explicitly smart contracts, bring trust once more by improving the insurance contract and, with the assistance of AI, mechanizing claims. No human mediation is required. SURETY.AI simplifies the buying procedure to get you the specific inclusion you need, while its AI calculation handles payouts without the requirement for recording a claim.
4. ***Smart contracts***: Smart contracts are programmable agreements connected to the blockchain. They are automated and, along these lines, don't require human mediation. For the insurance business, smart contracts empower miniaturized insurance arrangements to be given and guaranteed payouts to be computerized.
5. ***Tokens***: One explanation that the claim payout process is moderate is the requirement for fiat cash checks or bank transfers. Shoppers at times wait for a considerable length of time for the payout to show up in their account. Utilizing advanced tokens represented on the blockchain tackles this issue. Payouts can be made in an instant and afterward be re-used to purchase extra inclusion.
6. ***Extortion prevention***: Extortion is a significant issue in the insurance business, costing an expected US$80 billion every year (CAIF—Coalition Against Insurance Fraud, 2017). Blockchain, shrewd agreements and AI can help reduce this figure by mentioning data confirmed by AI from various sources before paying out a claim. What's more, the permanence and decentralization of blockchain permit insurance agencies to share extortion data.
7. ***Lower costs***: What the entirety of this indicates is lower premiums for purchasers. Customized insurance has never been so reasonable. Hearti is focused on giving the most creative and trouble-free insurance products to its clients. Blockchain is one of the innovations that will assist us.

Blockchain offers a progression of advantages that will catalyze the whole procedure of the insurance business. How about we look at some of them (Sharma, 2018)?

1. ***Blockchain in health insurance***: Blockchain is about informing executives, by interconnecting all the clinical administration offices, back-up plans, patients, doctors and so on, the blockchain can improve the degree of care the patients receive. Moreover, and it will smooth out the whole procedure as all the information is localized.
2. ***Blockchain in auto insurance***: There are two different ways through which blockchain can end up being valuable for the accident coverage industry. To begin with, it can interface all the clients and specialist co-ops; with the assistance of a shared record, all the data will be promptly accessible. It will help the auto insurance providers in decreasing the and extortion. Second, smart contracts will accelerate the process.
3. ***Blockchain in the life insurance industry***: Extra security may sound an extremely streamlined and simple procedure. Be that as it may, making a claim from the insurance agency is an onerous undertaking. It makes you face a progression of inquiries, endless administrative work and causes you to invest your time, cash and energy. In any case, with the assistance of blockchain, we can expect some alleviation here. By making a consortium of clinical offices, government offices and so forth, one can obtain all the data without any problem. Additionally, insurance agencies can utilize smart contracts to give programmed payouts to clinical offices and different recipients.

11.3.2.1 Blockchain in the Health Insurance Sector

A large number of the previously mentioned advantages of blockchain additionally apply to medical coverage, in addition to not many that are exceptional to this part of the business (Martin, 2020).

1. ***Clinical records***—DLT (appropriated record innovation) will be a help to clinical experts all over the place. By making a patient's clinical records unchanging, carefully available and straightforward, the clinical error will be a relic from days gone by. Since blockchain is extremely secure, clinical extortion and insurance fraud ought to likewise diminish significantly. For insurance specialists and policyholders, creating statements will be a simple, automatable procedure, with instant access to all the fundamental records to give precise rates.
2. ***Cases***—When a patient attends a clinic, treatment records will consequently be added to the blockchain, and the insurance agency will pay out. The requirement for complex structures and to-and-fro correspondence will be radically diminished.
3. ***Reduced costs***—Doctors, organizations and insurance providers will all observe huge proficiency support from the blockchain. With complete and confidential access to a patient's finished clinical history over all suppliers, specialists will have the option to see and use the results of tests made at different offices, without convoluted solicitations for data. They will have the option to consider the consequences of past methods, taking out the duplication of work that is so basic today. Medicines will take less time and include

less experimentation. The entirety of this implies clinical costs will go down, and that is to the advantage of everybody.

11.3.3 Blockchain Start-Ups in the Health Insurance Sector

The insurance industry could do with a significant redesign. Besides ever-increasing premiums with no additional value, the whole business is amazingly opaque and hard for customers to comprehend. Terms are regularly intricate, and individuals now and again overpay for protection they'll never require. Be that as it may, this isn't to imply that those insurance providers are fully to blame. Sadly, the accessible risk evaluation models and stages don't lend themselves to any sort of custom arrangements or imaginative risk-sharing models.

That is where blockchain comes in. Using frontline blockchain arrangements like smart contracts, decentralized installment systems and so on, new businesses and active participants are going to upset the insurance business by executing progressively custom, on-demand and distributed insurance arrangements. The accompanying organizations are for the most part attempting to execute blockchain to make better risk-sharing models while giving individuals increasingly custom and moderate insurance choices (Mire, 2019).

11.3.3.1 Category #1: Peer-To-Peer Insurance/Microinsurance

Existing insurance models need an update. The vast majority needn't bother with far-reaching inclusion for each expected setback, and a great many people pay high premiums for coverage they'll never require. Blockchain innovation makes it simpler for individuals to share inside a smaller network and look for insurance for explicit and restricted employments. These organizations are attempting to help decentralize insurance choices and obtain more focused insurance coverage that is customized to genuine customer needs.

1. ***SURETY.AI***: SURETY.AI, a venture from Hearti, is utilizing blockchain to offer microinsurance to unbanked populaces, especially in Asia. Their point is to use Hearti's AI programs, joined with another blockchain-fueled stage and Initial Coin Offering (ICO), to give an increasingly consistent experience to banks and insurance providers to generate more interest from unbanked and uninsured populaces and areas.
2. ***MediShares***: MediShares is a blockchain-based, decentralized, open source, shared guide commercial center. It utilizes smart contracts for clients hoping to enter mutual aid insurance services, and for insurance providers which need to offer these types of assistance.
3. ***Poleecy***: Poleecy is a blockchain-based microinsurance supplier in Italy. The foundation permits clients to look for and secure microinsurance arrangements for different requirements. It secures all insurance information through smart contracts on the blockchain, expanding trust in the exchange's veracity and practicality.
4. ***REGA***: REGA Risk Sharing is a worldwide programming firm that is creating blockchain answers for InsurTech and FinTech applications. It propelled a beta of a crowdsurance stage for protecting luggage when it gets lost, and it intends to launch additional blockchain-based crowdsurance choices later on.
5. ***Nexus Mutual***: Nexus is building blockchain-based answers for the insurance business. It will likely replace existing insurance models with smart contract-driven

shared markets. By helping individuals share risk across bigger networks, they would like to bring down insurance costs and substitute the requirement for greater insurance agencies.

6. ***iXLedger***: iXLedger is the innovation advancement arm of iX Technology Group. It will probably decentralize the current insurance worldview, excluding mediators that increase costs and move to a more distributed driven model. They are utilizing blockchain to consolidate insurance premiums.
7. ***Teambrella***: Teambrella is a social application that is intended to change existing insurance models. It will likely empower clients to impart dangers to friends and help individuals down in their luck. It uses blockchain innovation to control its distributed protection stage.

11.3.3.2 Category #2: On-Demand Insurance/Risk Sharing

Now and then you simply need insurance for a short period or a specific life occasion. At present, insurance markets are appropriate for on-demand protection or increasingly disseminated risk-sharing strategies. Blockchain can change that entirely, utilizing smart contracts and ground-breaking information to insure specific occasions or timeframes. These organizations are utilizing blockchain to give on-demand insurance policies, rebuild risk evaluation and give individuals progressively customized insurance alternatives.

1. ***RYSKEX***: RYSKEX is a blockchain-fueled platform and commercial center for B2B insurance markets. Their point is to help grow B2B back-up plans and mitigate risks quicker and easier. They influence smart contracts to deal with the end of insurance policies and future claims management and arbitration .
2. ***Buzzvault***: Buzzvault has manufactured an advanced resource vault utilizing blockchain to make it simpler for individuals to carefully compile inventories and record details of their assets. This blockchain-based information enables clients to access a modified smart insurance function for their unique home insurance needs, given their carefully recorded resources.
3. ***Kasko2Go***: Kasko2Go utilizes blockchain to make another "pay more only as costs arise" driving an insurance model that continuously rewards clients for better driving. They intend to welcome existing insurance providers to their blockchain platform as long as they consent to their model, which will be implemented by smart contracts.
4. ***Halos Insurance***: Supported by Techstars, Halos Insurance is attempting to make a completely computerized customer insurance platform intended to make insurance more straightforward for buyers, while making practical risk mitigation arrangements.

11.3.3.3 Category #3: Risk/Fraud Prevention

Insurance fraud is a crime with a long history. Also, it's hard for the two insurers and organizations to evaluate the danger of different accomplices or specialist organizations. By giving an increasingly straightforward history and a total record of exchanges on the system, blockchain can assist organizations with assessing new applicants and the veracity of insurance claims. They can likewise access thorough claim information, which should help detect extortion quicker. These organizations are discovering approaches to utilize the blockchain to reduce insurance fraud and assist organizations with evaluating the danger of new business opportunities.

1. ***VouchForMe***: VouchForMe is a platform utilizing blockchain to make a progressively decentralized distributed insurance product. Because of social evidence and individual associations, it would like to engage holders of crypto assets to put resources into P2P insurance premiums and make insurance advertisements all the more reasonable and customizable.
2. ***Piprate***: Piprate gives organizations in the (re)insurance space an opportunity to share information that creates trust, responsibility and simplicity. It uses blockchain information wallets and Application Programming Interfaces (APIs) to empower secure exchange and complete information recognition between colleagues. They will probably make insurance information sharing altogether increasingly secure and effective while adding to compliance initiatives.
3. ***Zillion***: Zillion is an InsurTech organization utilizing blockchain, smart information and smart contracts to provide insurance at lower rates.

11.3.3.4 Category #4: Insurance Data and Operations

Data analytics is the backbone of any insurance venture. Without great information, evaluation and conveyance become exceptionally dubious procedures. Blockchain is a useful device for protection information since it is a safe, appropriated database with progressively precise data. These organizations are utilizing blockchain to help improve the quality, availability and straightforwardness of protection information to upgrade tasks and decrease costs for the insurance provider.

1. ***CyStellar***: CyStellar is an intelligence provider that attempts to give real-time knowledge to the insurance, horticulture, and logistics sectors to support better information-driven dynamics. It coordinates a system of satellites, drones, ground sensors and venture programming to computerize information categorization, examination and analysis. It will probably make key information progressively valuable. CyStellar is building blockchain frameworks with expectations of conveying AI-fueled risk choice and guarantee appraisal for the insurance sector, alongside better provenance to maintain a strategic distance from risk in businesses like farming.
2. ***iChain***: iChain is turning out big business blockchain answers for the InsurTech business. It would like to digitize paper forms and improve transparency through its blockchain-fueled stage iChain Base. They are likewise executing a wallet to help insured people deal with their information safely from their cellphones.
3. ***B3i***: The Blockchain Insurance Industry Initiative (B3i) is a joint effort of insurers and reinsurers framed to investigate the capability of utilizing appropriated record advances inside the businesses to help all partners in the value chain. They are centered around creating and testing specialized improvements focused on better serving clients and upgrading exchange productivity, in this way stimulating competition.
4. ***Skyline Partners***: Skyline Partners is utilizing blockchain, smart contracts and real-time information investigation to reduce wasteful aspects in insurance models and open up increasingly customized solutions for the insured. Their priority is to limit the impact of natural disasters and weather on the world's uninsured and underserved.

5. ***Etherisc***: Etherisc is a decentralized insurance protocol to collectively build insurance products. It will likely form decentralized insurance applications, making the purchase and offer of insurance progressively proficient, delivering lower operational costs, expanding the transparency of protection compared with traditional practice and democratizing access to reinsurance products.

11.3.4 Billing Claim Management

Blockchain helps the insurance industry by addressing regularly occurring common problems. In the case of healthcare insurance, for instance, there are issues looked upon by both consumers and insurers which can be resolved utilizing blockchain.

11.3.4.1 Challenges for Health Insurance Providers

1. ***Trust issues***: Insurance clients, who are normally confused by the policy conditions, have become increasingly more careful about trusting insurance providers. This issue of trust is significant for insurance providers.
2. ***Silos***: The whole insurance industry works between different unique partners like controllers, insurance agencies, charge specialists, strategy holders, credit offices, specialists and emergency clinics. All these service providers work in their storehouses or silos and administration between them is challenging due to external factors on data sharing such as bureaucracy and state laws.
3. ***Managing patient information***: In most cases, insurance providers do not have access to patient data, which leads to increased processing expenses or allotting the wrong policy.
4. ***Wrong documentation***: Because of scattered documentation and filings among the different partners in the insurance network, document archives are either incorrectly filed or not recorded and occasionally lost.

11.3.4.2 Challenges for Health Insurance Consumers

1. ***Access to patient clinical history according to need and responsibility for information***: This happens frequently when the consumer tends to change the insurance policy type from the company. This situation can even happen when the client is on the same plan for a long time and the information is distributed in remote corners of the network. The patient information is stored by different suppliers instead of by the patient themselves. The end client has almost no control over their clinical history. So, during a crisis or during routine tests, the patient information won't be readily accessible to an alternate specialist doctor or emergency clinic without experiencing a cumbersome procedure to access the data. In this situation, the specialists offering assistance to the patients won't have a total perspective on the patient's clinical history leading to inappropriate/unnecessary tests, inaccurate conclusions or extended findings.
2. ***Processing/denying claims inside a predetermined timespan***: Insurance companies incorrectly processing past claims result in client disappointment. This again is connected to the significant issue of losing the client's trust.
3. ***Security***: Information regarding the identity of a client which is stored with the hospitals or insurance providers makes it prone to fraud, identity theft or leaks.

11.4 Building a Blockchain-Based Health Insurance Application using Hyperledger Fabric

Referring to blockchain, one will always hear a great deal about its decentralized nature. What makes this so attractive is that blockchain is unprotected by censorship, coercion or corruption. Decentralized applications are used on a peer-to-peer network, instead of on one computer. They are programs which are not governed by any entity on the web. All transactions across the network are stored at the core of a blockchain network: Distributed ledger. A Blockchain ledger is also categorized as decentralized as it is updated by several participants throughout the network, each contributing towards its maintenance.

11.4.1 Key Concepts Involved in Blockchain Application

A blockchain is mainly a mutual database loaded with sections that need confirmation and encryption. Every entry of a document depends on a logical connection with all its predecessors. The blockchain name alludes to the term "blocks" that will be appended to the recorded transaction chain. The code uses encrypted identifiers, called hashes, to accomplish this. The distributed ledger is a passage that will be decentralized to negate the requirement for a central authority to process, confirm or validate transactions. Organizations utilize distributed ledger technology for processing, validating or authenticating transactions or other data exchange types. Such documents are usually only ever maintained in the database when the parties concerned reach a consensus.

11.4.2 Architecture of Hyperledger Fabric

Linux Foundation introduced Hyperledger as an umbrella for open-source tools in 2015. Figure 11.2 shows the umbrella structure of Hyperledger.

All Hyperledger applications follow a design approach that includes a modular customizable approach, interoperability with a focus on a highly secure solution and the

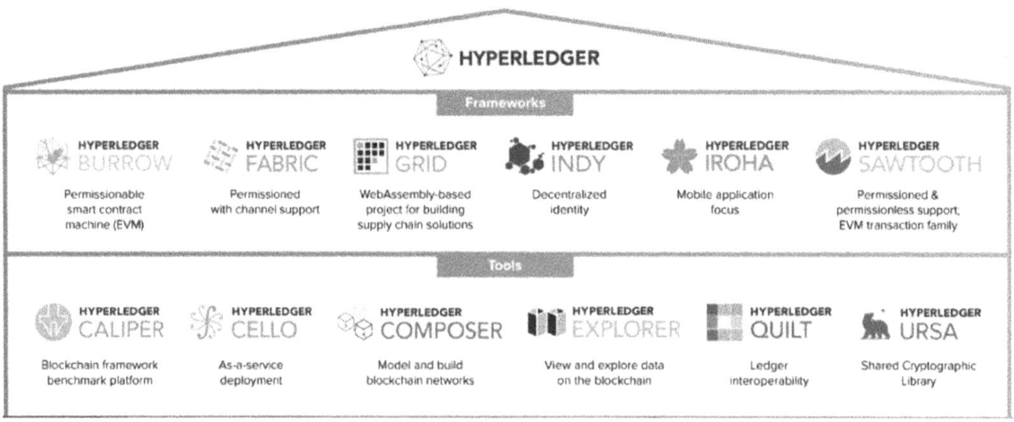

FIGURE 11.2
Hyperledger umbrella structure (image source: hyperledger.com).

development of a rich and easy-to-use API. The following are the minimum components for blockchain application development:

- ***Ledger***: A distributed ledger is an append-only structure that is shared across the business network.
- ***Smart contract***: A smart contract is a programming code with the set of business rules that have to be executed during the transaction.
- ***Consensus***: Consensus is known as a general agreement of a blockchain state. It makes sure that there is no fault in the state of the transaction and blockchain. There are different types of consensus mechanisms; commonly used mechanisms are Proof-of-Work (PoW) and Proof-of-Stake (PoS). There are many more mechanisms with variations in PoS such as Proof-of-Authority (PoA), Delegated Proof-of-Stake (DPoS), etc.
- ***Security and privacy***: The fundamental properties of blockchain i.e., immutability and append-only, provides security to the blockchain application. Also, Hyperledger Fabric is a private and permissioned blockchain which makes the system tamper-proof.
- ***Application Programming Interfaces (APIs)***: The APIs enable the users and applications to interface with blockchain.

As we are probably aware, Hyperledger by Linux foundation is a distributed ledger framework. Fabric is a blockchain framework under Hyperledger, presented by IBM. Fabric needs private authorization for blockchain, compared to a public permissionless mechanism that allows anonymous entities to work in the system (requiring conventional protocol such as PoW to authorize any transaction and protect the system). The members of the Hyperledger Fabric network are chosen by a Member Service Provider (MSP). Fabric uses decentralized ledger technology which utilizes smart contracts and is a platform through which members execute their transactions.

Hyperledger Fabric offers some plug-in options. For several organizations, ledger data can be stored, consensus structures can be moved in and out, Fabric supports different MSPs including internal and external MSPs. Hyperledger Fabric also provides the feature to create networks, enabling a group of participants to make another record of exchanges. This is an especially valuable alternative for systems where a few members that interact and do not need every exchange they make a specific value to some members and not others, for example, known to each member. On the off-chance that two members would create a channel, those members and no others would have duplicates of the record for that channel at that point.

Hyperledger Fabric has a two-part record subsystem: The World State and the Transaction Log. Each node has a duplicate of record, in which the world state represents the blockchain state at a given point in time. The world state is the record database. It's the database of transactions in the ledger. The transaction log records all transactions which have led to the current state of the blockchain; it's the historical data for the world state. The record is a blend of the world state and transaction log.

In Hyperledger Fabric smart contracts are known as chaincodes and are called to the blockchain by an external application when that application needs to connect with the record. By and large, a chaincode interacts only with the data section of the record, i.e., the world state and not the transaction log. Fabric provides the flexibility in programming languages to implement chaincodes. Chaincodes may be written in different languages, for example, Java, Python, Go, Node and so on.

11.4.3 Blockchain Application Development Using Hyperledger Fabric

Hyperledger Fabric is a distributed ledger record software programming framework backed by measured engineering giving high privacy, dependability, adaptability and versatility (Hyperledger Fabric, 2020). It is planned to help the pluggable execution of different segments and to overcome the subtleties and complexities of the whole financial atmosphere supporting customary instructive cautions.

The strategy for synchronizing record exchanges over the system to guarantee that records update when exchanges are acknowledged by the active members and that when records update in a similar request, they update with similar exchanges (Figure 11.3).

Since Fabric is a private blockchain, peers require permission to participate in the business network. The user has to be authorized by a certificate authority (CA) to interact with the blockchain application. The CA offers various certificate services to blockchain users. These services relate to user registration, transactions invoked on the blockchain, and transport layer secured (TLS) communications between different users or other components of the blockchain. After getting authorized, the user can access the Representational State Transfer (REST) server through REST APIs provided by the Hyperledger REST server. The application processes user requests to the network through a REST API. The REST API is used to retrieve the state of the database. It implements requests to the blockchain state database on Hyperledger Fabric. The decentralized application's interface can be built using any of the UI frameworks such as Angular framework. The UI retrieves the data through GET/POST calls to the REST API.

Blockchain is revolutionizing the way financial organizations conduct business with its distributed ledger, smart contracts and non-repudiation capabilities and the insurance industry is no exception. Here is an example to build a web-based blockchain application to facilitate insurance sales and claims using the Hyperledger Fabric platform.

Blockchain provides the insurance industry with an immense opportunity. It offers the opportunity to innovate in the way data are exchanged, claims are processed and fraud is avoided. To build a powerful new tool for insurance management, blockchain will put together developers from software firms, regulators and insurance companies.

Blockchain applications can be developed on cloud networks and local networks as well. The example discussed here is for the local network. This example demonstrates the use of blockchain for claims processing in the insurance sector.

There are five main components in the blockchain application which have to be decided before starting to build the application.

- Peers.
- Certificate authorities.

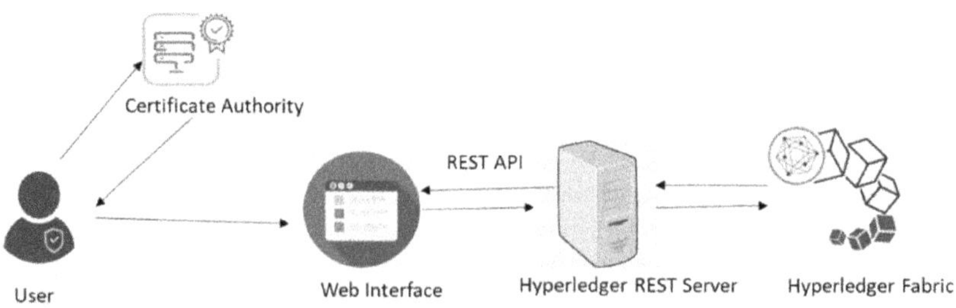

FIGURE 11.3
Hyperledger Fabric application control flow.

- Endorsement policy.
- Distributed ledger.
- Smart contract.

Peers. Peers are the participating nodes in the blockchain network. There are four types of participating peers in the claims insurance application: Patient, insurance provider, endorser and committer.

- Patient peer is the one who claims for the insurance.
- Insurance provider peer is an insurance company that provides insurance and is responsible for processing the claims.
- Endorser peer is responsible for verifying the accuracy of the claims. The endorser is a peer who receives a transaction request to be endorsed. The endorser node must have the chaincode. This node gives its endorsement as approve or reject.
- Committer peer is responsible for validating and committing the transaction against the endorsing policy. The committer node will have the distributed ledger and the world state. This node may not hold chaincode.

Certificate authorities. The peer has to get certified by the MSP either by internal Fabric-CA or external-CA. A simple way to get authorized is by using GIT. A peer can be authenticated through the Github account.

Endorsement policy. Endorsing is important to avoid double-spending. An e-policy may be decided based on the requirement of the application. Let's consider there are three endorsing peers, say E1, E2, E3. The client sends a request for endorsement/approval. Each endorser executes the proposed transaction. But none of these executions will be updated in the ledger. After checking the consistency, the endorser approves or denies the transaction. Now let's consider different sample endorsing policies.

- Endorsing Policy 1: All three nodes E1, E2, E3 must sign.
- Endorsing Policy 2: Any two endorsers' approval is sufficient.
- Endorsing Policy 3: At least two approvals are required; E1 and E3 must sign.

After collecting the endorsements, clients send the endorsement status to the organizing peer. The organizer organizes the transactions. Organizing happens in parallel with all the transactions submitted by other applications, across Fabric. Ordering is done by applying different algorithms such as SOLO, Kafka, etc. Ordering of the transactions is required to maintain consistency in the data.

The organizing peer sends ordered transactions to all committing peers. A committer will commit the transaction based on the endorsing policy. If the transaction succeeds the endorsing policy, then it is committed and blocks are added to the ledger.

Distributed ledger. A distributed ledger is a database of electronic records. It is shared and coordinated across several nodes through consensus. It is replicated, shared and synchronized among various nodes in the business network.

Smart contract. A smart contract (called chaincode in Fabric) is a set of business rules that are executed automatically when a transaction takes place between two clients. It contains the terms that are mutually agreed upon by partners. For example, in insurance applications, chaincode may include terms and conditions for the list of hospitals for cashless payment, the conditions that are claimable, the ceiling amount on each type of condition, etc. A smart contract gives transparency in the transaction and avoids fraud.

11.4.4 How to Create a New Blockchain Application

1. Install the prerequisite software—Docker, Docker Compose, Git client, npm, Node .js, Python and Hyperledger composer.
2. Build Hyperledger Composer REST server.
3. Create the insurance Business Network Administration (BNA).
4. Generate certificates for peers.
5. Build Docker images for network.
6. Start the insurance network (BNA).
7. Start the Fabric.
8. If deployment is successful, start the composer-rest-server.
9. Call the composer-rest-server API in the frontend for integration.

11.5 Conclusions and Future Work

Blockchain leverages the insurance industry's performance, security and transparency. Distributed ledger technology has beneficial applications to automate the processing of insurance claims, improve cybersecurity standards and even speed up the payment process. The potential of blockchain to build confidence in a trustless environment through the use of public ledgers and robust cybersecurity protocols will have a significant impact on the future growth of the insurance industry. Slowly, the initial perception that blockchain is for cryptocurrencies has changed and blockchain is revolutionizing various sectors such as finance, energy, insurance etc. Soon, a drastic change is expected in all the business processes using blockchain.

References

ACFE. (2018). Insurance fraud handbook. *Acfe*, *1*(1), 1–20. https://doi.org/10.1093/oxfordjournals.bjc.a047785

Beers, B. (2019). A brief overview of the insurance sector. *Investopedia*. https://www.investopedia.com/ask/answers/051915/how-does-insurance-sector-work.asp

Bolton, RJ and Hand, DJ. (2002). Statistical fraud detection: A review. *Statistical Science*, *17*(3), 235–255. https://doi.org/10.1214/ss/1042727940

Brown, S. (2020). 7 ways you're getting ripped off by insurance companies how fullled are you in your life? https://www.lifehack.org/458575/7-ways-youre-getting-ripped-off-by-insurance-companies

CAIF—Coalition Against Insurance Fraud. (2017). *By the numbers: Fraud statistics*. Coalition Against Insurance Fraud. https://www.insurancefraud.org/statistics.htm

Chen, J. (2019). Insurance fraud. *Journal of Risk and Insurance*, *69*(3). https://doi.org/10.1111/1539-6975.00026

Derrig, RA. (2002). Insurance fraud. *Journal of Risk and Insurance*, *69*(3), 271–287.
Ghezzi, SG. (1983). A private network of social control: Insurance investigation units. *Social Problems*, *30*(5), 521–531. https://doi.org/10.2307/800269
Hamer, L. (2018). Here's how health insurance companies ripped off people for years. https://www.cheatsheet.com/money-career/heres-health-insurance-companies-ripped-off-people-years.html/
Hernandez, A. (2020). Insurance industry trends 2020: Growth, stats, and forecast. https://policyadvice.net/blog/insurance-industry-trends/
Hyperledger Fabric. (2020). *A blockchain platform for the enterprise*. Hyperledger Fabric. https://hyperledger-fabric.readthedocs.io/en/latest/
Kumari, K, Mrunalini, M, Kumar, M, Talasila, V and Dixit, PK. (2020). *Design model for energy trading on blockchain*. 2019 4th International Conference on Electrical, Electronics, Communication, Computer Technologies and Optimization Techniques (ICEECCOT), 2019, pp. 336–341, doi: 10.1109/ICEECCOT46775.2019.9114816
Lim, K. (2020). How blockchain benefits the insurance industry. https://link.medium.com/A8LwSTRab6
Lincoln, R. (2003). *An exploration of automobile insurance fraud an exploration of automobile insurance fraud Robyn Lincoln Helene Wells & Wayne Petherick*.
Liu, S. (2019). Size of the blockchain technology market worldwide from 2018 to 2023. *Statista.Com*. https://www.statista.com/statistics/647231/worldwide-blockchain-technology-market-size/
Komarovsky, M. (2016). 5 ways health insurance can rip you off. https://www.thrillist.com/health/nation/ways-insurance-companies-rip-you-off
Means, WI, Did, W and Begin, I. (2020). Overview: Insurance. https://www.encyclopedia.com/finance/encyclopedias-almanacs-transcripts-and-maps/overview-insurance
Mire, S. (2019). 19 startups using blockchain to transform insurance [Market Map].
Morley, NJ, Ball, LJ and Ormerod, TC. (2006). How the detection of insurance fraud succeeds and fails. *Psychology, Crime and Law*, *12*(2), 163–180. https://doi.org/10.1080/10683160512331316325
Mrunalini, M. and Kumar, DP (2020). Energy trading using Ethereum blockchain. ICTIS 2020.
NY Criminal Defense. (2020). *Home insurance fraud*. NY Criminal Defense. https://nyccriminallawyer.com/fraud-charge/insurance-fraud/home-insurance-fraud/
PA Insurance Fraud Prevention Authority. (2020a). *Automotive insurance fraud*. PA Insurance Fraud Prevention Authority.
PA Insurance Fraud Prevention Authority. (2020b). *Health insurance fraud*. PA Insurance Fraud Prevention Authority. https://www.helpstopfraud.org/Types-of-Insurance-Fraud/Health
Parker, J, January, AS and Binning, C. (2020). Representing individuals in interviews: The UK Perspective. 1–11.
Podgor, E. (1999). Criminal fraud. *American University Law Review*, *48*(4), 1.
Martin, R. (2020). The complete guide to blockchain for insurance companies. https://igniteoutsourcing.com/blockchain/blockchain-and-insurance-industry/
Sachon, L. (2018). Types of life insurance fraud. https://www.policygenius.com/life-insurance/types-of-life-insurance-fraud/
ScaleFocus. (2018). 9 insurance industry technology trends in 2020 [Updated].
Sharma, TK. (2018). How are insurance companies using blockchain technology for their benefits? https://www.blockchain-council.org/blockchain/how-are-insurance-companies-using-blockchain-technology-for-their-benefits/
Tropea, J. (2019). Insurance disruption: How blockchain is transforming the industry. 13 Listopada. https://www.bankrate.com/insurance/blockchain-disruption/
Viaene, S, Dedene, G and Derrig, RA. (2005). Auto claim fraud detection using Bayesian learning neural networks. *Expert Systems with Applications*, *29*(3), 653–666. https://doi.org/10.1016/j.eswa.2005.04.030
WNS Global Services. (2018). Top 5 trends in the insurance industry. https://www.wns.com/Portals/0/Documents/Articles/PDFFiles/600/195/Top-5-Trends-in-the-Insurance-Industry.pdf
Wargin, J. (2020). 8 insurance technology trends transforming the industry in 2020. https://www.duckcreek.com/blog/insurance-technology-trends/

12

Blockchains in the Pharmaceutical Sector

Muralidhar Kurni, Saritha Kuppala, Somasena Reddy K and Manorama Devi B

CONTENTS

12.1 Introduction

In the pharmaceutical industry, the market value of counterfeit drugs is billions of dollars annually. It is currently the most critical issue in the world, particularly in developing countries. Aside from the above, interoperability, drug traceability and data security are among the urgent concerns that are putting immense pressure on the pharmaceutical industry. Blockchain can introduce drastic improvements to the industry through transparency and simpler traceability of processes. Here are some of the advantages blockchain can offer (Akeo, n.d.):

- ***Increase trust***: Blockchain can monitor the entire supply chain for producers, wholesalers and retailers. This not only increases the visibility but also maintains a high level of confidence among the parties.
- ***Enhanced security***: The immutable ledger is considered one of the most secure systems in the world. Blockchain can ensure that the ledger's recorded drug information maintains secure and unmodified medical records for the patient.

DOI: 10.1201/9781003133179-12

- ***Visibility added***: Visibility and privacy are among the most critical issues in the pharmaceutical supply chain. Blockchain is the most vital tool to make stored data available to all parties.
- ***Avoid drug counterfeiting***: Registering drug details on blockchain is intended to track, trace and authenticate drugs at all levels by manufacturers and regulatory authorities. It would make it impossible to counterfeit products.

12.2 Pharmaceutical Industry Overview

In the last few decades, the pharmaceutical industry has developed a research-based strategy, enhanced technology and facilities in the bioscience sector to develop new formulations and cures for diseases.

12.2.1 Pharmaceutical Industry

The pharmaceutical industry plays an essential part in developing vaccines and medicines to prevent and minimize the prevalence of diseases, treat illness and improve quality of life through groundbreaking research and technical progress to respond to the population's complex healthcare requirements (James Lind Institute, 2019). This industry's main objective is to provide pharmaceutical products to sustain health or avoid infections and diseases that affect the global population. The pharmaceutical industry covers various subsectors of drug development, manufacturing or distribution and selling by drug producers or marketers and biotechnology firms in the medical sector. The discovery, production, manufacture and marketing of pharmaceutical drugs or vaccines for patients aims to prevent, cure or alleviate various disease symptoms. Health supplements decrease the risk of disease and fulfill the regular dietary needs of vitamins and minerals.

The discovery and development of new pharmaceuticals with reduced side-effects and increased therapeutic activity accelerate emerging innovations and scientific achievements. Pre-clinical development, clinical trials and safety surveillance or monitoring for most of the drugs evaluated for use in humans are carried out to assess their safety and effectiveness before approval and market launch. The industry comprises various regulatory bodies monitoring patents, drug safety, drug quality and pricing. The pharmaceutical industry is influenced by several complex research, legislative, regulatory, political, social and economic factors. The pharmaceutical industry can be affected by practicing physicians, pharmacists, researchers, government and industry scientists in hospitals, clinics, pharmacies and private organizations. The advantages of pharmaceutical drugs can be improved by medical chemists, molecular biologists and pharmacists.

12.2.2 Classification of Pharmaceutical Industry

For an easy understanding of the industry, the current pharmaceutical industry can be divided into three groups (Reddy, 2018). They are the following:

1. Bulk drugs.
2. Formulations.
3. Biotechnology.

This classification provides a basis for the industry summary in all respects. Let us dive into each segment.

1. ***Bulk drugs***: Bulk drugs are the material used in pharmaceutical production, i.e., pharmaceutical drugs such as pills, ointments and syrups. This is also called the "Active Pharmaceutical Ingredient (API)." The manufacture of bulk drugs is essential and costly at the same time. It needs a lot of technical skills and money. It is not as straightforward as we assume to create a standardized method for producing a particular drug. Meeting the quality needed while preserving safety measures is a significant challenge for the bulk pharmaceutical industry. Since this is a chemical industry, it is, of course, often related to environmental protection. Hazardous waste disposal, manufacturing of quality medicines and protection of the green ecosystem are the industry's core obligations. Fermentation, organic synthesis and natural extraction are the methods used in this global drug industry.
2. ***Formulations***: The formulation is a procedure used to make medicinal products by combining APIs and inert substances (excipients) according to predefined ratios. In this pharmaceutical industry division, finished dosage forms are prepared. The main challenge here is the quality, safety and efficiency of the finished dosage form. The key factors influencing the formulation sector's efficiency and performance are the maintenance of production facilities in compliance with regulatory requirements and the design of a robust process with a robust quality system. Since the finished dosage forms are final drugs and are taken as tablets, syrups, etc., patient safety is crucial. Acceptable manufacturing practices and a robust investigative system to investigate defects are necessary to maintain this sector.
3. ***Biotechnology***: Biotechnology deals primarily with the techniques used in biopharmaceutical processing. The main tools for the preparation of biopharmaceuticals are living microorganisms. The method used in this technique modifies the live organisms according to human usage requirements. In recent years, this industry has shown rapid growth. More than 270 items for human consumption are now available. In the new electronic era, biotechnology plays a critical role in enhancing people's healthy lifestyles. The biggest obstacle is to raise funds for this segment. Research and development costs are too high, as 36 percent of medicines fail during development before the preliminary stage. Biotech drug prices are, therefore, very high compared to a common pill. Regulatory compliance for this industry is also a major challenge. Regulatory agencies conduct thorough examinations to avoid future disasters.

12.2.3 Pharmaceutical Market Overview

With a projected growth of US$1.3 trillion by the end of 2020, a clear increase in many major infections and diseases would affect the global pharmaceutical market (James Lind Institute, 2019). Increased pressure on the healthcare budget imposed by an increasing incidence of chronic disease is part of a trend visible in the pharmaceutical industry; emerging economies have seen demand for medicinal products more than in industrialized economies; the regulator is becoming more cautious approving new and innovative medicines. The pharmaceutical market's growth reflects an expansion in health infrastructure, doubling disposable incomes among many middle-class households, greater insurance coverage, rising disease prevalence, aggressive market penetration and product patents by relatively smaller companies.

The average human is exposed to more illnesses and diseases that need preventive approaches to preserve health and increased study to enhance the population's quality of life. Hectic daily schedules, lack of sleep and exercise, bad food and other lifestyle choices have to led poor digestion, high obesity rates, breathing problems, and other health problems. Rising demand for health supplements and better drugs is driven by globalization and urbanization. The increasing number of chronic diseases has increased people's dependence on medication and health supplements. The benefits of medication and diagnosis impact pharmaceutical firms' research and development, providing patients with the correct dosage, comfort and compliance with drug regimens that increase the incidence and technology of chronic diseases.

12.2.3.1 Size of Pharmaceutical Business

Since health is a concern for everyone, the availability of medicines everywhere is a necessity. Supply needs are also vital. The size of the sector is therefore also large. Almost all developed and emerging countries have seen a major expansion of the pharmaceutical industry. This, along with other big industries, is also one of the main sources of employment.

Advancing computer technology has brought tremendous business shifts. Automation in production units increased the market volume and decreased drug preparation lead time. This reality is expressed in the global sales of the pharmaceutical industry.

Revenue growth in the pharmaceutical industry has risen to an appreciable amount in recent years. For the first time in 2014, sales exceeded US$1 trillion (Reddy, 2018).

This rapid growth contributes to the assumption that the industry will hit US$1.4 trillion by 2022 (Reddy, 2018). After 2020, many patents will expire. Market analysts, therefore, expect growth levels to decrease slightly after 2020.

The US, Switzerland and China are the biggest players in the industry. Many countries import large quantities of raw materials from China.

12.2.4 Challenges of the Pharmaceutical Industry

A vital aspect of healthcare is the pharmaceutical industry. Without it, drug production, delivery or exploration will not take place. When we talk about the pharmaceutical industry, we say these three things: Distribution, development and discovery.

The pharmaceutical industry is actually not in good shape. The fact is that nine out of ten medications do not pass the clinical trial process. This also means that the FDA rarely approves a new drug. This is largely due to a shortage of patient data on which pharmaceutical companies base their testing and approval process.

Let us take a quick look at the challenges (Singh, 2020) to better understand the pharmaceutical industry.

1. ***Differences in pharmaceutical data***: Data is at the heart of the pharmaceutical sector as it helps firms experiment, understand and invent new medicines for various diseases. When attempting to address specific illnesses, pharmaceutical firms often find that the data gap is a major issue. This difference in data is derived from the silos which store the data. The silos work by connecting to various platforms. The reliance on multiple sources and the inability to validate the data uploaded

and exchanged are real issues for data discrepancy. Data discrepancy also comes about because of the data sources and divisions of various data systems and models.

2. ***Generic drugs have increased competition***: Generic drug competition has increased. It is the rationale behind the FDA's decision to smoothly and quickly market low-cost generic drugs. This makes it impossible for new medicines to be licensed. New medicines usually have an exclusivity duration of 180 days. However, the backlog of generic applications is massive, and thus the concept of exclusivity is difficult to uphold.
3. ***Rising consumer expectations***: Every day, consumers become more knowledgeable. Consumers demands are rising. With increased scrutiny, pharmaceutical firms need to take better economic and clinical steps to offer consumer care in poor and affluent countries.
4. ***Time-consuming and resource-heavy data analytics***: The data analytics aspect becomes very time consuming and resource-packed, as data are accessed from various sources using different models and frameworks. Companies must first ensure that the data they collected is reliable and thorough before analyzing them. They must also ensure that they use sophisticated data analytics techniques to find out what they are searching for.
5. ***Supply chain***: Supply chain management is one of the pharmaceutical industry's major challenges. The supply chain for pharmaceuticals is complex and risky. Any breach in the supply chain means that the pharmaceutical industry loses lots of money because of fraud and falsification. In the healthcare global survey, pharmaceutical firms are predicted to lose about US$200 billion annually because of counterfeit drugs.
6. ***Poor research productivity***: The scientific community in pharma has achieved nothing remarkable in the last decade. The production rate remained the same, contributing to the conviction that the research and creation process is inherently flawed. When you compare it to other science fields, scientific research in the pharmaceutical industry is nowhere.
7. ***Stagnation***: The last challenge facing the pharmaceutical industry is stagnation. That is because the methods, management culture and mental models do not change. All is achieved in a conventional way that does not challenge any of pharmaceutical industry's present pressure points.

In terms of management culture and procedures, almost every industry has changed. However, health and pharmaceuticals seem to be influenced by the cut-throat competition beyond many pharmaceutical competitors' reach.

12.3 Blockchain Solutions to Pharmaceutical Industry

Now that we understand the problems of the pharmaceutical industry let us explore the solution. Blockchain is a new technology that holds the key to all of this. Some challenges go beyond the capability of blockchain but indirectly affect them. Blockchain is a peer-to-peer solution for which a centralized organization does not have to work properly. It uses a consensus model to achieve consensus on network transactions and other operations. The blockchain networks are immutable, stable and transparent as well.

Blockchain will revamp the pharmaceutical industry by incorporating three main elements: Privacy, transparency and traceability. It will respect the regulations, procedures, privacy and global rules of the industry. Clinical studies, for example, would benefit greatly from access to greater clarity and accurate facts.

12.3.1 Blockchain Can Add Value to the Pharmaceutical Industry

The current health crisis affects us all: It is a global struggle that gives companies and producers a special responsibility in the pharmaceutical sector. These days, the essential requirement for doctors, physicians, patients, drug manufacturers and medical devices is product availability, safety and reputation.

Technology is an engine in the manufacture and delivery of these goods. It has a major presence in both upstream and downstream production: Data analysis and research, innovation, quality, manufacturing, logistics and management. As we applaud these life-saving efforts, it is worth seeing how new technologies like blockchain add value (Samuga, 2020).

1. ***The global process must be transparent***: Pharmaceutical supply chains are extremely diverse and are produced and distributed internationally by many international manufacturers, regulatory agencies, distributors, hospitals, insurance firms and producers. With new diseases such as Covid-19, this dynamic chain must be flexible and receptive to the marketing of new medicines. This means that manufacturers must be creative and rapidly adapt to the current market requirements. Suppliers must also comply with additional or updated legislation on transport. To do this, a producer must ensure the consistency of each ingredient and ensure that products are delivered in time and under optimum conditions of storage and transport. These problems are more critical than ever in a crisis such as the current one: After all, it concerns the timely delivery of life-saving agents for human life. Technology can help multi-company business processes in many fields operate more smoothly.
2. ***It begins with trust***: Blockchain would be a potential alternative to the pharmaceutical supply chain's formidable problems. Blockchain technology is particularly predestined as it no longer includes two or three partners, but several partners, such as vendors, distributors and so on, as part of a network. Blockchain offers traceability through data, storage and delivery through an entity in product life cycles. For highly regulated industries such as pharmaceuticals, this is particularly relevant. This industry needs accountability in clinical trials, control over a lot from scale-up, validation and quality assurance before the final approved product is marketed. Many pharmaceutical firms use contract production systems to manage the acquisition and production processes. Documentation is produced and follows products from raw material to finished goods and distribution phases. These documents can include regulatory requirements, specifications of ingredients or contractual details. Blockchain enables the correlation and audit of information such as packaging materials, established proof and regulation integrity, through collaboration with other parties, of all related commercial content certifications. This means that different parties must create trust to orchestrate the flow of content, knowledge and finance. There is a large amount of time and money

spent on contracts, auditing expenditures, reconciliation and legal proceedings. Blockchain technology essentially makes a reliable environment of distributed data ownership.

3. ***Privacy and Innovation***: Institutions share and extend their information and data worldwide, especially when people's lives are at risk, as with Covid-19. Blockchain offers the capacity to exchange safe and unchanging data, enabling businesses to join forces in an innovative spirit more easily. By separating, people can access blockchain data, patient data can be secured sustainably. It is crucial that when it comes to medical data, nobody wants to give up their right to personal privacy, even in the run-up to this pandemic. The general use of patient data for the advancement of clinical research is, however, indispensable. For example, this is at stake in clinical trials: Patients must be advised and give consent at any clinical trial stage. This consent shall be properly registered and stored safely, including in compliance with existing data protection regulations. It is also important how these systems treat historical patient details. The patient can then determine knowledge can be "unlocked." Furthermore, only data related to the disease under review should be made available. This separation of access permissions can be carried out using distributed ledger technology. Different parties retain an unlimited number of essentially equal copies of the ledger (or transaction and process step). Proper steps ensure that all the ledger copies accept new transactions and reach a consensus on the ledger's current status. Depending on the access options for participants on a network, distributed ledgers may be divided into "approved" or "open" ledgers. While the latter is available to all, access to the account directory in the former is controlled.
4. ***Product quality traceability***: In pharmaceutical manufacturing and distribution, process step traceability plays an important role. The products' flows must be reviewed from the outset and unambiguously defined to minimize counterfeit merchandise and quickly retrieve the faulty product's source. Smart contracts are a significant added value offered by blockchain. These may be added automatically to the deliveries and ensure that the goods themselves disclose a breach of these rules or substitutes if storage conditions are not suitable. Trust in the visibility and traceability of the supply chain is the basis of Smart contracts. This activates those actions automatically during predefined events. Processes involving the approval of many participants in the supply chain may be automated. For example, a logistics company's verified proof of delivery will automatically activate digital invoicing and payment through the banking system.

12.3.2 Blockchain Will Revolutionize the Pharmaceutical Industry

According to Statista, pharmaceuticals are a US$466 billion industry (Zahreddine, 2018). However, privacy issues and transparency in clinical trials can delay potential drug development and increase costs. To address these privacy issues, new technologies such as blockchain should be explored. Blockchain will revolutionize the pharmaceutical industry, and it would be the perfect way to deal with some transparency, privacy and traceability initiatives (Zahreddine, 2018).

Blockchain is, at its very core, a distributed ledger system with verifiable transactions. The ledger is encrypted and verifiable across the entire chain for any subsequent transaction. For example, when there is a record of 100 transactions, every transaction can be checked in its previous and subsequent transactions. Blockchain, in short, will provide anonymity and trust to verify and audit activities.

This contributes to forward integrity and privacy for a transaction. For example, a supermarket could easily recognize which farm a broccoli head came from in food traceability. A medication could be traced to pharmaceutical firms in the same way.

1. ***Blockchain applications in pharmaceutical firms***: One might argue that for the pharmaceutical industry, blockchain has been constructed because of the industry's stringent privacy policies, legislation and global regulations. Blockchain can help to solve inherent problems due to this. The technology can improve the confidentiality of information in clinical trials, opening the door to more information. This can also lead to shorter cycles for drug production and discovery periods. A BioMed Central report explores how clinical trials reproducibility has been a problem for some time and how blockchain technology can combine data security with secure, decentralized monitoring of all data. Different applications for blockchain use in clinical trials are also accessible, such as building public registers. According to a Pistola Alliance study, the revealing of clinical trial data rapidly became top priority for large and small pharmaceutical firms, with 60 percent of pharmaceutical companies either using or experimenting with blockchain. This would allow an individual to participate in an unknown clinical trial. Using blockchain will help alleviate concerns that certain people will risk their data when participating in a clinical trial. If more people are more comfortable with these details, better life-changing treatments will save more lives. In the healthcare sector, in general, patients can trust their verifiable information to be safeguarded.
2. ***Scandal in China stimulates support for blockchain***: In July 2018, a Chinese producer of vaccines was forced to stop production after artificial data was detected, making some manufactured vaccines unsuitable for children. This created public outrage. Crypto investors in China have used this investigation as a soapbox to debate freely why the whole supply chain should be tracked and traced via blockchain. A group of companies in the US founded the MediLedger project last year and building an industry-owned blockchain network for the pharmaceutical sector based on open standards and specifications. In October 2018, the company launched the saleable returns protocol for directory and verification services as the first of several initiatives. It is interesting for a more conservative industry to see a solid, early adoption to test blockchain uses.
3. ***Transparency is blockchain's future in pharma***: Patients want reliable results and want to know what they did is useful in future studies. Using blockchain, up-to-date data may be open to all stakeholders at any time. Creating a greater sense of confidence through blockchain and ensuring patients are safer would create a stronger relationship between the pharmaceutical industry and the public. Also, medication recalls would make it possible to return drugs much more effectively than ever before through the supply chain. The initiatives built in the pharmaceutical industry through blockchain are vast, far more than any other industry. In the future, blockchain will have a huge effect on many industries. If they are not yet, all pharmaceutical industry stakeholders should regard blockchain as an enormous opportunity to boost every aspect of the lifecycle, including sponsors, service producers, the supply chain and patients.

12.3.3 The Ways Blockchain Benefits the Pharmaceutical Industry

Some businesses have adapted rapidly to emerging technologies such as cloud and blockchain. The pharmaceutical industry is one of them. Blockchain safety is very appealing for the pharmaceutical industry because it relies on encryption; few other industries do. A ledger cannot be manipulated at the core of blockchain technology, making it so valuable to the pharmaceutical industry.

Since there are thousands of computers in the blockchain, any transaction is sealed into a block which cannot be hacked. To modify each device where the chain is stored, a hacker must hack and modify it individually. This is unlikely, in other words.

This section addresses some aspects that the blockchain benefits the pharmaceutical industry (FINSMES, 2020):

1. ***Secure documents***: Since the internet was established, the safe transmission of confidential documents has been a problem for businesses. The cloud has solved some of the issues, and the best online fax service will send documents safer than email. However, the design of the blockchain makes it the perfect option for data storage and document transmission. With ledgers that document each transaction and cannot be modified, there are far fewer chances of committing a cybercrime.
2. ***Supply chain logistics***: A phase in the pharmaceutical process from research and development to shipping demands a lot of attention and visibility. Incompatible computer applications and shipping visibility contribute to many headaches. The blockchain will eradicate these headaches because the ledger is fully transparent and can be seen every step of the way. It does not matter what sort of computer system is used. The blockchain operates on different platforms. As the blockchain is decentralized, several intermediaries who inject themselves into the process can be removed. This saves a lot of time and money. MediLedger is a project introduced in 2017 by Chronicled to simplify supply chain operations using blockchain technology.
3. ***Safety of drugs***: Also, how the drugs are created is being disrupted by the blockchain. The traceability method from compound centers to other parts of the supply chain is more traceable. This increases the accountability of the development process and can avoid many deaths by the administration of incorrect prescriptions. The supply chain to the point of sale is clear so that nothing is missing when the drug is manufactured. Checamed, a 2017 smartphone app, helps customers verify medicines and general information by scanning a QR code.
4. ***Control of clinical trials***: It is a logistic nightmare to perform various clinical trials for pharmaceutical companies' medications. The data are complex, and reliable results are evident in the blockchain management of this system. The digital and immutable ledger will more thoroughly classify and verify many of the various studies than ever before. Patientory INC is a fine example of blockchain's utility in allowing patients, researchers and health organizations to store and access data securely.
5. ***Provenance***: The global size of the counterfeit drugs market ranges from US$75 to 200 billion and is rising rapidly. The epidemic of counterfeit and fake medicines is a concern that the pharmaceutical industry has not overcome. By allowing manufacturers and customers to monitor the medicine from source to point of sale, blockchain will help minimize the problem to a significant extent. The package stored in the blockchain can be given a unique code, making it easily traceable

over the entire supply chain. Dokchain is a platform that allows industry people and consumers to maintain transactions, access the data and automate paperwork using blockchain technology.

12.4 Blockchain Use-Cases in Pharma

There are several use cases of blockchain in pharmaceuticals. Below are some of the notable ones (Singh, 2020):

1. ***The authenticity of returned drugs***: Pharmaceutical firms must regularly deal with returned drugs. This is because of wholesalers' over-stocking. That is why the unused stock must be returned to the manufacturers. At any point in time 2–3 percent of the drugs are returned. However, if it is expressed in terms of money, it can hit US$7–10 billion. The key concern, however, is that the returns are counterfeit medicines. The difficulty for pharmaceutical firms lies in identifying and separating them before they can sell the returned drugs. Briefly, pharmaceutical firms need to check the details on authenticity before releasing their drugs back to the market. Each drug must be barcoded and serialized to ensure that it happens. A centralized authority achieves this. However, this could mean that another vendor manages the authentication of drugs. In the US, a centralized database regulator is missing. A decentralized blockchain is a solution. This helps the pharmaceutical companies to conveniently record the serial number of the package on the blockchain. This ensures that the drug can be tested anywhere. It enables consumers and wholesalers to verify authenticity without having to rely on a central authority. The SAP Pharma Blockchain POC application is one of the proof-of-concept solutions to the problem. It has a decentralized blockchain that both consumers and wholesalers can use.
2. ***Compliance with the pharmaceutical supply chain***: The pharmaceutical supply chain is one of the most significant issues for pharmaceutical companies. The task is not only to efficiently control the supply chain but also to adhere to the standards. Some of the challenges that can be addressed by a blockchain-powered pharmaceutical supply chain are:
   - Reduction in falsified drugs.
   - Improved visibility.
   - Compliance with regulations.
   - Better cold chain shipping.
   - *Sensitive drugs*: Drugs often need to be monitored by several parameters. It includes the collection of information such as air quality, humidity, temperature range, etc. If one of these criteria is not preserved, the drug will go wrong and will not benefit the end user. Vaccines are one of the best examples. During the journey through the supply chain, a carefully managed environment is required. By integrating with the supply chain and the IoT, blockchain can help solve this problem. The supply chain can be prepared with devices that track humidity, temperature and other essential factors. Once registered, the parties involved can easily be contacted to take the required action as needed. It solves the problem of handling and synchronizing a separate directory.

- *Compliance*: Blockchain is equally useful to incorporate management and supply chain compliance. The main features of blockchain, including immutability, distributed design and transparency, make this possible. All of these should be used to enforce the supply chain process so that transport authorities can comply with the guidelines.
- *Automation*: Blockchain also includes smart contracts. Smart contracts include the power to automate blockchain activities. This is very useful since smart contracts will create alerts if they do not comply. When completed, all drug-related parties will be informed.

3. ***Better clinical trials***: As blockchain is used to store patient records, it can also provide ways to enhance clinical trials performed by pharmaceutical companies. Blockchain can be used by organizations to connect with patients and access information at each phase of the clinical trial process. This decreases patient anxiety and allows them to understand the risks better. The clinical guidelines for both clients and patients are much clearer. This is a vital step because it is often difficult to obtain informed consent satisfactorily and comprehensively. Ten percent of the trials, including unapproved forms, have not been signed with a consent document, lack guidelines and do not inform the patient of a review of the procedure, etc. according to the FDA. The incorporation of blockchain enhances clinical trials as it increases consent transparency and traceability. The consent forms can be reviewed with a timeline. Often, no-one can modify the information once it is processed.
4. ***Quality and efficiency of clinical trial data***: Efficiency and quality of clinical trial data can increase with blockchain. The decentralized design enables the clinical laboratories to use a clear, immutable data source where the data cannot be disturbed. The clinical trial data is stored in the public blockchain, where data can be reviewed whenever required. It is tamper-proof, and clinical laboratories should fully trust the data to conduct their test results. In the end, both the consistency of the patient's experience and the researchers will be enhanced. Pharmaceutical firms may also use the system to encourage more patients to take part in the trials.
5. ***Inventory management***: Pharmaceutical companies can handle their inventories much better with the tight integration with the supply chain. The inventory may also be automated to activate a supply or demand scenario. For example, if the demand is on the rise, the system will simply warn of the demand and request further drug production. It will also give wholesalers proper exposure and how their inventory is handled in various circumstances.

12.5 Premier Companies Using a Blockchain Solution with Healthcare and Pharma

Many businesses in the pharmaceutical and healthcare sectors use blockchain technology. Some of the most notable are given below (Singh, 2020):

1. ***Pfizer***: It engages actively in the MedilLedger project. The project aims to create an environment that will enable the drug industry to get to the last detail. It also means that counterfeiting is not possible. Ensuring that only manufacturers

can process serial numbers and apply single identifiers to products (noted in the header) makes accessing the chain on a random basis much harder for a fake product. The blockchain system uses zero-knowledge proofs to ensure compliance without actually exchanging data.

2. ***NMC Healthcare***: The UAE-based private healthcare provider has been focusing on developing its internal infrastructure with blockchain startups. NMC announced a collaboration with Du in January 2017 to introduce electronic health records via blockchain.
3. ***United Healthcare***: United Healthcare and Optum are both seeking to take part. The consortium in which they participate comprises Multiplan, Humana and Quest Diagnostics. The key goal of the project is to reduce the total costs of administrative activities. Using blockchain, the whole process can be streamlined, and the database can be modified more often than conventional systems.
4. ***Roche***: Roche is one of the major pharmaceutical giants. Currently, Abbvie and Pfizer are testing the pilot of the supply chain via their Genentech division. The Roche diagnostics division in Asia said it intends to collaborate with PwC Singapore and a startup named Dex to provide a pilot to submit patient blood data in real time. The blockchain project can help clinicians access more up-to-date data rather than measuring outcomes between doctor appointments for weeks or months.

12.6 Startups and Emerging Companies That Develop Blockchain Solutions for the Pharmaceutical Industry

We highlight five startups and emerging companies that are developing blockchain solutions for the pharmaceutical industry (Startus Insights, n.d.):

1. ***StaTwig***: Vaccine supply chain: StaTwig is an Indian startup that provides vaccine supply chain improvement solutions. VaccineLedgerTM facilitates end-to-end vaccine tracing through the vaccine supply chain. The blockchain solution collects tamper-resistant data in real time to increase accountability for all stakeholders. It assigns a unique ID and alphanumeric code to track its lifecycle from manufacture to distribution at hospital pharmacies.
2. ***FarmaTrust***: Clinical trials: FarmaTrust, a UK-based startup, develops Ethereum's blockchain-based pharmaceutical solutions. It uses blockchain to ensure protected anonymity and, therefore, true double-blind testing. The startup uses mobile applications to alert patients when they should take the medicines in trails and wearables to track how they respond to medicines. The solution enables pharmaceutical companies to receive faster regulatory approval and gives interested parties direct access to data.
3. ***BlockMedx***: Electronic prescribing: BlockMedx is a US-based startup that offers electronic prescription solutions using blockchain. The startup sends and receives electronic prescriptions safely via blockchain technology and also records them.

BlockMedx also uses drug analytics to predict risk behaviors for patients. The approach is free of charge for both patients and pharmacies and delivers medical care through multiple doctors and healthcare facilities.

4. ***Hypertrust Patient Data Care***: Real-world data: German startup Hypertrust Patient Data Care offers blockchain solutions for patient information safety. The startup uses blockchain to produce more relevant data during the process. The approach facilitates a deeper understanding of a patient's condition and better treatment care. It also helps the method of drug discovery in personalized medicine.
5. ***Humanscape***: Rare diseases: Humanscape is a South Korean company that offers personalized information on rare diseases. To protect patients' health records, *Rarenote* uses blockchain technology, including its genetic test results, symptoms and medical treatment information. The anonymized data is accessible by pharmaceutical firms and research institutes to advance new medicine production if the patient agrees.

12.7 Conclusion

Many blockchain innovations are still pilot projects, and deployment over the entire supplier network could take a long time. An example of this is the MediLedger project created in 2017 to test a closed blockchain system to determine who was using a drug. Experts agree that blockchain could revolutionize industries like pharmaceuticals. Moreover, in many ways, the current crisis impressively demonstrates that technology can offer high added value. The bottom line is: Modern blockchain technology is just as important as greater numbers of people are taking part in it.

Glossary

Blockchain: Blockchain is an immutable digital ledger that is programmed to record transactions and anything that has a value.

Clinical trials: Clinical trials are scientific studies conducted to find efficient ways to prevent, screen for, diagnose or cure diseases.

Decentralized: To transfer the control of an organization or government from a single entity to several smaller ones.

Interoperability: Ability of a product or a system for an unrestricted sharing of resources and exchange information.

Provenance: The chronology of the origin, ownership, custody or location of a product.

Supply chain: Supply chain is the sequence of processes involved in the production and distribution of goods from manufacturers to consumers.

Traceability: Ability to verify the history and location of an item using documented recorded identification.

References

Akeo. (n.d.). Blockchain in Pharmaceutical. https://akeo.tech/wp-content/uploads/2018/11/Blockchain-in-Pharmaceutical.pdf

FINSMES. (2020). How the Pharmaceutical Industry is Using Blockchain. *Physiology News*. https://doi.org/10.36866/pn.92.27

James Lind Institute. (2019). Pharmaceutical Industry Overview. *Pharmaceutical Processing*. https://doi.org/10.4135/9781412953979.n481

Reddy, RK. (2018). Overview of Pharmaceutical Industry. https://www.pharmatimesnow.com/2018/10/overview-of-pharmaceutical-industry23.html

Samuga, A. (2020). How Blockchain Can Add Value to the Pharmaceutical Industry. https://www.epmmagazine.com/opinion/how-blockchain-can-add-value-to-the-pharmaceutical-industry/

Singh, N. (2020). Blockchain in Pharma: Will Pharmaceutical Industry Evolve? https://101blockchains.com/blockchain-in-pharma/

Startus Insights. (n.d.). 5 Top Blockchain Solutions Impacting the Pharma Industry. https://www.startus-insights.com/innovators-guide/5-top-blockchain-solutions-impacting-the-pharma-industry/#:~:text=StaTwig%2C%20FarmaTrust%2C%20BlockMedx%2C%20Hypertrust,our%20Global%20Startup%20Heat%20Map!&text=Our%20Innovation%20Analysts%20recently%20looked,solutions%20for%20the%20pharma%20sector.

Zahreddine, M. (2018). How Blockchain Will Revolutionize the Pharmaceutical Industry. *Forbes*. https://www.forbes.com/sites/forbestechcouncil/2018/11/14/how-blockchain-will-revolutionize-the-pharmaceutical-industry/#11dfc6d726e5

13

Blockchain in the Pharmaceutical and Healthcare Ecosystem

Arnab Banerjee

CONTENTS

13.1 Introduction

The pharmaceutical industry always focused on the developed economies of Europe and the US for its research and new drugs. But in the last few years governments in developing economies have focused and funded a lot on healthcare, making it a priority. The result is that emerging markets have a bigger pharma spend, of around US$281 billion compared to US$196 billion for the top five EU countries [1]. Due to this radical change

DOI: 10.1201/9781003133179-13

in the outlook of healthcare, the nature, ways of research and opportunity of the pharma business are changing tremendously and globally. It is becoming global in nature and the supply chain is becoming more complex by the day. To prove a point, the key ingredients of drug manufacturing, the active pharmaceutical ingredients (APIs) and bulk drugs are mainly supplied by India and China to all major pharma manufacturers the world over. Today, clinical trials are global in nature and products are sold specifically to a market. It is like a consumer-packaged product and that makes its supply chain, safety of products and purity so important for patients. All these make the industry vulnerable and ask for stricter measures and control with higher standards of protocols. The same is evident with the security acts and medicine directives in the US and Europe. This is where the need for mature technology comes into the picture to chart the unexplored path.

13.1.1 An Overview of the Pharma and Healthcare Ecosystem and Their Challenges

The global healthcare sector is valued at close to US$11.9 trillion globally and is growing close to 7 to 8% annually since 2014 [9]. The global pharmaceuticals market is worth approximately US$934.8 billion in 2017 and will reach US$1.17 trillion by 2021, growing at 5.8% [10]. These numbers show the scale of the sector and are indicative that it holds a major share of the global economy apart from being of importance to humanity. Due to its importance, sensitivity and impact on individuals and society the industry is highly regulated. It is one of those industries which touches the economic, demographic and social fabric of society and has deep impact on each of them. Due to its nature, reach and sensitivity of impact the pharma companies and regulators are both risk averse and relentlessly seek safety, transparency and traceability of the products. They try to be as impartial as possible, working at the forefront of science and management. Healthcare and pharma both look divergent and dependent but have the same core values of cure, passion and humanity. Both have a concentrated effort for the benefit of society and a passion for accuracy. Their association is very close and highly dependent. Their challenges are shared and revolve around cost, resources, process, access and quality.

13.2 Challenges in Pharma Companies and Healthcare Ecosystems

The drug development process is always cost and time sensitive. It is a stressful, research oriented, intensive process with many unknowns, limited chances of success and is highly dependent on talent. The pharma supply chain is considered one of the most challenging in the world. With the potential to adversely affect human life the supply chain is critical. It needs to ensure safety, security and foster resilience. The pharma industry today also covers the medical devices industry which has a lot of connected devices. Though there are many challenges in this industry, this section highlights the most prominent challenges faced by pharma companies:

1. Fake, substandard, counterfeit, devices and medicines. As per some studies these account for up to US$200 billion annually [2]. This is also known as pharmaceutical falsification.
2. Cold chain shipping in the pharma industry. Many drugs have living organisms or contain components of living organisms. Such products are sensitive to temperature and susceptible to contamination if they deviate from prescribed limits

of temperature. Maintaining a desired temperature range is an essential part of product stability and efficacy. Having transparency in the cold chain is very important in such products.

3. Compliance: Compliance is an integral part of the pharma industry. The ability to comply with all rules laid down by the respective countries' medical authorities is an important aspect of this industry. As an example, suppliers and distributors need to abide by the norms set by the Food and Drug Administration (FDA) in the US. This is a basic compliance for pharmaceutical companies to adhere to for existence.
4. Disruption: Supply chain disruption is a perennial risk for any business. The same is applicable for pharma industry as well. With globalized businesses traversing countries, the supply chain is opaquer today than before. This is a formidable challenge, especially for the pharma supply chain.
5. Drug development process: The drug development process involves time, talent and materials, with multiple stakeholders. The process is talent-driven, cost and time intensive, has limited chances of success and multiple unknowns. The result of the effort is an ability to generate a new drug or generate a new method of drug production. It is a highly competitive environment in a highly collaborative atmosphere. Today research findings are protected by patents. There are chances that competitors or organizations with criminal intent can reproduce the clinical research with low-cost products and process thus undermining years of work by research firms. Protection of information in the drug development process is crucial for its sustenance and future development.
6. Pharma clinical trials: The clinical trials are spread across four entities. It involves pharma companies, clinical research organizations, trial sites and patients. The two other aspects we cannot lose sight of are the doctors/physicians and the data generated while doing these trials. The process of a trial involves data exchanges across systems and most of the information is confidential. This includes patient records, protocols, results, medicine doses, etc. Safe and secure information sharing but maintaining transparency for regulators is a challenge in today's clinical trials.
7. Recall management. Many times a situation arises where pharma companies need to recall their products (medicines or devices). Achieving a full recall is a challenge due to the lack of visibility from manufacturers all the way to the end consumer primarily due to lack of technology.

There are various other challenges in the pharma and healthcare industry. But the above highlighted are the most prominent and impacts overall drug availability, the consumption of it and the general healthcare industry.

With time people are getting more and more health conscious but the nature and kind of diseases are dramatically changing and getting more complicated. The Covid-19 pandemic is a very good example and the lack of a vaccine until the end of 2020 has made this focus even more pertinent. Due to this, the focus of society is moving from cure to prevention. This section of the chapter focuses on challenges that impact the general healthcare system. The supply chain, which includes inventory management and disposal, is considered one of the biggest cost centers for healthcare providers [3]. Healthcare needs to maintain a lot of patient records which are personally identifiable and have considerable personal information. The medical care system needs to share a lot of critical information (including personal data) across different entities (like imaging, diagnostics, labs, public health, legal) and needs to be done securely. Today healthcare companies work in silos and cross-company collaboration is through the traditional methods of reports, phone, and/or emails. Another example of collaboration is between the hospitals and insurance providers, and it is primarily driven through emails (in developing nations like India). There are cases of insurance fraud and rejection of valid insurance claims due to information mismatch. In either of the cases either the insurance company or the consumer suffers for lack of a transparent system. In many of the medico-legal cases the information needs to be shared between the legal system, judiciary, public safety offices, police and care-givers/hospitals. Collaboration in most of these cases is by means of manual processes, devoid of any system. These leads to information leaks and misuse.

The healthcare system needs to integrate with a host of systems for routine patient care and information sharing. The basic system used by most hospitals are called an electronic medical record (EMR). But today information needs to be shared across systems and hospitals and thus it becomes more of an electronic health record (EHR). Most hospitals use an Enterprise Resource Planning (ERP) system like Oracle or SAP, and it needs to integrate with the EMR/EHR. Today healthcare records also integrate with the Maintenance Management Information System for Medicaid known as MMIS and/or Oncology Research Information System (ORIS). There is a lot of critical and personally identifiable information shared with host of systems for this purpose. Transparency, authenticity and safety of these information is always a challenge. It is evident such a huge system with a complicated network and volume cannot be managed or secured manually!

These processes in the pharma and healthcare ecosystem need a mature technology for medical systems to operate safely and serve humanity.

13.3 The Need For a Mature Technology in Pharma and Healthcare

The healthcare system and the EHR today interface a highly complicated system of systems. The EHR traverses through multitude of systems, thus getting exposed to vulnerability and prone to misuse. EHR data are interfaced to labs, hospitals, diagnostic imaging centers, patient monitoring devices, pharma companies, MMIS and ORIS. The hospital also has a lot of internal systems like ERP and other supply chain systems where the patient health record (EHR) interfaces. This evidently asks for information audit, tracking and monitoring. The distributed ledger technology (DLT) driven blockchain network is a good fit for these purposes. It is a mature technology which can overcome the challenges faced by pharma and healthcare companies and benefit the overall industry. The blockchain network can introduce radical changes in the way stakeholders are managed and has implications for the entire ecosystem. The system can bring a secure network infrastructure, cutting across different stakeholders, geography and systems. The impact of blockchain will be similar for both pharma and the healthcare system but the application will be different for healthcare and pharma.

Pharma Companies

The application of blockchain in pharma is more diverse, driving a lot of benefits across a lot of stakeholders in the value chain spectrum of the industry. It will not only benefit the pharma companies but also the end consumers. It will bring transparency to drug distribution, drug development and help with the tracing and trackability of products all the way to consumers. Another great benefit which the blockchain system can bring to the pharma companies is in meeting compliance and regulation requirements. As the US FDA brings in the Drug Supply Chain Security Act (DSCSA) and Europe follows the Falsified Medicines Directive (FMD), meeting such compliance requirements will only be possible with blockchain technology.

Healthcare System

The application of blockchain in the healthcare system will be oriented towards clinical trials and information transparency while sharing patient medical records across systems/organizations. It will play a major role in clinical trials and in ascertaining the transparency of consent and reduce exploitation of the subjects in clinical trials. Apart from that the safety, security and operation of medical devices can also benefit from the blockchain system. First, these devices, being costly products, benefit from being track and trace enabled with the blockchain solution. For wearable devices it also assures the patients of its authenticity and origin.

Blockchain technology will be useful in pharma and healthcare but the interoperability of the blockchain network is going to be one of the key factors for its success. The features of blockchain, like those of immutable, transparent, consensus, chronological data links will enhance the security and trust factors in the overall pharma and healthcare ecosystem. The ability to write smart contracts and ability to make the process digital and contactless is an added advantage which blockchain brings as a technology

13.4 Blockchain for Drug Supply Chain

The pharma and health systems today are significantly digital. The Organisation for Economic Cooperation and Development (OECD) has estimated that around 2.5% of global pharmaceutical drugs are counterfeit [4]. It is estimated the numbers in developing countries are far worse. It is expected to be around 10–30% counterfeit [5]. The pharma and drug supply chain needs to be secure, integrated and should have the ability to provide provenance of product (medicine and devices). The data for provenance must be transparent, immutable and auditable to generate trust.

As discussed above a DLT-powered blockchain network is a solution to look forward to and it can provide visibility, regulatory compliance and supply chain integrity. The blockchain network system must be organized by the manufacturer to derive the most benefit. Manufacturers must bring in the key supply chain partners to form the chain of ownership, thus establishing provenance and traceability.

Apart from traceability and provenance (to combat counterfeiting) there are a few other areas where blockchain can play a crucial role in pharma and healthcare, and these are drug development/discovery, clinical trials, genomic data management and patents and intellectual property.

US Drug Supply Chain and Blockchain Technology

The US Food and Drug Administration, also popularly known as the FDA, in 2013 passed rules to regulate and monitor the manufacturing of drugs. This act is called the Drug

Supply Chain Security Act (DSCSA). The intent of DSCSA is to have an electronic system of records to track, trace and provide the provenance of prescription drugs in the US. In other words, the law makes drugs traceable to improve anti-counterfeiting. The law regulates transactions making it transparent between dispensers and pharmacies and with manufacturers, distributors (stockists) and Third-Party Logistics Providers (3PL). The idea is to make drugs available on prescription which are also traceable throughout the pharma supply chain, thus establishing provenance. The act will become fully applicable in 10 years, i.e., 2023. There are three main goals to accomplish by 2023, these are:

1. The system should be able to verify a legitimate drug down to the package level. The anti-counterfeiting check should be at the package level.
2. The system and infrastructure should be developed such that fake or counterfeit drugs should be easily detectable.
3. The system should aid in a successful drug recall situation.

The DSCSA needs the data to be verified among the partners. There is no centralized database or system having any centralized record keeping. The law enforces a track and trace solution for medicines and warrants that the product is traceable through all the supply chain partners. This makes the DLT-based blockchain network a tailor-made solution for this requirement.

Pharma companies are coming together to form networks on blockchain technology to make themselves ready for the DSCSA by 2023. Twenty-four companies have joined together in the US to form a pharmaceutical supply chain network named MediLedger, built by a company named Chronicled a blockchain startup. It can also be called as a blockchain consortium. The solution proposes an interoperable blockchain-based track and trace system for US prescription drugs. The blockchain system tracks the change of ownership in the supply chain, authenticates the drug manufacturer and establishes provenance. The MediLedger network members comprises of manufacturers like Novartis, Novo Nordisk, Pfizer, Sanofi, Gilead, GSK, wholesalers like McKesson and AmerisourceBergen as well retailers like Walgreens and Walmart [6].

So, it can be seen that governmental rules are forcing pharma companies to adopt technologies like blockchain. MediLedger is creating permissioned blockchain for pharma companies, bringing in the partners (manufacturer, distributor, 3PL, dispenser) into the network and tracking the change of ownership and establishing provenance. Companies like IDLogiq, Rymedi and TraceLink are also exploring blockchain for the DSCSA-focused project and trying to get approval from the FDA.

SAP has a solution named Advanced Track and Trace for Pharmaceuticals (ATTP) which can uniquely mark and identify a transaction for tracking pharma products. The ATTP solution helps in regulatory reporting of pharmaceutical products as required by various countries. This solution is not related to blockchain technology. SAP also has Information Collaboration Hub for Life Sciences which connects pharmaceutical organizations and their supply chain partners on a secure network that is owned and managed by SAP. SAP has integrated the ATTP with the SAP Information Collaboration Hub for Life Sciences. SAP has launched its blockchain pharmaceutical traceability solution, specially purposed to meet DSCSA requirements. For this purpose SAP uses MultiChain, the blockchain platform developed by Coin Sciences. The ATTP solution generates a unique ID which is stored in the blockchain system (MultiChain) and the ID is verified from blockchain as and when needed. The SAP solution based on blockchain technology empowers end customers to check various drug related product attributes like product code, batch/lot numbers, expiration date based on batch/lot numbers, authenticating manufacturer's data. All these data are originally created into the blockchain network by manufacturers at the time of shipment from the manufacturing facility. Because the DSCSA needs verification among the participants there is no need for a centralized database.

European Drug Supply Chain and Blockchain Technology

In order to protect its people the European Union (EU) has adopted certain rules for tracking medicines and averting fake products. This set of rules is known as the Falsified Medicines Directive (FMD). These rules were legalized by the European Union Parliament in 2016. The aim of the directive is to provide safe medicines to European patients which includes anti-counterfeiting, anti-tampering security on packages, tracking and delivery of medicines. Drugs, as well as medical devices, have ingredients and components which travel through the complex, global supply chains in which documentation is manual and paper-driven with lot of handovers and border crossings. The EU regulation maintains a centralized data of all medicine produced so that it can be verified at any time by anyone. The centralized data are with the European Medicines Verification Organisation (EMVO) and all manufacturers are supposed to share it. This regulation is targeted to solve the problems of counterfeiting in the drug supply chain. With government-backed mandates, the manufacturers are required to provide features on medicine packages to enable a systematic means to verify the authenticity of the medicine from its batch/lot number at the time of dispensing it to a patient. This will prevent fake/counterfeit medicines from entering the supply chain. As per the EU FMD the safety features expected on the prescription medicine are standardized. There are two features requested, namely:

1) Unique identifier in the form of a 2D data matrix (barcode): A pharmacy, while dispensing the medicine to consumer/public, will have to scan the 2D barcode and authenticate the product.
2) An anti-tamper device (ATD): A pharmacy, while dispensing the medicine to consumer/public, will physically check the anti-tamper device.

These process and infrastructures will reduce the fake and/or tampered products. Also, as per the directive the manufacturers will be required to contribute financially to establish the IT verification system to enable the authentication.

Though the law seems to be very similar to the DSCSA there is a subtle difference. In the DSCSA the verification of data is based on partners but in the EU FMD the data are to be verified with a central authority, EMVO. EMVO stores product data and enables verification at the time of dispensing. Thus, the FMD makes sure the product is traceable throughout the pharma supply chain from manufacturing to the end customer with a single custodian of authentic information. As EMVO is a single custodian of information the solution can be achieved without blockchain. But having the DLT-based blockchain network provides possibilities of security, trust, consensus, smart contracts and nonrepudiation, making it a more tailor-made solution for this requirement.

PharmaLedger is a blockchain consortium comprising of 29 members including 12 global pharmaceutical companies. This blockchain solution is specially designed for the EU FMD solution. For EU FMD, the solution offered by SAP is a combination of ATTP along with SAP Information Collaboration Hub for Life Sciences. In the solution, once the manufacturer produces the medicine the unique identifier of the batch/lot number is registered, stored and shared with EMVO. The SAP Information Collaboration Hub for Life Sciences system acts as a facilitator for message routing, verification and connectivity to EMVO.

India Drug Supply Chain and Blockchain Technology

India is also mandating pharma companies to introduce the barcoding of pharmaceutical products. This is to encourage traceability of products which can be invoked through a bar code scan on the medicine packages. This will also help in anti-counterfeiting. The National Institution for Transforming India (NITI) has partnered with Oracle Corp and Apollo Hospitals to develop the solution on the Oracle blockchain platform which is built on Hyperledger Fabric to advance the traceability of pharmaceutical products [7]. The Indian government's drug control arm, the Central Drugs Standard Control Organization, known as CDSCO, is also partnering in this project to use technology to solve the problem of counterfeiting. The blockchain-based solution will provide real-time visibility into the drug supply chain and improve traceability of all drugs produced in and exported from India.

All these three countries/continents (US, Europe, India) drug security aspect helps us understand that the drug supply chain is going to change and be impacted drastically. Figure 13.1 shows a high level but simple representation of how the different aspects of pharma companies is going to reorient with the US DSCSA, EU FMD and Indian drug controls. Figure 13.1 depicts that the process which was more linear and disjointed will become more connected and centralized. This transformation will happen with the adoption of DLT-driven blockchain.

13.5 Clinical Trials and Blockchain Technology

Drug development is a phased project. A new drug development enters a clinical trials stage when there are enough reasons to believe that the new drug being developed will improve the care of patients or cure the disease.

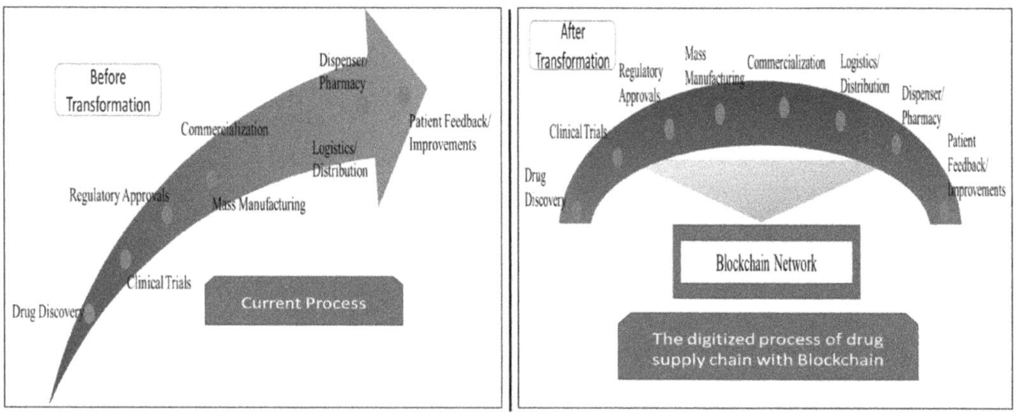

FIGURE 13.1
Digital transformation of the drug development and supply chain with blockchain.

There are four major stake holders in a clinical trial:

1) Sponsor: Sponsors are the organizations which fund the trial. They are generally the pharma companies, but can also be an academic institution or a hospital.
2) Clinical Research Organization (CRO): The CRO is the umbrella organization that provides the pharmaceutical and biotechnology aspect of the trial and hosts the Principal Investigators and the panel of doctors administering the dosage.
3) Participant/Subject/Patient: Persons or patients participating in the trial, who have provided their consent to be a part of the trial.
4) Ethics Review Board (ERB): This is the board which reviews the protocols to be followed for the trial and provides its approval. The board also protects the rights, safety, security, welfare, health and over all wellbeing of patients/subjects taking part in the trial.

Before the clinical trial stage, a drug is assessed for its impact and effectiveness in preclinical research. The protocol to be followed must be approved by the ERB. The clinical trials are a four-phased process.

Phase-0: In this phase a small sample of people/subjects (say 10–15) gets a very small amount of drug dose. This phase is designed to see the holistic effect of the drug on the body and its affect. This encompasses a check for negative reaction, degradation of health and over all wellbeing. It is generally administered on a healthy body. Based on a favorable phase-0 results, a drug can get into phase-1 trial. ERB reviews the results and provides consent for phase-1. If results are unsatisfactory, the drug may not proceed to phase-1.

Phase-1: With success in phase-0 the trials move to phase-1 where the drug is tested for side effects. The people/ patient/ subject group and dosage both increase. The drug may or may not help patients, but it is mainly to test the drug's safety on a patient. It is mostly to determine the negative effects on the subject and see for reactions. Based on a favorable phase-1 results, a drug can get into phase-2 trial. ERB reviews the results and provides consent for phase-2.

Phase-2: With success in previous trials the drug enters this phase and the number of people/ patient/ subject increases and it can go up to 500. This phase checks drug combinations, drug efficiency and dosage identification. Based on a favorable phase-2 results, a drug can get into phase-3 trial. ERB reviews the results and provides consent for phase-3.

Phase-3: This phase tests the drug's efficacy, effectiveness and safety on many people/ subjects; it can be several hundred patients (sometimes even 1000's). Often, these tests are randomized to test the performance against the standard drug. The phase-3 trial is considered critical as positive and favorable results in this phase lead to approval for use by most of the drug administrators like the FDA or CDSCO. Phase-3 decides whether there are more improvements needed to make it suitable for use or not.

Phase-4: Drugs approved in phase-3 is available to the general public as a prescribed drug. But still there is more research needed which is mainly to check the therapeutic dosage and its long-lasting side effects and safety. This happens in phase-4 trials where it is tested in several hundreds or thousands of patients. This phase is also known as Post Marketing Surveillance Trials.

The development process takes several years, and the outcomes are critical. The drug research and development process are a high investment business and a non-conclusive trial result can have huge negative consequences on pharma companies. Due to this reason, there are a lot of chances for data manipulation, forgery and fraud in clinical trials. For the safety of patients and the accuracy of results, having a system aided by technology to produce fair and just clinical trial results is the need of the hour.

The following are the challenges in clinical trials:

Data management: The process of clinical trials generates a lot of data. It starts from patient records and then spans out to reports, blood tests, surveys, medical imagery, clinical records, etc. to name a few. It also has records for the sponsor organization, the CRO, apart from patients and what is approved by the ERB. In order to get approval from drug administrators it is prone to fraud, which is at times unintentional as well. The frauds can range from modifying data, hiding data, changing patients records or removing observations to guide the administrators to make favorable decisions. There is different access to the data like blinding data, nonblinding data, locked data, etc. The data are stored in siloed systems in individual companies and most of the trials today are globalized. This leads to data duplication and access issues. Due to the globalization of the trials, the drug development data aggregation is a big challenge. The data across systems and organizations are also required to be compliant with regulatory authorities. All these call for a system that cuts across geography, systems, organizations and people. A system which can foster trust and efficiency.

Data sharing: As the trials are global, with the involvement of multiple organizations, teams, systems and people, sharing (of data) faces a lot of challenges. Due to these the data are vulnerable to misrepresentation for favorable decisions. The challenge is not just restricted to data leaks but also to frauds and abuse of confidential data. Many a times companies warrant the need for a third party data verification. Sharing of data in a controlled way and complying with all federal and local laws makes it challenging.

Regulatory requirements: For drug approval all systems which store data relevant to drugs and trials and which will aid the FDA in deciding must be compliant with 21 CFR 11. 21 CFR 11 is a FDA regulatory requirement that needs the collection of technological and procedural controls to protect data within a closed computer system. Open computer systems must also include controls to ensure that all records are authentic, incorruptible and (where applicable) confidential. Audit trials are required on data for its change. All data must be an electronic record and require electronic signatures.

Subject/patient confidentiality: At the start of a trial all subjects/patients/volunteers are enrolled, and their data are to be retained once the trial is over. The subject identity must be protected as it is highly confidential data and an oversight in such cases can have adverse effect or life risk. The system of having and managing the data should not only be secure but also robust and trustworthy.

The data can be segregated into four categories. The data are of interest to sponsors, principal investigators of research organizations, ERBs and subjects. Sponsors needs to know the protocol limitations, trial sites and demographics of subjects and the entire detail of the trial. ERBs should be aware of the protocol details, limitations and approvals on the specifics of the protocol. Principal investigators of research organizations need to be aware of trial design, inclusion/exclusion criteria and subject types. While the subjects need to be aware of protocols, consents are provided along with risks and compensations. These are a kind of tripartite agreement and information needs to be transparent, and everyone needs to be aware of his or her role. Special information relating to compensation should be transparent but should also be confidential, based on who needs to have access to the information.

All these challenges and requirements hint at a strong use case for a DLT-based blockchain network. Before the clinical trial begins, consents, clinical trial protocols, patient record and data during the trial like reports, blood tests, surveys, medical imagery and clinical records, including details of primary and secondary outcomes, can be bundled into data structures and stored on the blockchain. This data in the blockchain system will be immutable, linked and provide a robust proof of their existence which can be accepted by the regulatory authority. The blockchain will make sure the data are not owned by any individual or organization and is completely decentralized. The blockchain system will show the robustness, security and have a consensus mechanism which will ensure data provenance and public auditability. Another powerful feature of blockchain which can be widely used for clinical trials is smart contracts, where rules can be set for data or validation of it. All these requirements point to a private blockchain network design. The creator (originator) of the private blockchain network will control who can join the network and with what privileges and will mostly be initiated by the sponsors of the trials.

Blockchain technology can improve the patient engagement with more transparency and overcome recruitment challenges with more informed subjects. It can help aggregate data, improve analytics and access to clinical trials. It can help improve on the access to data and drive transparency. It can close clinical research gaps and accelerate drug development, be more cost effective and improve patient safety and care. Figure 13.2 shows a bird's eye view of the stakeholders or the members in a clinical trial and how they can all be brought together and get connected into the blockchain. As per Figure 13.2, the data generated by all stakeholders can be submitted to the blockchain. The regulators can then refer to and review the blockchain data rather than asking different organizations to submit their data. This will significantly reduce the time for approval and also improve the authenticity if the data.

Figure 13.3 shows the different entities of data which are generated as a part of clinical trials. These data are generated by different members, and all of these are required by

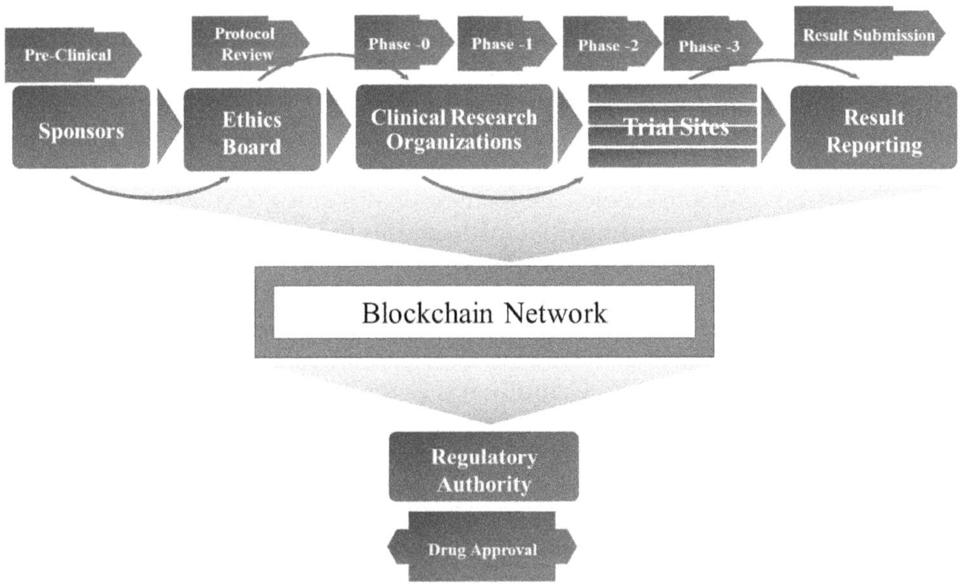

FIGURE 13.2
Stakeholders and blockchain network in clinical trials.

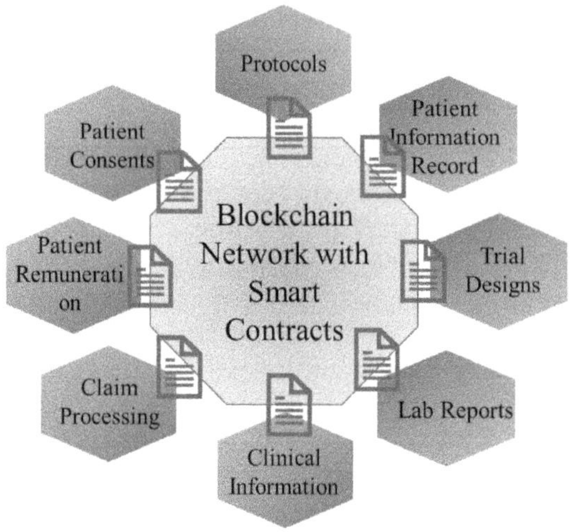

FIGURE 13.3
Different entities of data for clinical trials and the unified platform driven by blockchain.

regulators for the review of the trial. As the trials involve different groups/establishments, spread around different sites/locations, patients and data sources, there are multiple challenges faced by research organizations. These are issues like keeping track of their documentation, keeping track of progress, accuracy of data and authentication of data. Rigorous and strict regulations from the FDA and other regulatory authorities ask for meticulous documentation of all clinical trial stages, any change in the data is well captured and auditable at any time. So, bringing the partners together along with documentation is key for a trial's success and approval.

For a regulator like the FDA in the US or the European Medicines Agency the blockchain will be a game changer. If regulators are made a part of the blockchain network and they have access to data as it is being generated, then they can see the real-time information and be able to conduct ongoing reviews and assessments. This would change the whole process not only for pharma companies/sponsors, researchers and CROs but also the regulatory bodies and ERBs. It will drastically reduce the approval time and along with improved transparency. This will thus save a lot of cost and crucial time to market for a drug.

There are several companies which are focused on designing and using blockchain for clinical trials. One of the best examples in this regard is the German company Boehringer Ingelheim and IBM Canada coming together to use blockchain for clinical trials [8]. The trial being tried will aid in collaboration over patient consent, secure health data and patient engagement. There are other companies also attempting to plug into the DLT-driven blockchain network in various aspects of clinical trials like health data, patient records, protocol management, etc. Guardtime is a company offering patient engagement for clinical trials using blockchain technology. Synonymous with blockchain it can provide transparency of the data being used in trials. This also helps in a better audit of the data as required by regulators and drug control agencies. Also due to the features of blockchain it can control the authenticity, security and transparency of patient health data. Using blockchain it can access and pull health data from multiple sources. ClinTex uses a hybrid approach to combine blockchains and other technologies to help researchers create and maintain a successful clinical trial. It provides a platform based on blockchain and driven by smart contracts to drive quality and operational improvements in clinical trials. BioPharma Ledger is another platform based on blockchain technology which was launched by ALTEN Calsoft Labs.

13.6 Other Uses of Blockchain in the Pharma Industry

Blockchain technology has positively helped the pharma industry in the drug development process and clinical trials management. Apart from these two areas there are other aspects where blockchain as a technology is making significant impact in the pharma and healthcare industry. It is still evolving in the areas of patents, intellectual property and consortia for trial patients in the pharma and healthcare industry. But in the area of genomic data management, the development of consortia for helping pharma manufacturers is gaining more ground and getting close to reality. These are explored in brief in this section.

13.6.1 Genomic Data Management

Genomics is the study of genes and the entire DNA concept. It involves the sequencing of genes along with their structure and function. The human genome project is considered as the world's largest collaborative biological project. The success of the project and subsequent research have led to the generation of large volumes of genomic data, which is extensively used in biotechnology, forensic biology, medical diagnosis, virology and medical research. These data are also used in clinical trials and drug development research. Though having and using the data seems promising, the huge volume of data and its accessibility remain a challenge. The question is about having a system or platform for reliable and secure management of these genomic data which are to be stored securely, exchanged seamlessly and transacted flawlessly across any medical research and drug development system. There are other aspects of challenges in genomic research. Drug development for rare genetic disorders needs patients who are difficult to get, especially in a specified city or country. Obtaining a list of such accredited patients is challenging. Genomic data are required by many organizations (for the purpose of research), so they must be shared. Secure sharing of data with authenticity and access is always a challenge. The need for genomic data is also different for different types of research; for example, pharma companies need the data to develop personalized medicines, research organizations need the data to identify disease-specific genomics, government needs the data to forecast mass disorders in a location or ethnic group or to forecast epidemics, the data are even needed by insurance companies.

All these challenges and requirements point to having decentralized data which are available as designed, yet secure and verifiable. The data are expected to be electronically stored and shared. The large volume of genomic data along with the need for secured storage makes blockchain technology an obvious choice. The storage of information in a blockchain enables the purpose of sharing the genome data securely, exchanging the information seamlessly and transacting it across organizations flawlessly. The cryptographically stored data in blockchain technology is a proven and powerful tool for peer-to-peer (members of blockchain network) data exchanges (transactions) without a third party. Blockchain features like decentralized data, data security, authentication and smart contracts can be highly beneficial in the field of genomics. A blockchain network can enable secure transactions between various user groups like research groups/pharmaceutical companies. The blockchain platform will make the data access and security for genomic data easy to its members. This will improve the information access as needed for research studies. It will reduce the cost and time of procuring the data. The buyer of the data (pharma companies, research institutes) can gain access to genomic data or set of genomic data as per a grant . Blockchain can also maintain the anonymity of both users during data exchange.

But as there are many blockchain networks coming up, the interoperability of blockchain is going to be a fundamental need for the usage of genomic data management. There are companies exploring blockchain technology for genomic data exchange and management. Zenome is a company specializing in the storing, processing and exchanging of genetic information in a blockchain-based distributed architecture. It enables genetic information monetization for the data owner by providing a platform to make data available for the sake of scientific research. The biotechnology company, DNAtix is also providing a platform using blockchain to analyze, store and transfer of digitized DNA sequences for research and invention. It is a smart platform to anonymously share an encrypted genetic service. Shivom, is a genomics and personalized medicine company, and uses blockchain technology to provide the platform. It helps people to sequence their genes, store them and make them available to research companies. So, these are examples of how companies are exploring the use of the technology of the blockchain network for genomic data management and utilization.

13.6.2 Supplier Consortia and Preventive Maintenance Powered by Blockchain

The globalization of the supply chain and the global sourcing of ingredients (from low-cost economies) for drug manufacturing has introduced many complications. Unethical players and noncompliant suppliers along the supply chain can introduce counterfeited and adulterated materials, often with tragic consequences. This can lead to product license cancellation or product recall and will have a detrimental impact on brand image. It will also attract a lot of ire from public, health authorities and policymakers. The suppliers are needed to adhere to the guidelines of the product they provide and ensure its quality and consistency. This is to ensure patient safety by eliminating substandard, falsified and improperly packaged medicines.

Apart from ingredients, suppliers are also a partner in pushing the supply chain forward through logistics and manufacturing. In most of the cases the partners of plant maintenance, third party logistics providers, plant component suppliers are common (the same) for multiple companies in the industry. Pharma companies are highly regulated and compliance-driven and are thus extremely selective of their partners. The machines or components must meet the Good Manufacturing Practice (GMP), FDA norms (cGMP) and biological safety standards. One of the key challenges they face is that of a reliable partner having an experience of a similar industry and a proven track record. The pharma companies put lot of clauses, compliance and certification requirements on their suppliers/partners.

These two requirements put the focus on the need for an authentic and reliable supplier who can provide the required product or service as desired across the pharma industry. This is where the blockchain-driven supplier consortium can be very helpful. A blockchain consortium will provide a platform where it can bring all the suppliers (for their specified specialty) into a single platform. The platform will hold their sensitive information without breaching privacy laws and making it available to interested members. The members

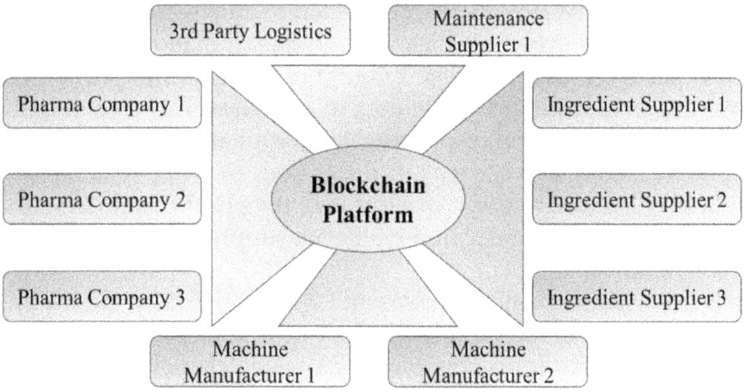

FIGURE 13.4
A representation of a blockchain consortium bringing partners together.

(like pharma manufacturers) can authenticate supplier data like compliance certificates or feedback from a similar pharma manufacturer and help them chose the best supplier for their purpose. It will benefit the suppliers as they will not need to furnish their data to every manufacturer. They will just need to ensure the data availability centrally. The blockchain-driven consortia will act as a central platform to help facilitate the data sharing with smart contracts for verification of the certificates, its authenticity and its validity. The platform will also help pharma manufacturers to compare suppliers, select them as per their suitability, along with their track-record. Figure 13.4 represents an elaboration of how a blockchain can provide a platform and bring both manufacturer and supplier (partners) together. The figure shows how information for these suppliers/participants can be fed into the blockchain which can then be used by the pharma company for its purpose.

Consortia can be set up by any pharma manufacturer, or it can also be by a third party. The first attempt should be to onboard the suppliers so that profiling of a group of suppliers can be achieved. Based on the profile of the consortia the pharma manufacturers can be onboarded as per their needs and benefits. For example, there can be a consortium of API suppliers or manufacturing services in a specific country and then based on the value proposition leads to onboarding pharma manufacturing companies. The members of the consortium need to have close coordination, established agreements, shared vision, purpose and above all the clear definition of success. This will help in the verification and authentication of suppliers and their validity. The governance rules of the consortium are to be laid down transparently and smart contracts need to be there to validate transactions. This will drive, consensus mechanisms, access and permission criteria.

13.7 Blockchain with IoT: A New Paradigm for Drug Manufacturing and Transparency

Blockchain has a lot of applications in the drug development process, pharma supply chain and helps the manufacturing process. Blockchain essentially provides a platform to serve data among partners securely and enables transparency. The clinical trials are revolutionized with the blockchain technology as discussed before. But blockchain is a standalone platform where data must be fed to drive the benefits. This section of the chapter looks at the aspects of bridging the cyber–physical gap of data. It explores what are the different options available to bridge the gaps. The Internet of Things (IoT) provides that bridge of the cyber–physical gap and can bring the data to any system. The combination of the IoT with blockchain is very powerful, especially for the pharma industry as it can help to drive the compliance, safety and security of drugs and, above all, patient care. Blockchain with the IoT will play a major role in two aspects of the pharma industry, first in the drug manufacturing process and secondly in the pharma supply chain. These are elaborated in detail in later subsections.

An integrated IoT with blockchain approach: Characteristically the IoT and blockchain can be treated and discussed separately. The IoT system is primarily involved in transforming data from the physical to cyber worlds. The key element of this is to be real time and uninterrupted capture of data from a source (using sensors) and securely transfer it to a database or cloud server. The cost of data capture must be cost-effective and it must be completely human, system, operations and process agnostic. IoT systems need to have the ability to capture data in offline modes (when not connected to the internet). But the most important aspect is the security of the data as it gets captured, transmitted and used. Lastly, there must be a seamless mechanism to share this data in almost real time (minimal latency) across partners/supply chain channels without any process dependency and minimal operating cost. The key to such needs at an enterprise scale indicates solutions beyond traditional means. Traditionally, the data exchanges are through point-to-point interfaces like B2B messaging, Electronic Data Interchange (EDI messaging), etc. This is where the blockchain system along with the IoT plays a decisive role.

13.7.1 Combining IoT and Blockchain for Pharma Manufacturing

The use of the IoT in pharma manufacturing is picking up quite rapidly. IoT sensors and trackers can enable data capture for various scenarios like handling materials, equipment operations, monitoring manufacturing environment, preventive maintenance and managing process variability and yield. This concept and idea can be extended to medical device manufacturing, wearable devices, body embedded device manufacturing and drug manufacturing.

The IoT can help in capturing data on machine performance. These can be the physical attributes like vibration, pressure, temperature during the manufacturing process. There can be other physical aspects related to drug manufacturing like media Ph, compressed air pressure, humidity, state of liquids, viscosity, density, etc. The information gathered by the IoT sensors can be used to detect anomalies which can indicate or help prepare for proactive maintenance, minimizing downtime and ensuring workplace safety. The use of the IoT can be further extended by feeding these IoT data to blockchain as a platform where the maintenance suppliers are a party to the data. These data feeds can help suppliers to prepare for maintenance (preventive) or safety preparation thus reducing downtime and communication overheads. The IoT can capture data during drug production and storage which can help bring transparency of conditions and help in monitoring and identifying root causes in case of problems. These attributes can be temperature, humidity, light exposure, radiation, pressures or other vital parameters as applicable to a manufacturing environment. At a later stage or during recall the capture of these environmental parameters can be of great help in identifying the root cause of a problem with a particular lot or batch number. Feeding these captured data from the IoT into a blockchain can help the data to be maintained centrally and can be made available to regulatory authorities. Trust in the data in the blockchain will be very high and can be shared across partners to help diagnose a manufacturing problem.

13.7.2 IoT and Blockchain in the Pharma Supply Chain

The products manufactured in a factory get shipped out into the complex world of the drug supply chain, comprising multiple partners across different countries and geographies. The products get shipped and transit through a multi-modal supply chain before they reach a patient or consumer. There can be many changes happening in the physical environment during transportation, in-transit storage, retail or hospital storage and at the time of dispensing. The IoT can offer an invaluable insight and visibility into the supply chain process conditions in real time. This can allow for immediate actions if there are anomalies or deviations from standards during storage or transportation. To enable this, it will need a lot of infrastructure investments like tags or labels on the packages being transported, the transit vehicles need to have sensors and transmission capabilities, vehicles need to have GPS capabilities. The in-transit storage (warehouses) and ocean freight also need IoT sensor capabilities as also the last mile delivery and storage before dispensing to customer. Having these provides a 360-degree view of the supply chain which has unprecedented transparency and insight for the manufacturer.

13.8 Prescription Drugs Transparency

Most US states are passing a law for transparency in prescription drug pricing. By 2019, 33 states in the US had enacted several laws to address drug prices, affordability and access. The law impacts multiple stakeholders like pharma companies, health insurance companies, pharmacy benefit managers and the state regulatory authority to control drug prices. There are numerous factors playing a role in the drug price increase and it is difficult to understand the reasons for it but at the same time it does adversely affect the patients and Medicare spending. Public attention focuses on drugs' list prices (wholesale price) but the actual cost charged to insurance companies and the applicable rebates, discounts and fees are completely off limits to the outside world. So, increases in drug prices are mostly considered unreasonable. Drug price transparency helps states gain an accurate understanding of the factors driving pharmaceutical companies to increase drug prices. The transparency also helps states gain a better understanding of precisely which drugs and types of drugs will need to increase and how that would create affordability challenges for consumers. This will also help states understand the impact on premiums as set by insurance companies.

Blockchain can help drive the transparency desired by state authorities to solve the problem for pharma manufacturers. As it needs to bring multiple agencies together and drive transparency, a blockchain network can be an ideal fit. On a blockchain network pharmaceutical manufacturers can disclose the relevant information related to the cost incurred. These can be, but not limited to, research and development costs, clinical trial costs, production costs and advertising costs. The pharmacy benefit managers disclose the utilizations, rebates and discounts, preference of drugs, incentives information and information on contracts, while the health insurers provide information on prescription drug cost-sharing and other information. This information on the blockchain will help all the parties immensely in getting access to information and decision-making. The platform will drive transparency and will help the pharma manufacturers, pharmacy benefit managers and health insurers to better understand the cost and price structures and negotiate prices. This will also help pharma manufacturers in increasing prices with complete transparency and rationale. The issues of rising drug prices and pricing strategies are complex for manufacturers. The solution to the problem lies in bringing all interested parties to a single platform enabled by blockchain and to be transparent about pricing and the reasons for hiking the prices. There can be smart contracts in blockchain which can help determine the unusual spikes in price which can get the attention of pharmacy benefit managers or state regulators and can help bring all the key parties to the table and discuss details with shared data.

13.9 Pandemics like Coronavirus and the Advent of Blockchain Technology

As discussed in previous subsections, blockchain technology is driving transparency in drug supply chain for the FDA-guided US DSCSA or European Union's FMD. Blockchain is also driving a lot of transparency in clinical trials and genomics data management and its monetization. Blockchain is also helping provide a transparent platform with its suppliers thus helping the manufacturing and supply chain to a great extent. But the Covid-19 pandemic has given another aspect to think about for the pharma supply chain, the one that has an integrated supply chain view.

The Covid-19 pandemic caused a lot of issues for pharma companies due to ingredient non-availability, material stuck in ports, logistics issues, reduced manufacturing operations and manpower non-availability, to name a few. Due to lockdown, even within a country the movement of goods (interstate) was badly impacted. Due to the lack of visibility to tertiary level suppliers, last-mile deliveries, real-time logistics information, many of the supply chain actions were left to guess work or tremendous amount of follow up efforts. Any disruptions during these transits or beyond primary suppliers create havoc due to lack of visibility. This pandemic brought these problems to the fore as due to lockdowns and sudden disruptions, suddenly pharma companies were struggling with their supplies or logistics and had no clue of their whereabouts.

This pandemic thus brings the issue of supply chain transparency, visibility and trackability to the forefront and blockchain are suitably placed to solve this problem as we have seen before. The Covid-19 does not add any new dimension to transparency as this is required for the EU FMD or US DSCSA. But the pandemic does hint in bringing the logistics and last-mile delivery partners into the network or tertiary suppliers into consideration of visibility. The aspect brought forward by the blockchain is the transparency and visibility of an extended and operational supply chain. The blockchain-driven network will eliminate manual reconciliations among various supply chain trading partners like buyers and suppliers. These manual processes will make the process slow and prone to errors. The system will also reduce the need for control towers or arrays of reports. Blockchain technology makes the supply chain resilient and promotes seamless and contactless transactions. The pandemic and scarcity of the vaccines/medicines and the sheer volume of need will make any of these things be required more than ever: Supply chain trust, transparency and resilience. As we move ahead, and beyond the Covid-19 crisis, blockchain can contribute in helping a system which is reliable and decentralizes the information by making every member equitable and responsible.

It is now known that there are certain brands of Covid-19 vaccine will need ultra-low temperature freezing before being administered to patients. This means the Covid-19 vaccine will be stored and managed at a temperature range of –50 to –70 degrees Celsius. Due to this the vaccine administration, storage, distribution becomes critical, and traceability becomes an important aspect for effective immunization. Blockchain will play a key role in making this traceability transparent and possible. The vaccine batches produced by the manufacturer will need to be entered into the blockchain system at the time of shipment. From that point onwards there will be an integration to blockchain for every transaction/ change of ownership of the batches. This will enable the blockchain system to trace and track the flow of goods to the pharmacy/ end customer. An IoT-enabled solution can trace and track the physical conditions during transportation and storage. The vaccine is expected to reach the furthest part of a country in the same condition and at the temperature prescribed by the manufacturer. It is well known that the remotest part (specially in a developing or under developed country) has the maximum chance of getting counterfeit products or stale products due to lack of infrastructure or information. This traceability of vaccines will ensure the right product is administered to the patients with the utmost effectiveness of the vaccine and prevent counterfeiting. This is critical for the success of vaccination programs and the safety of citizens of a country.

13.10 Conclusion

Being one of the largest industries in the world, pharma and healthcare is extensive, complex and immensely important. It is regulated and thrives on safety and quality. Today, to remain competitive and ensure product safety at the industrial scale it needs the support of technology more than before. The compliance of regulators for traceability of products to the consumer for the US DSCSA or EU FMD is only possible with mature technology like blockchain. These are also being adopted in other countries like India. To ensure a cost-effective, transparent and safe drug development and testing process the blockchain will be very effective for clinical trials. Other aspects of the pharma industry like genomic data management, supplier consortia for preventive maintenance and prescription drug transparency can be achieved through a blockchain network. The problems of counterfeiting, compliance and safety of patient records (EHR) are possible to solve through blockchain. The interfacing and sharing of data across systems like MMIS and labs can be done more safely with blockchain. Having blockchain will drive a more precise evaluation of data by review boards and enable a faster drug approval. The IoT and blockchain in the pharma supply chain can bring a lot of capabilities like a 360-degree view of the supply chain which has unprecedented transparency for patients, manufacturers and hospitals. Pandemics like Covid-19 also demonstrate the need for more transparency and blockchain can rightly provide this. Overall blockchain (and the IoT in some cases) together as a technology capability can make a significant difference to the pharma industry. It can make it more safe, secure, reliable and cost effective.

Key Terminology and Definitions

Clinical Trials—They can be defined as trials to evaluate the effectiveness, impact and safety of medications or medical devices by monitoring their effects on large groups of people.

Consortium—A private blockchain network run by a company or a group of companies. Consortium is a blockchain network that is setup by a company or a third party and has devised its own consensus mechanism. It also controls the companies who can join this network.

European Falsified Medicines—The Falsified Medicines Directive is a legal framework and set of rules regarding features for the packaging of medicinal products for human use within the European Union. It covers wide aspects of record-keeping for wholesale distributors, inspections norms for pharmaceutical producers, an EU-wide quality mark to identify online pharmacies and obligatory safety features on packages.

European Medicines Verification Organisation—Established by the European Commission to administer the Falsified Medicines Directive to secure the drug supply chain

FDA—US Food and Drug Administration. It is the federal drug regulator and approver in the US.

GPS—Global Positioning System. This system tells where exactly on earth (latitudes and longitudes) the object is and can show it in a map.

IoT—Internet of Things. It is a network of objects which can transfer data from a source to database or server over internet following some protocols.

Node—A participant in a blockchain network is referred to as a node. A full node is a computer/ participant that can fully validate transactions and download the entire data of a specific blockchain.

Pharmacy benefit manager—Pharmacy benefit manager handle some or all of the pharmacy benefit for health plans (formulary design, cost sharing and tiers, pharmacist networks and contracts, price concession negotiation with manufacturers). Pharmacy benefit manager is generally not a part of the drug distribution/supply chain.

Private blockchain—A closed blockchain network where participants are controlled by a single entity or founding member. A private blockchain will have its own verification process for new participants. A private blockchain may also limit which individuals are able to participate in consensus of the blockchain network.

US Drug Supply Chain Security Act—The Drug Supply Chain Security Act (DSCSA) outlines requirements for manufacturers, repackagers, wholesale distributors, dispensers and third-party logistics providers. This mainly revolves around product tracing and serialization of products. Manufacturers and repackagers must verify products at the package level, using a standardized numerical identifier.

References

1. Ascher, J, Bogdan, B, Dreszer, J and Zhou, G. (2015). Pharma's Next Challenge. https://www.mckinsey.com/industries/pharmaceuticals-and-medical-products/our-insights/pharmas-next-challenge (Accessed 18 March 2020).

2. United States Department of Commerce. (2016). *2016 Top Markets Report Pharmaceuticals*, International Trade Administration. http://trade.gov/topmarkets/pdf/Pharmaceuticals _ Executive_Summary.pdf (Accessed 9 June 2020).
3. LaSalle Solutions. (2019) What are the Biggest Challenges in Healthcare Supply Chain? https://lasallesolutions.com/2019/07/30/healthcare-supply-chains/ (Accessed 15 June 2020).
4. Takyar, A. (2019). Blockchain in Pharma Supply Chain-Reducing Counterfeit Drugs. https://www.leewayhertz.com/blockchain-in-pharma-supply-chain/ (Accessed 18 June 2020).
5. Petre, A. (2017). Blockchain Use Cases in Healthcare. https://www.linkedin.com/pulse/blockchain-use-cases-healthcare-anca-petre/ (Accessed 22 June 2020).
6. Mediledger. (2019). FDA DSCSA Pilot Project. https://www.mediledger.com/fda-pilot-project (Accessed 22 June 2020).
7. Venkatasubramanian, KV. (2018). India to Combat Fake Drugs with Blockchain, *Chemical & Engineering News*. https://cen.acs.org/pharmaceuticals/India-combat-fake-drugs-blockchain/96/i34 (Accessed 26 June 2020).
8. Lunch, M. (2019). Boehringer Ingelheim and IBM bring Blockchain to Clinical Trials. https://www.outsourcing-pharma.com/Article/2019/02/14/Boehringer-Ingelheim-and-IBM-bring-blockchain-to-clinical-trials (Accessed 2 July 2020).
9. Wood, L. (2019). The $11.9 Trillion Global Healthcare Market: Key Opportunities & Strategies, *Businesswire*. https://www.businesswire.com/news/home/20190625005862/en/11.9-Trillion-Global-Healthcare-Market-Key-Opportunities (Accessed 7 July 2020).
10. Business Research Company. (2018). The Growing Pharmaceuticals Market: Expert Forecasts and Analysis, *Market Research.com*. https://blog.marketresearch.com/the-growing-pharmaceuticals-market-expert-forecasts-and-analysis# (Accessed 7 July 2020).

Index